Risk Factors in Atrial Fibrillation: Appraisal of AF Risk Stratification

Editors

MOHAMMAD SHENASA
PRASHANTHAN SANDERS
STANLEY NATTEL

CARDIAC ELECTROPHYSIOLOGY CLINICS

www.cardiacEP.theclinics.com

Consulting Editors
RANJAN K. THAKUR
ANDREA NATALE

March 2021 • Volume 13 • Number 1

ELSEVIER

1600 John F. Kennedy Boulevard • Suite 1800 • Philadelphia, Pennsylvania, 19103-2899

http://www.theclinics.com

CARDIAC ELECTROPHYSIOLOGY CLINICS Volume 13, Number 1
March 2021 ISSN 1877-9182, ISBN-13: 978-0-323-82774-4

Editor: Joanna Collett
Developmental Editor: Arlene Campos

Cardiac Electrophysiology Clinics (ISSN 1877-9182) is published quarterly by Elsevier Inc., 360 Park Avenue South, New York, NY 10010-1710. Months of issue are March, June, September, and December. Subscription prices are $238.00 per year for US individuals, $502.00 per year for US institutions, $249.00 per year for Canadian individuals, $535.00 per year for Canadian institutions, $303.00 per year for international individuals, $535.00 per year for international institutions and $100.00 per year for US, Canadian and international students/residents. To receive student/resident rate, orders must be accompanied by name of affiliated institution, date of term, and the signature of program/residency coordinator on institution letterhead. Orders will be billed at individual rate until proof of status is received. Foreign air speed delivery is included in all Clinics subscription prices. All prices are subject to change without notice. **POSTMASTER:** Send address changes to Cardiac Electrophysiology Clinics, Elsevier Health Sciences Division, Subscription Customer Service, 3251 Riverport Lane, Maryland Heights, MO 63043. **Customer Service: 1-800-654-2452 (US and Canada). From outside of the US and Canada, call 314-477-8871. Fax: 314-447-8029. E-mail: JournalsCustomerService-usa@elsevier.com (for print support); JournalsOnlineSupport-usa@elsevier.com (for online support).**

Reprints. For copies of 100 or more of articles in this publication, please contact the Commercial Reprints Department, Elsevier Inc., 360 Park Avenue South, New York, NY 10010-1710. Tel.: 212-633-3874; Fax: 212-633-3820; E-mail: reprints@elsevier.com.

Cardiac Electrophysiology Clinics is covered in *MEDLINE/PubMed (Index Medicus)*.

Contributors

CONSULTING EDITORS

RANJAN K. THAKUR, MD, MPH, MBA, FHRS
Professor of Medicine and Director, Arrhythmia
Service, Thoracic and Cardiovascular Institute,
Sparrow Health System, Michigan State
University, Lansing, Michigan, USA

ANDREA NATALE, MD, FACC, FHRS
Executive Medical Director of the Texas
Cardiac Arrhythmia Institute, St. David's
Medical Center, Professor, Dell Medical

School, University of Texas at Austin, Austin,
Texas, USA; National Medical Director,
Cardiac Electrophysiology, Consulting
Professor, Division of Cardiology, Stanford
University, Stanford, California, USA; Clinical
Professor of Medicine, Case Western Reserve
University, Cleveland, Ohio, USA; Director,
Interventional Electrophysiology, Scripps
Clinic, San Diego, California, USA

EDITORS

MOHAMMAD SHENASA, MD, FACC, FAHA, FHRS
Department of Cardiovascular Services, Heart
and Rhythm Medical Group, Monte Sereno,
California, USA

PRASHANTHAN SANDERS, MBBS, PhD
Centre for Heart Rhythm Disorders, The
University of Adelaide and Royal Adelaide
Hospital, Adelaide, Australia

STANLEY NATTEL, MD
Department of Medicine, Montréal, Heart
Institute and Université de Montréal,
Department of Pharmacology and
Therapeutics, McGill University, Montréal,
Québec, Canada

AUTHORS

MARTIN AGUILAR, MD, PhD
Department of Medicine and Research Center,
Montreal Heart Institute and Université de
Montréal, Montréal, Québec, Canada

BAHA'A AL-AZAAM, MD
Division of Cardiology, Departments of
Medicine and Pharmacology, University of
Illinois at Chicago, Chicago, Illinois, USA

JONATHAN P. ARIYARATNAM, MB BChir
Centre for Heart Rhythm Disorders, The
University of Adelaide and Royal Adelaide
Hospital, Adelaide, Australia

RISHI ARORA, MD
Feinberg Cardiovascular and Renal Research
Institute, Northwestern University Feinberg
School of Medicine, Chicago, Illinois, USA

ADRIAN BARANCHUK, MD, FRCPC, FCCS
Division of Cardiology, Queen's University,
Kingston, Ontario, Canada

RAIMUNDO BARBOSA-BARROS, MD
Coronary Center of the Hospital de Messejana
Fortaleza, Ceará, Brazil

SHIH-ANN CHEN, MD
Professor of Medicine and Vice President,
Division of Cardiology and Cardiovascular
Research Center, Taipei Veterans General
Hospital, Taipei, Taiwan

YI-JEN CHEN, MD, PhD
Professor of Medicine, Division of
Cardiovascular Medicine, Department of

Internal Medicine, Wan Fang Hospital, Taipei Medical University, Taipei, Taiwan

HARRY J.G.M. CRIJNS, MD, PhD
Department of Cardiology, CARIM School for Cardiovascular Diseases, Maastricht University Medical Center+, Maastricht, the Netherlands

DAWOOD DARBAR, MBChB, MD
Chief, Division of Cardiology, Co-Director, Center for Cardiovascular Research, Division of Cardiology, Departments of Medicine and Pharmacology, University of Illinois at Chicago, Department of Medicine, Jesse Brown Veterans Administration, Chicago, Illinois, USA

DOBROMIR DOBREV, MD, PhD
Institute of Pharmacology, West German Heart and Vascular Center, University Duisburg-Essen, Essen, Germany

HANI ESSA, MRes, Mrcp
Liverpool Centre for Cardiovascular Science, University of Liverpool and Liverpool Heart and Chest Hospital, Liverpool, United Kingdom

N.A. MARK ESTES III, MD
Heart and Vascular Institute, University of Pittsburgh Medical Center, Pittsburgh, Pennsylvania, USA

CELINE GALLAGHER, RN, MSc, PhD
Centre for Heart Rhythm Disorders, The University of Adelaide, Royal Adelaide Hospital, Adelaide, South Australia, Australia

GAIL ELIZABETH GEIST, DVM
Feinberg Cardiovascular and Renal Research Institute, Northwestern University Feinberg School of Medicine, Chicago, Illinois, USA

YUTAO GUO, MD, PhD
Liverpool Centre for Cardiovascular Science, University of Liverpool and Liverpool Heart and Chest Hospital, Liverpool, United Kingdom; Department of Cardiology, Medical School of Chinese PLA, Chinese PLA General Hospital, Beijing, China

MASAHIDE HARADA, MD, PhD
Associate Professor, Department of Cardiology, Fujita Health University School of Medicine, Kutsukakecho, Toyoake, Japan

JEFF S. HEALEY, MD, MSc
Population Health Research Institute, McMaster University, Hamilton, Ontario, Canada

JORDI HEIJMAN, PhD
Department of Cardiology, CARIM School for Cardiovascular Diseases, Maastricht University Medical Center+, Maastricht, the Netherlands

JEROEN M. HENDRIKS, RN, MSc, PhD
Centre for Heart Rhythm Disorders (CHRD), South Australian Health and Medical Research Institute (SAHMRI), The University of Adelaide, Royal Adelaide Hospital, Adelaide, South Australia, Australia; Caring Futures Institute, College of Nursing and Health Sciences, Flinders University, Bedford Park, South Australia, Australia

SATOSHI HIGA, MD, PhD, FHRS
Vice President and Executive Director, Chairperson, Cardiac Electrophysiology and Pacing Laboratory, Division of Cardiovascular Medicine, Makiminato Central Hospital, Urasoe City, Okinawa, Japan

ANDREW M. HILL, MSc, FRCP
Liverpool Centre for Cardiovascular Science, University of Liverpool and Liverpool Heart and Chest Hospital, Department of Medicine for Older People, St Helens and Knowsley Teaching Hospitals NHS Trust, Liverpool, United Kingdom

RODDY HIRAM, PhD
Postdoctoral Researcher in Cardiology, Department of Medicine, Montreal Heart Institute (MHI), Université de Montréal, Montréal, Quebec, Canada

SUGAKO ISHIGAKI, MD
Chief, Cardiac Electrophysiology and Pacing Laboratory, Division of Cardiovascular Medicine, Makiminato Central Hospital, Urasoe City, Okinawa, Japan

BOBBY JOHN
Associate Professor, James Cook University, Townsville, Australia; Townsville University Hospital, Douglas, Queensland, Australia; Christian Medical College, Vellore, India

SØREN PAASKE JOHNSEN, MD, PhD
Department of Clinical Medicine, Aalborg
University, Aalborg, Aalborg, Denmark

JONATHAN M. KALMAN, MBBS, PhD
Department of Cardiology, Royal Melbourne
Hospital, Department of Medicine, University
of Melbourne, Melbourne, Australia

PAUL KHAIRY, MD, PhD
Electrophysiology Service and Adult
Congenital Heart Center, Montreal Heart
Institute, Université de Montréal, Montreal,
Quebec, Canada

ALEC KHERLOPIAN, MD, MPH
Division of Cardiology, Tufts Medical Center,
Boston, Massachusetts, USA

ANDRES KLEIN, MD
Arrhythmia Service, Division of Cardiology,
Department of Medicine, University of
Ottawa Heart Institute, Ottawa, Ontario,
Canada

CHU-PAK LAU, MD
Honorary Clinical Professor, Department of
Medicine, Queen Mary Hospital, The University
of Hong Kong, Central, Hong Kong

DENNIS H. LAU, MBBS, PhD
Department of Cardiology, Centre for Heart
Rhythm Disorders, The University of Adelaide,
Royal Adelaide Hospital, Adelaide, Australia

DOMINIK LINZ, MD, PhD
Centre for Heart Rhythm Disorders, South
Australian Health and Medical Research
Institute, The University of Adelaide and Royal
Adelaide Hospital, Adelaide, Australia;
Department of Cardiology, CARIM School for
Cardiovascular Diseases, Maastricht
University Medical Centre+ and
Cardiovascular Research Institute, Maastricht,
the Netherlands; Department of Cardiology,
Radboud University Medical Centre, Nijmegen,
the Netherlands; Department of Biomedical
Sciences, Faculty of Health and Medical
Sciences, University of Copenhagen,
Copenhagen, Denmark

GREGORY Y.H. LIP, MD, FRCP
Professor, Liverpool Centre for Cardiovascular
Science, University of Liverpool and Liverpool
Heart and Chest Hospital, Liverpool, United

Kingdom; Aalborg Thrombosis Research Unit,
Department of Clinical Medicine, Aalborg
University, Aalborg, Denmark; Department of
Cardiology, Medical School of Chinese PLA,
Chinese PLA General Hospital, Beijing, China;
Department of Internal Medicine, Diabetology
and Nephrology, Faculty of Medical Sciences
in Zabrze, Medical University of Silesia,
Katowice, Poland

JUSTIN G.L.M. LUERMANS, MD, PhD
Department of Cardiology, CARIM School for
Cardiovascular Diseases, Maastricht
University Medical Center+, Maastricht, the
Netherlands

CHRISTOPHER MADIAS, MD
Division of Cardiology, New England Cardiac
Arrhythmia Center, Tufts Medical Center,
Boston, Massachusetts, USA

AKIRA MAESATO, MD, PhD
Chief, Cardiac Electrophysiology and Pacing
Laboratory, Division of Cardiovascular
Medicine, Makiminato Central Hospital,
Urasoe City, Okinawa, Japan

RAJIV MAHAJAN, MD, PhD
The University of Adelaide, South Australian
Health and Medical Research Institute, Lyell
McEwin Hospital, Adelaide, Australia

JASON D. MATOS, MD
Instructor of Medicine, Department of
Medicine, Division of Cardiology, Beth Israel
Deaconess Medical Center, Harvard Medical
School, Boston, Massachusetts, USA

MELISSA E. MIDDELDORP, PhD
Centre for Heart Rhythm Disorders, The
University of Adelaide, Royal Adelaide
Hospital, Adelaide, South Australia, Australia

KATARZYNA NABRDALIK, MD, PhD
Liverpool Centre for Cardiovascular Science,
University of Liverpool and Liverpool Heart and
Chest Hospital, Liverpool, United Kingdom;
Department of Internal Medicine, Diabetology
and Nephrology, Faculty of Medical Sciences
in Zabrze, Medical University of Silesia,
Katowice, Poland

STANLEY NATTEL, MD
Department of Medicine, Montréal, Heart
Institute and Université de Montréal,

Department of Pharmacology and Therapeutics, McGill University, Montréal, Québec, Canada

KJELL NIKUS, MD, PhD
Heart Center, Tampere University Hospital and Faculty of Medicine and Health Technology, Tampere University, Finland

JEAN JACQUES NOUBIAP, MD, MMed
Centre for Heart Rhythm Disorders, The University of Adelaide, Adelaide, Australia

ANDRÉS RICARDO PÉREZ-RIERA, MD, PhD
Centro Universitário Saúde ABC, Laboratório de Metodologia de Pesquisa e Escrita Científica, Santo André, São Paulo, Brazil

RAJEEV KUMAR PATHAK, MBBS, PhD
Australian National University and Canberra Hospital, Canberra, Australian Capital Territory, Australia

LUCIANO EVARISTO PEREIRA-REJÁLAGA, MD
Sanatorio Medicordis

ANNA PFENNIGER, MD, PhD
Feinberg Cardiovascular and Renal Research Institute, Northwestern University Feinberg School of Medicine, Chicago, Illinois, USA

STEEVE PROVENCHER, MD, MSc
Professor of Medicine, Pulmonologist, Centre de Recherche de l'Institut Universitaire de Cardiologie et de Pneumologie de Quebec, Department of medicine, Université Laval, Quebec, Canada

SREEVILASAM PUSHPANGADHAN ABHILASH, MD, DM
Australian National University and Canberra Hospital, Canberra, Australian Capital Territory, Australia

PRASHANTHAN SANDERS, MBBS, PhD
Centre for Heart Rhythm Disorders, The University of Adelaide and Royal Adelaide Hospital, Adelaide, Australia

ROOPINDER K. SANDHU, MD, MPH
Mazankowski Alberta Heart Institute, University of Alberta, Edmonton, Alberta, Canada

FRANK W. SELLKE, MD
Karl E. Karlson, MD and Gloria A. Karlson Professor of Cardiothoracic Surgery, Professor of Surgery, Department of Cardiothoracic Surgery, Brown Medical School and Lifespan Hospitals, Providence, Rhode Island, USA

HASSAN A. SHENASA, BS
Heart and Rhythm Medical Group, Monte Sereno, California, USA

MOHAMMAD SHENASA, MD, FACC, FAHA, FHRS
Department of Cardiovascular Services, Heart and Rhythm Medical Group, Monte Sereno, California, USA

MARIA STEFIL, BSc, MBBS, MRes
Department of Cardiology, Royal Liverpool Hospital, Liverpool Centre for Cardiovascular Science, University of Liverpool and Liverpool Heart and Chest Hospital, Liverpool, United Kingdom

KAZUYOSHI SUENARI, MD, PhD
Chief, Department of Cardiology, Hiroshima City Hiroshima Citizens Hospital, Hiroshima City, Hiroshima, Japan

ISABELLE C. VAN GELDER, MD, PhD
Department of Cardiology, University Medical Center Groningen, University of Groningen, Groningen, the Netherlands

VICTOR WALDMANN, MD, PhD
Electrophysiology and Adult Congenital Heart Disease Unit, Hôpital Européen Georges Pompidou, Université de Paris, Paris, France

SHAYNA WEINSHEL, BS, MS
University of Central Florida College of Medicine, Orlando, Florida, USA

CHRISTOPHER X. WONG, MBBS, MSc, PhD
The University of Adelaide, South Australian Health and Medical Research Institute, Adelaide, Australia

JUQIAN ZHANG, MBBS, MSc, PhD, MRCP (Edinburgh)
Liverpool Centre for Cardiovascular Science, University of Liverpool and Liverpool Heart and Chest Hospital, Liverpool, United Kingdom

PETER ZIMETBAUM, MD
Richard A. and Susan F. Smith Professor of
Cardiovascular Medicine, Department of
Medicine, Division of Cardiology, Harvard
Medical School, Center for Cardiovascular
Outcomes Research, Beth Israel Deaconess
Medical Center, Boston, Massachusetts,
USA

Contents

Atrial fibrillation is the most common arrhythmia globally. The global prevalence of atrial fibrillation is positively correlated with the sociodemographic index of different regions. Advancing age, male sex, and Caucasian race are risk factors; female sex is correlated with higher atrial fibrillation mortality worldwide likely owing to thrombo-embolic risk. African American ethnicity is associated with lower atrial fibrillation risk, same as Asian and Hispanic/Latino ethnicities compared with Caucasians. Atrial fibrillation may be heritable, and more than 100 genetic loci have been identified. A polygenic risk score and clinical risk factors are feasible and effective in risk stratification of incident disease.

Inflammation and fibrosis have been implicated in the pathophysiology of atrial fibril-lation. Atrial fibrosis causes conduction disturbances and is a central component of atrial remodeling in atrial fibrillation. Cardiac fibroblasts, the cells responsible for fibrosis formation, are activated by inflammatory mediators and growth factors associated with systemic inflammatory conditions. Thus, inflammation contributes to atrial fibrosis; the complex interplay of these maladaptive components creates a vicious cycle of atrial remodeling progression, maintaining atrial fibrillation and increasing thrombogenicity. This review provides up-to-date knowledge regarding inflammation and fibrosis in atrial fibrillation pathophysiology and their potential as therapeutic targets.

Risk Factors

Hypertension (HT) confers the highest population-attributable risk among factors leading to atrial fibrillation (AF). Data also are accumulating regarding the associa-tion between pre-HT, aortic stiffness, and increased incident AF or AF recurrence. Atrial remodeling due to HT is progressive but also reversible. Although inhibition of the renin-angiotensin-aldosterone system has shown the greatest promise in improving AF outcomes, optimal blood pressure targets in individuals with HT and AF remain elusive. AF management demands an integrated care approach. HT is best treated alongside a comprehensive risk factor management program where other AF risk factors are targeted, with involvement of a multidisciplinary team.

Atrial fibrillation (AF) and heart failure (HF) have similar risk factors, frequently coexist, and potentiate each other in a vicious cycle. Evidence suggests the presence of AF in both HF with reduced ejection fraction (HFrEF) and HF with preserved ejection fraction (HFpEF) increases the risk of all-cause mortality and stroke, particularly when AF is incident. Catheter ablation may be an effective strategy in controlling symptoms and improving quality of life in AF-HFrEF. Strong data guiding management of AF-HFpEF are lacking largely due to its challenging diagnosis. Improving outcomes associated with these coexistent conditions requires further careful investigation.

Risk factors including cardiometabolic and endocrine disorders have a significant impact on atrial remodeling causing atrial fibrillation (AF). Diabetes mellitus and hyperthyroidism are strong independent risk factors for AF and worsen outcomes of rhythm control strategies. An early diagnosis and intervention for these risk factors combined with rhythm control strategies may improve the overall cardiovascular mortality and morbidity. This review summarizes the current state of knowledge about the AF risk factors diabetes mellitus and thyroid disease, and discusses the impact of the modification of these risk factors on primary and secondary prevention of AF.

Obesity and metabolic syndrome are both associated with atrial fibrillation (AF). Recent research has revealed new insights into the effects of cardiac and noncardiac adipose tissue in mediating these associations. Cardiac adipose tissue, such as epicardial fat, is a powerful predictor of AF and leads to myocardial fatty infiltration and adipokine-induced fibrosis. Increases in noncardiac adipose tissue cause deleterious metabolic, neurohormonal, hemodynamic, and structural changes. Weight loss leads to a regression of adiposity-related fibrosis, structural abnormalities, conduction abnormalities, and reduction in AF burden. As a result, weight loss and risk factor treatment is now an established pillar of AF management.

Obstructive sleep apnea (OSA) creates a complex and dynamic substrate for atrial fibrillation (AF), which is characterized by structural remodeling as a result of long-term OSA as well as transient and acute apnea-associated transient atrial electrophysiological changes. OSA is present in 21% to 74% of patients with AF, and nonrandomized studies suggest that treatment of OSA by continuous positive airway pressure may help to maintain sinus rhythm after electrical cardioversion and improve catheter ablation success rates. Management of OSA in patients with AF requires a close interdisciplinary collaboration between the electrophysiologist/cardiologist and sleep specialists.

mortality associated with AF in the general population is not shared by athletes, clinically significant morbidities exist (eg, reduced exercise capacity, athletic performance, and quality of life). Additional research is needed to fill current gaps in knowledge pertaining to the natural history, pathophysiologic mechanisms, and management strategies of AF in the athlete.

Atrial fibrillation (AF) is the most commonly diagnosed arrhythmia and eludes an efficacious cure despite an increasing prevalence and a significant association with morbidity and mortality. In addition to an array of clinical sequelae, the origins and propagation of AF are multifactorial. In recent years, the contribution from the autonomic nervous system has been an area of particular interest. This review highlights the relevant physiology of autonomic and neurohormonal contributions to AF origin and maintenance, the current state of the literature on targeted therapies, and the path forward for clinical interventions.

A confluence of clinical and epidemiologic factors has provoked a steep increase in the prevalence of atrial fibrillation in adults with congenital heart disease. Atrial fibrillation is the most common presenting arrhythmia. Much remains to be unraveled about the mitigating role congenital heart disease, residual hemodynamic defects, surgical ramifications, and shunts and cyanosis on new-onset and recurrent atrial fibrillation in this population. Catheter ablation is increasingly performed for atrial fibrillation. This synopsis provides an overview of current knowledge on atrial fibrillation in adults with congenital heart disease, addresses clinical management, and discusses knowledge gaps and areas for future research.

Atrial fibrillation is a chronic, progressive condition that presents a major health burden. This review summarizes recent studies assessing atrial fibrillation progression and its associated risk factors, describes the mechanisms underlying atrial fibrillation progression, and discusses the clinical implications of the progressive nature of atrial fibrillation. Progression of atrial fibrillation burden, and clinical progression from paroxysmal to more advanced (persistent/permanent) forms is common, but progression rates are variable. Atrial fibrillation progression parallels progressive atrial remodeling induced by atrial fibrillation risk factors and atrial fibrillation itself, and is associated with worse clinical outcomes.

Diagnostic Tests

The electrocardiogram and various echocardiography modalities are important risk markers for atrial fibrillation (AF). Electrocardiographic criteria of left atrial enlargement, advanced interatrial block, and PR-interval prolongation are atrial risk markers for AF. Transthoracic echocardiography is elementary for risk stratification of AF. Transesophageal echocardiography is a valuable tool to detect cardiac sources of embolism if early cardioversion is necessary. Intracardiac echocardiography is a real-time tool for guidance of percutaneous interventions, including radiofrequency ablation and left atrial appendage closure in patients with AF.

importance. There are nonmodifiable, modifiable, and reversible risk factors for AF. The modifiable risk factors include hypertension, obesity, coronary artery disease, heart failure, diabetes mellitus etc. These risk factors should be screened and adequately treated to prevent occurrence of AF at the primary care level itself. This will reduce recurrence rates of AF and will treat underlying conditions predisposing to AF.

The growing burden of atrial fibrillation health care resource utlization has created an urgent need to develop preventative strategies and opportunities to improve outcomes in the prevalent population. Modifiable risk factors contribute to both disease development and progression. In the prevalent atrial fibrillation population, modifying cardiovascular risk factors has decreased disease burden and progression. However, further research is required to determine the role of comprehensive cardiovascular risk factor modification programs in primary prevention. An understanding of strategies required to facilitate health behavior change is crucial to the effective implementation of cardiovascular risk factor management programs.

CARDIAC ELECTROPHYSIOLOGY CLINICS

Foreword
Atrial Fibrillation Risk Factors

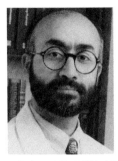
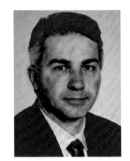

Ranjan K. Thakur, MD, MPH, MBA, FHRS   Andrea Natale, MD, FACC, FHRS

Consulting Editors

Atrial fibrillation (AF) is the most common sustained cardiac arrhythmia seen in clinical practice. When we started our clinical careers about 25 years ago, electrophysiologists were usually consulted for other arrhythmia issues, such as syncope, ventricular tachycardia, implantable cardioverter defibrillator implantation, supraventricular tachycardia management, and AF management was not a very prominent part of our clinical practice. Then came Haissaguerre's seminal paper showing that AF can be triggered by rapid electrical firing from the pulmonary veins. This incited worldwide interest in trying to understand and successfully ablate AF. Concerted effort by basic scientists, clinicians, and industry has brought us to the point where the majority of an electrophysiologist's clinical effort is exerted on managing AF.

Our understanding has grown tremendously. Patient selection is more informed. Safety of the ablation procedure has improved. We are better informed about progressively sequencing the right lesion sets in a patient. But unfortunately, the clinical results of catheter ablation have remained more or less the same.

We need to develop other approaches to tackling AF to improve outcomes. A deeper understanding of AF risk factors, risk factor modification, and lifestyle modification may be beneficial. Research has demonstrated that multiple risk factors predispose to AF. Among these are family history (genes), hypertension, heart failure, diabetes, obesity, sleep apnea, smoking, pulmonary disease, cardiomyopathies, endocrine abnormalities, valvular heart disease and coronary artery disease, alcohol consumption, and air pollution. Although these predisposing factors are well discussed individually, an amalgamated comprehensive review by experts in the field was absent.

We congratulate the editors, Drs Shenasa, Nattel, and Sanders, for a timely issue on this important approach to deepen our understanding of AF, and it is hoped, improving future therapeutic outcomes. This issue will be of interest to clinicians and researchers. We hope that the readership will enjoy reading the individual articles.

Ranjan K. Thakur, MD, MPH, MBA, FHRS
Sparrow Thoracic and Cardiovascular Institute
Michigan State University
1440 East Michigan Avenue; Suite 400
Lansing, MI 48912, USA

Andrea Natale, MD, FACC, FHRS
Texas Cardiac Arrhythmia Institute
Center for Atrial Fibrillation at
St. David's Medical Center
1015 East 32nd Street, Suite 516
Austin, TX 78705, USA

E-mail addresses:
epthakur@gmail.com (R.K. Thakur)
andrea.natale@stdavids.com (A. Natale)

Preface

Risk Factors in Atrial Fibrillation: Appraisal of Atrial Fibrillation Risk Stratification

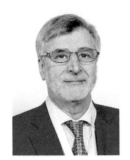
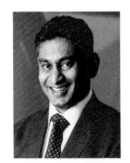
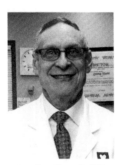

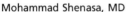

Mohammad Shenasa, MD Prashanthan Sanders, MBBS, PhD Stanley Nattel, MD

Editors

Atrial fibrillation (AF) remains the most common sustained arrhythmia encountered in clinical practice, with an increasing incidence related to increasing survival of patients with AF-promoting comorbidities as well as population aging. Accordingly, the prevalence of important AF-associated morbidities, like stroke and heart failure, is increasing, along with the related social and economical burden. Despite significant progress in understanding the pathophysiologic mechanisms of AF on one hand and the advances in the catheter ablation of AF on the other, the present management options are still far from perfect.

Comprehensive management of AF requires a multidisciplinary approach beyond catheter ablation.

Over the past couple of decades, a large body of evidence has demonstrated that multiple risk factors predispose to AF occurrence. Among these are well-established risk factors, like genetic predisposition, hypertension, heart failure, diabetes, obesity, sleep apnea, cigarette smoking, pulmonary disease, cardiomyopathies, endocrine abnormalities, valvular heart disease, and coronary artery disease. There are also some novel risk factors associated with AF, such as alcohol consumption, air pollution, social and recreational habits, and infectious diseases, like COVID-19.

Recent work has demonstrated that the effective targeting of AF risk factors with a multidisciplinary approach is a potentially important therapeutic intervention, with the potential to reduce AF burden, increase the long-term success of ablation therapy, and in some cases, even obviate ablation.

Although these risk factors are individually discussed in several textbooks and articles, a collective and comprehensive text is overdue.

In this issue of *Cardiac Electrophysiology Clinics*, we dive into the depth of AF risk factors by inviting leaders in each area to provide their current perspective on the state-of-the-art.

We have arranged the Table of Contents according to specific risk factors.

We are confident that this first collective text on the management of AF risk factors will be useful to those who take care of patients with AF.

Card Electrophysiol Clin 13 (2021) xix–xx
https://doi.org/10.1016/j.ccep.2020.12.001
1877-9182/21/© 2020 Published by Elsevier Inc.

We wish to thank Ms Mona Soleimanieh for her superb assistance in finishing this project.

Mohammad Shenasa, MD
Heart and Rhythm Medical Group
18324 Twin Creeks Road
Monte Sereno, CA 95030, USA

Prashanthan Sanders, MBBS, PhD
Centre for Heart Rhythm Disorders
South Australian Health and
Medical Research Institute
University of Adelaide and
Royal Adelaide Hospital
Adelaide, Australia

Stanley Nattel, MD
Montreal Heart Institute and
Université de Montréal
Montréal, Quebec, Canada

Department of Pharmacology and Therapeutics
McGill University
3655 Promenade Sir William Osler
Montreal, Quebec H3G 1Y6, Canada

E-mail addresses:
mohammad.shenasa@gmail.com (M. Shenasa)
prash.sanders@adelaide.edu.au (P. Sanders)
stanleynattel@gmail.com (S. Nattel)

Epidemiology of Atrial Fibrillation
Geographic/Ecological Risk Factors, Age, Sex, Genetics

Juqian Zhang, MBBS, MSc, PhD, MRCP (Edinburgh)[a],
Søren Paaske Johnsen, MD, PhD[b], Yutao Guo, MD, PhD[a,c],
Gregory Y.H. Lip, MD, FRCP[a,b,c],*

KEYWORDS

• Atrial fibrillation • Epidemiology • Risk factors • Genetics

KEY POINTS

- Atrial fibrillation is the most common arrhythmia with increasing public health burden worldwide.
- The prevalence of atrial fibrillation is positively correlated with sociodemographic index globally and income level among different regions.
- Advancing age, male sex, and Caucasian race are risk factors for atrial fibrillation; female sex is associated with higher atrial fibrillation mortality, likely owing to thromboembolic risk.
- Atrial fibrillation may be a heritable disease.
- Currently there are more than 160 genetic loci discovered in common atrial fibrillation, and polygenic risk score combined with clinical risk factors are effective in risk stratification for incident atrial fibrillation.

INTRODUCTION

Atrial fibrillation (AF) is the most common arrhythmia with ever-increasing public health impact.[1] Over 50 years of observation in the Framingham Heart Study (FHS), there is a 4-fold increase in prevalence and more than 3 times increase in the incidence of AF.[2] The estimated prevalence of AF in United States is 5.3 million in 2009.[3] In the European Union, 8.8 million adults over 55 years of age were estimated to have AF in 2010, which is projected to increase to 17.9 million by 2060.[4] The worldwide prevalence of AF in 2017 is estimated at 37.6 million cases, which is projected to increase by more than 60% by 2050.[5]

According to the Global Health Data Exchange database, AF is related to loss of 6.0 million disability-adjusted life-years worldwide in 2017, which is a 77% increase from 1997, and it consists of 0.24% of total disability-adjusted life-years globally.[5] Between 2000 and 2010, there were 3,960,011 AF-related hospitalizations in United States, with the mean cost of each admission increasing from $6410 in 2001 to $8439 in 2010.[6] The total annual cost for treatment of AF in 2001 is estimated to be $6.65 billion in the United States. In Denmark, the average 3-year cost related to AF is estimated to be €20,403 to €26,544 per patient, and €219 to 295 million nationwide between 2001 and 2013.[7] AF is

[a] Liverpool Centre for Cardiovascular Science, University of Liverpool and Liverpool Heart and Chest Hospital, Liverpool, L14 3PE, UK; [b] Department of Clinical Medicine, Aalborg University, Søndre Skovvej 15, Aalborg, Aalborg 9000, Denmark; [c] Department of Cardiology, Medical School of Chinese PLA, Chinese PLA General Hospital, Beijing, China
* Corresponding author. Liverpool Centre for Cardiovascular Science, University of Liverpool and Liverpool Heart and Chest Hospital, Liverpool, L14 3PE, UK.
E-mail address: Gregory.Lip@liverpool.ac.uk

Card Electrophysiol Clin 13 (2021) 1–23
https://doi.org/10.1016/j.ccep.2020.10.010

associated with significantly increased risk of all-cause mortality (relative risk [RR], 1.46), cardiovascular mortality (RR, 2.03), and stroke (RR, 2.42).[8] In 2018, AF is registered as the cause of death in 25,845 death certificates in the United States.[9] Worldwide, AF-related mortality is 0.3 million in 2017, and it is likely to reach 0.4 million by 2050.[5]

AF is influenced by multiple risk factors, which can be categorized into modifiable (eg, sedentary lifestyle, smoking, alcohol use, obesity, hypertension, diabetes, heart failure) and nonmodifiable risk factors (eg, age, sex, ethnicity, and genetics). This review aims to summarize the epidemiologic features of AF with a focus on the nonmodifiable risk factors.

GEOGRAPHIC AND SOCIODEMOGRAPHIC VARIATION OF ATRIAL FIBRILLATION

The prevalence of AF varies among geographic regions (**Figs. 1** and **2**, **Table 1**). In rural Uganda, the prevalence is 0 in a community-based cohort,[10] yet in an urban area of Jimma in Ethiopia, the prevalence is 4.3%.[11] The reported prevalence is between 0.63% and 2.87% in females, and 0.91% and 5.66% in males in China,[12–14] 1.4% and 2.2% in Japan,[15,16] 1.4% in Belgium,[17] 2.4% in Italy,[18] 2.9% in Sweden,[19] 1.4% in Australia,[20] 1.1% in the United States,[21] and 1.8% and 2.2% in Brazil.[22,23] There is a positive correlation

between AF prevalence and area-based socioeconomic status among different regions in China.[12] In national screening of AF in Korea, the highest prevalence of AF is noted in the lowest socioeconomic group, which gradually increases with increasing income levels following a "J" shape.[24] The most deprived areas had a higher percentage of elderly people; with age adjustment, the prevalence is positively correlated with income level.[24] In the United States, income and education level are inversely associated with cumulative incidence of AF before 80 years of age.[25] However, the lifetime risk of AF increases with higher income and education in most ethnic and sex groups, except in white women.[25] The observation could be due to shorter life expectancy of people with a lower income and educational level, leaving them a lesser chance to survive into later stage of life to develop AF; however, white women have a relatively lower mortality rate and longer life expectancy; therefore, this trend is minimized in their group.[25]

When ranked into low, low-middle, middle, high-middle, and high sociodemographic index (SDI) regions based on average income per person, educational level, and total fertility rate of each region, there is a clear trend that with increasing SDI, there is increase in AF prevalence according to data from the Global Burden of Disease Study 2017 (GBD 2017) (**Fig. 3**).[26] The mean prevalence in high SDI regions (1212.6 per 100,000

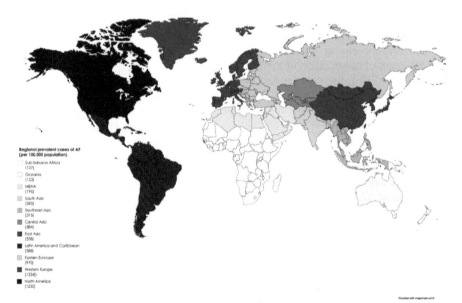

Fig. 1. Global map of AF prevalence. Prevalent cases of AF per 100,000 population in both sexes in 2017 in different geographic regions, including sub-Saharan Africa, Oceania, Middle East and North Africa (MENA), South Asia, Southeast Asia, Central Asia, East Asia, Latin America and Caribbean, Eastern Europe, Western Europe and North America. Each geographic region is color coded depending on its prevalent cases Map created by Mapchart.net available from https://mapchart.net/world.html. (*Data from* GBD 2017 data visualization available from http://vizhub.healthdata.org/gbd-compare.)

Prevalence of AF in different regions

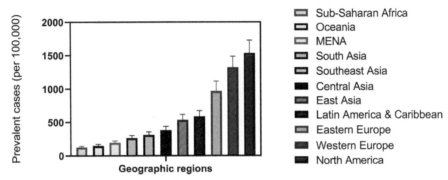

Fig. 2. Prevalent cases of AF in geographic regions. Bar chart of prevalent cases of AF per 100,000 population in both sexes in 2017 in different geographic regions. MENA, Middle East and North Africa. Graph generated by GraphPad Prism. (*Data from* GBD 2017 data visualization available from http://vizhub.healthdata.org/gbd-compare.)

population) is almost 7-fold higher when compared with low SDI regions (175.0 per 100,000 population).[26]

For patients diagnosed with AF, the income level positively correlates with level of health-related quality of life,[27] and lower socioeconomic status are associated with decreased access to medical care and undertreatment with anticoagulation, resulting in a higher risk for thromboembolic event.[24,28,29] There is concern in underreporting of AF burden and its stroke risk in Africa, where there is large disparity in published studies.[28] AF is more prevalent in younger patients in Africa, with a higher percentage of rheumatic valvular disease compared with developed countries, which poses further challenges for stroke prevention owing to difficulty in getting access to regular monitoring of oral anticoagulation treatment.[29]

AGE

Fifty years of follow-up in the FHS noted advancing age as the strongest risk factor for developing AF as compared with sex, smoking, alcohol, body mass index, hypertension, left ventricular hypertrophy, significant heart murmur, heart failure, and myocardial infarction.[2] Large-scale combined European cohorts noted marked increase in the AF incidence in men from 50 years of age, whereas women tend to develop AF after 60 years of age, a decade later than men.[30] However, the lifetime risk of AF is similar in both sexes, likely owing to longevity of women.[30] The incidence of AF almost doubles with every 10-year increment in age above 60.[2]

Although the prevalence of AF varies in countries and regions of different sociodemographic characteristics, aging is consistently found to be associated with increased prevalence and incidence of AF.[2,4,15,22,31–35] In data published from the GBD 2017 study, there is a stepwise increase in the global prevalence of AF with advancing age: 0.07% in 30 to 34 years, 0.72% in 55 to 59 years, 6.52% in 80 to 84 year, and 8.18% in 95 years and older (**Fig. 4**).[26]

Advancing age is not only a risk factor for AF; it is also a strong risk factor for stroke in AF.[36,37] Age 65 years and older is associated with a more than 3-fold increase in stroke risk (RR, 3.33),[38] and odds ratio for stroke in age greater than 75 years is 1.76.[39]

Elderly patients with AF (>65 years) comprise two-thirds of the AF hospitalizations in the United States; they have longer average length of stay (3.7 days vs 2.9 days), higher in-hospital mortality (1.0% vs 0.3%), and share different clinical profiles compared with younger patients. Elderly patients have higher chances of kidney disease (14% vs 7%), whereas the younger patients tend to be obese (21% vs 8%) and use more alcohol (8% vs 2%).[40]

SEX

Male sex is associated with higher prevalence of AF across different socioeconomical and ethnicities (**Fig. 5**, see **Table 1**). The GBD 2017 dataset noted 516 (95% confidence interval, 449–586) global prevalent cases of AF per 100,000 population in male sex as compared with 467 (95% confidence interval, 404–530) cases per 100,000 in women.[26] In the Multi-Ethnic Study of Atherosclerosis (MESA),a higher circulating level of endogenous bioavailable testosterone is associated with higher risk of AF in men with a hazard ratio of 1.32; however, it is negatively correlated with AF

Table 1
Overview of the global prevalence of AF in the general population

Nation/Region	Study Period	Source	Age	Population	Definition of AF	Prevalence			Reference
						Overall (%)	Male (%)	Female (%)	
Africa									
Ethiopia	2017	Community based cross-sectional	≥40	634 Male: 43.2%	Cardiovascular examination and 12-lead ECG	4.3	2.9	5.3	Tegene et al,[11] 2019
Ghana	2009–2010	Community based	≥50	924 Male: 51.9%	12-lead ECG	0.3			Koopman et al,[65] 2014
Tanzania (elderly)	2009–2010	Community based cross-sectional	≥70	2232 Male: 43.7%	12-lead ECG	0.7	0.3	1.0	Dewhurst et al,[31] 2012
Uganda	2015	Community based cross-sectional	≥18	856 Male: 37.5%	12-lead ECG	0			Muthalaly et al,[10] 2018
Asia									
China	2006–2011	Population based	≥60	3922 Male: 43.8%	12-lead ECG	1.8	2.0	1.6	Li et al,[66] 2015
China	2014–2015	National cross-sectional	≥40	726,451 Male: 46.7%	Self-reporting of symptoms and 12-lead ECG	2.3			Wang et al,[12] 2018
China	2017–2019	Regional cross-sectional	≥40	18,796 Male: 39%	12-lead ECG	1.1	1.5	0.9	Wang et al,[13] 2020
China (elderly)	2013–2015	Community based cross-sectional	≥80	1056 Male: 49.8%	12-lead ECG	5.3	5.8	4.8	Huang et al,[32] 2018
Hongkong	2014–2015	Community based	≥18	13,122 Male: 28.5%	Smartphone single-lead ECG and self-reporting of symptoms	8.5	10.6	7.6	Chan et al,[33] 2017
Taiwan	2015–2016	Pharmacies	>50	3563 Male: 43%	Blood pressure device with specific algorithm for AF	2.6			Chao et al,[67] 2017
India	2016–2017	Population-based selective screen in rural area	≥40	2100 Male: 47.8%	Mobile ECG	1.6	2.3	1.0	Soni et al,[68] 2019
Japan	2008–2015	Annual health check-up by national health insurance	40–81	~123,030	12-lead ECG	0.8 in 2008 1.4 in 2015	1.7 in 2008 2.9 in 2015	0.2 in 2008 0.4 in 2015	Kodani et al,[15] 2019

Country	Years	Source/Setting	Age	Sample size	Diagnosis method	Prevalence			Reference
Japan	2014–2017	National insurance database	40–74	~1100 Male: 70%	12-lead ECG	1.9 in 2014 2.2 in 2017			Narita et al,[16] 2020
Malaysia	2007–2014	Selective screen from 18 urban and 22 rural communities	≥30	10,805 Male: 44%	12-lead ECG	0.49 at baseline 0.54 at 3 y			Lim et al,[69] 2016
South Korea	2015	National cross-sectional	≥20	41,505,679	Diagnosis on discharge or outpatient visits	0.67			Lee et al,[24] 2018
South Korea	2006–2015	National cross-sectional	≥20	~40,000,000	Diagnosed on discharge or outpatient	0.7 (in 2006) 1.5 (in 2015)			Kim et al,[70] 2018
Thailand (elderly)	2016	Community based, cross-sectional	≥65	1277 Male: 42.6%	12-lead ECG	1.9			Phrommintikul et al,[71] 2016
Europe									
Belgium	2010–2014	Population-based	≥20	65,747 Male: 41.4%	12-lead ECG	1.4	1.8	1.1	Proietti et al,[17] 2016
Denmark	2015–2016	Population based	65–74	1318 Male: 51.4%	Single-lead ECG during CT	3.1	5.2	0.9	Kvist et al,[72] 2017
Germany	2007–2017	Population based	35–74	5000 Male: 49.4%	12-lead ECG	2.5	4.6	1.9	Schnabel et al,[73] 2012
Ireland	2014	37 GP clinics in rural area	≥60	7262 Male: 45.3%	Radial pulse pulsation confirmed by ECG	10.9			Smyth et al,[74] 2016
Italy	2002–2013	Administrative health database	≥40	~35,000	Hospital diagnosis of AF	2.4	2.7	2.1	Marzona et al,[18] 2020
Italy (elderly)	2016–20	Population based	≥65	6016 (4528 eligible) Male: 47.2%	12-lead ECG and report of diagnosis, interrogation of pacemaker	7.3	8.6	6.2	Di Carlo et al,[75] 2019
Netherland	2002	Community-based cohort	≥55	6934 Male: 37.2%	12-lead ECG	7.7	8.6	7.1	Krijthe et al,[4] 2013
Netherland	2013	Population-based, during vaccine with GP	≥60	3269 Male: 49%	Single-lead ECG	3.7	4.4	3.1	Kaasenbrood et al,[76] 2016
Norway	2012–2015	Population based cross-sectional	63–65	3706 Male: 51.2%	12-lead ECG or documentation of diagnosis	4.5	6.4	2.4	Berge et al,[77] 2018
Portugal	2013	Health system registry	No restriction	383,000 Male: 49.2%	Documented diagnosis	2.1			Rodriguez-Manero et al,[78] 2019
Portugal (elderly)	2013–2015	National recruited	≥65	7500 Male: 41.1%	12-lead ECG, Holter and event recorder	9.0	8.9	9.1	Monteiro et al,[79] 2018

(continued on next page)

Table 1
(continued)

Nation/Region	Study Period	Source	Age	Population	Definition of AF	Prevalence Overall (%)	Male (%)	Female (%)	Reference
Russia	Published 2020; Survey: 2006–2009	Population based, cross-sectional	≥55	1732 Male: 46.4%	12-lead ECG and 24-h Holter	6.6	5.8	7.4	Shkolnikova et al,[80] 2020
Spain	2010–2012	Population based, cross-sectional	≥40	8343 Male: 47.6%	12-lead ECG	4.4	4.4	4.5	Gomez-Doblas et al,[81] 2014
Spain (elderly)	2015	Community based cross-sectional	≥90	59,423 Male: 25.9%	Documented diagnosis of AF	16.9			Lahoz et al,[82] 2019
Spain (elderly)	2015–2016	Community based	≥65	7065 Male: 41.1%	Pulse check, confirmed by 12-lead ECG	2.3			González Blanco et al,[83] 2017
Sweden	2005–2010	National registry	≥20	307,476 Male: 55%	Documented diagnosis of AF	2.9	3.3	2.5	Friberg et al,[19] 2013
Sweden (elderly)	2001–2003	Population based	≥60	6904 Male: 41.2%	12-lead ECG	4.9	5.2	4.8	Lindberg et al,[84] 2019
United Kingdom	2000–2016	16 sequential cross-sectional cohorts from GP registry	≥35	5,058,699 Male: 51.8% (in 2000)	Documented diagnosis	2.0 (in 2000) 3.2 (in 2016)			Adderley et al,[85] 2019
United Kingdom (elderly)	2001–2003	Population-based, cluster randomized controlled trial	≥65	14,802 Male: 42.6%	Hospital diagnosis or ECG	7.3 at baseline			Fitzmaurice et al,[86] 2007
Oceania									
Australia	1999–2000	National, population-based survey	≥25	8273 Male: 48.4%	12-lead ECG	1.4	1.5	1.4	Diouf et al,[20] 2016
Australia	2000–2009	Cross-sectional from database of tertiary center	No restriction	204,668 in total Indigenous: 5892 (male: 51.7%) Nonindigenous: 198,776 (Male: 53.8%)	Documented diagnosis of AF	Indigenous: 3.7 Nonindigenous: 7.1			Wong et al,[34] 2014

Country (region)	Years	Study design/setting	Age	Sample size/Male	Method of diagnosis	Prevalence			Reference
Australia (elderly)	2012–2013	Community based, cross-sectional (pharmacies)	≥65	1000 Male: 44%	Single-lead iPhone ECG	6.7			Lowres et al,[87] 2014
New Zealand	2010–2014	Retrospective cohort from 170 GP clinics	No restriction	73,900 Male: 57.1%	Documented diagnosis of AF	1.7	2.1		Tomlin et al,[88] 2017
North America									
Canada (elderly)	2014–2015	Community based (pharmacies)	≥65	1145 Male: 40.9%	Single-lead ECG	2.5	3.6		Sandhu et al,[89] 2016
Canada (elderly)	2015–2016	Population-based GP clinics	≥65	2054 Male: 46.6%	Initial screen by pulse check, single-lead ECG and blood pressure device with AF algorithm, confirmed by 12 lead ECG ± 24-h Holter	2.7	3.7		Quinn et al,[90] 2018
United States	2004–2005	Insurance database	≥20	21,648,481	Inpatient diagnosis of AF or outpatient claims	1.1			Naccarelli et al,[21] 2009
United States	1958–2007 (50-y follow-up)	Community-based cohort (Framingham study)	50–89	Original cohort: 4420 Offspring cohort: 5091	12-lead ECG, Holter, telemetry, monitor	(Age-adjusted period prevalence) 1958–1967: 2.0 1998–2007: 9.6	(Age-adjusted period prevalence) 1958–1967: 1.4 1998–2007: 4.9		Schnabel et al,[2] 2015
United States (Hispanic/Latino)	2008–2011	Population based	18–74	16,415 Male: 40% Hispanic/Latino only	12-lead ECG and self-report of physician diagnosis	1			Linares et al,[91] 2019
United States (elderly, African American)	2014–2016	Community-based	White: 78 ± 8; African American: 77 ± 6	1193 62% African American Male: 36%	48-h ambulatory ECG, discharge diagnosis of AF, ECG	White: 11.0 African American: 5.8	White men: 12.7 African American men: 4.7	White women: 9.4 African American women: 6	Loehr et al,[92] 2019
United States (elderly)	2014–2017	5 outpatient clinics	≥65	2286 Male: 60%	Single-lead ECG	5.1			Keen et al,[93] 2017

(continued on next page)

Table 1
(continued)

Nation/Region	Study Period	Source	Age	Population	Definition of AF	Prevalence			Reference
						Overall (%)	Male (%)	Female (%)	
United States (elderly)	2016–2017	Community-based cross-sectional	75–94	2616 Male: 42%	Ambulatory ECG monitor, reporting of symptoms	16.4			Rooney et al,[94] 2019
South America									
Brazil	2009–2016	ECG screen from 125 GP clinics	No restriction	676,621 Male: 42.5%	12-lead ECG	2.2			de Moraes et al,[22] 2019
Brazil	2011	Primary care center of 658 municipalities	≥5	262,685 Male: 40.4%	12-lead ECG	1.8	2.4	1.3	Marcolino et al,[23] 2015
Ecuador	2017	Population-based	≥60	298 Male:41.9%	24-h Holter	2.3	3.2	1.7	Del Brutto et al,[95] 2019

Abbreviations: CT, computed tomography; ECG, electrocardiogram; GP, general practitioner.

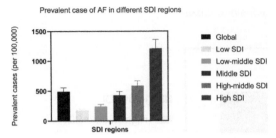

Fig. 3. Prevalent cases of AF in different sociodemographic regions. Prevalent cases of AF per 100,000 population globally (*black*) and in different sociodemographic index (SDI) regions (*in different colors*) in 2017. Graph generated by GraphPad Prism. (*Data from* GBD 2017 data visualization available from http://vizhub.healthdata.org/gbd-compare.)

risk in women (hazard ratio, 0.81).[41] Male sex is also associated with higher incidence of AF with age and race adjusted odds ratio of 1.61 during approximately 9 years of follow-up in 11,806 candidates in the Reasons for Geographic and Racial Differences in Stroke study.[42] The GBD 2017 study noted a male to female ratio in AF incidence in 2017 of 1.09, very similar to the ratio in 2007 (1.09) and 1997 (1.07).[5] Although both sexes share some risk factors such as age, white race, height, weight, use of blood pressure–lowering medications, and history of cardiovascular disease. However, diabetes is only correlated with incident AF in women and not in men.[42]

Female sex is associated with substantially higher mortality rates in the AF population across

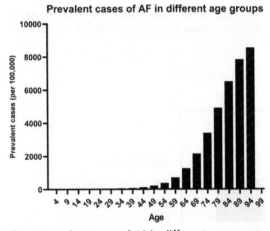

Fig. 4. Prevalent cases of AF in different age groups. Prevalent cases of AF globally per 100,000 population in different age groups with 5-year increments in both sex globally in 2017. Graph generated by GraphPad Prism. (*Data from* GBD 2017 data visualization available from http://vizhub.healthdata.org/gbd-compare.)

different socioeconomic regions (**Fig. 6**).[26] The FHS noted a risk factor-adjusted odds ratio of death of 1.5 in men and 1.9 in women with AF compared with those without.[43] A Korean national cohort study of 15,411 patients with AF showed 3.81-fold increased mortality risk in women compared with general population, as compared with 3.35-fold increase in men,[44] and the higher mortality risk in women remains across all age groups.[44] In GBD 2017, AF global mortality is significantly lower in men at 2.87 (2.56–3.26) per 100,000 compared with women of 4.66 (4.99–4.83) per 100,000 population.[26] Meta-analysis of 30 studies showed 12% higher risk of all-cause mortality, 55% increased risk of cardiovascular mortality and 2-fold increase in stroke risk associated with AF in women as compared with men.[45]

Some prior studies have shown that women tended to be undertreated with anticoagulation[46,47]; however, the recent GLORIA-AF study noted no significant sex difference in anticoagulant prescription globally.[48] Another possible explanation for the observed difference in mortality is sex predisposition to thromboembolism, as female sex is an independent strong risk factor for thromboembolism in AF.[49,50] However, the exact mechanism(s) underlying the higher mortality in women with AF is unclear.

ETHNICITY

Caucasian ethnicity carries a higher risk for incident AF. Numerous studies have demonstrated that African Americans, despite an overall higher risk factors for AF, have a significantly lower prevalence of AF compared with Caucasians.[35,51–55] Meta-analysis of these studies demonstrated African Americans have almost half the risk of AF compared with Caucasians (odds ratio, 0.51; 95% confidence interval, 0.44–0.59).[56] In a meta-analysis of 2 large community cohorts— the Cardiovascular Health Study (CHS) and the Atherosclerosis Risk in Communities (ARIC) study—European ancestry is identified to be positively correlated with incident AF after adjustment for other risk and confounding factors; using genetic admixture analysis, the risk of AF increases by 13% in African Americans with every 10% increase in European ancestry.[51] The lifetime risk of AF is higher in Caucasians (33%) than in African Americans (21%).[25] Similar trend is also found in Hispanics/Latinos and Asians. The lifetime risk of AF is approximately 1 in 5 among Chinese adults, and increases with advancing age.[57] MESA found a significantly decreased overall AF incidence in Hispanics, Chinese, and non-Hispanic black patients as

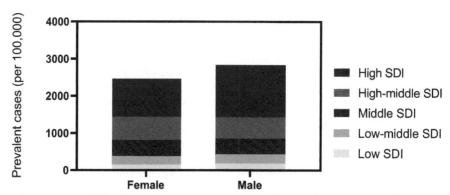

Fig. 5. Prevalent cases of AF in different sociodemographic regions and genders. Prevalent cases of AF per 100,000 population in different SDI regions in male and female in 2017. Graph generated by GraphPad Prism. (*Data from* GBD 2017 data visualization available from http://vizhub.healthdata.org/gbd-compare.)

compared with non-Hispanic white patients hospitalized for AF: the age- and sex-adjusted incidence rate per 1000 person-years for non-Hispanic whites is 11.23, as compared with 6.07 in Hispanics, 5.77 in non-Hispanic blacks, and 3.94 in Chinese.[58] Similar finding is noted by another large-sized hospital cohort, which also identified more pronounced risk associated with Caucasians in the absence of acquired cardiovascular risk factors.[59] In menopausal women, African American and Hispanic ethnicity is also negatively correlated with incidence of AF as compared with Caucasians.[60,61]

There are variations in ethnic predisposition to AF in indigenous populations. Indigenous Australians have reduced AF prevalence as compared with nonindigenous population (3.7% vs 7.1%)[34];

however, a survey of male veterans in the United States showed almost similarly raised age-adjusted AF prevalence among Caucasian (5.7%), Native American/Alaskans (5.4%), and Pacific Islanders (5.2%) as compared with Africans (3.4%), Hispanics (3.0%), and Asians (3.6%).[62] A higher prevalence of AF is noted in the Aboriginal Métis population in Canada (2.1%) compared with the general population (1.4%),[63] as well in Maori octogenarians in New Zealand (21% in Maori vs 13% in non-Maori).[64]

GENETICS OF ATRIAL FIBRILLATION
Heritability of Atrial Fibrillation

A community-based cohort in the Framingham Offspring Study found that the risk of AF in offspring with at least one parental AF is 1.85 times

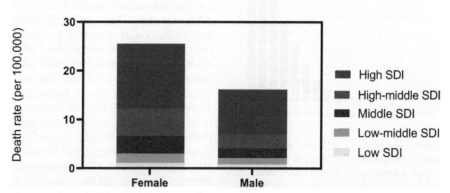

Fig. 6. Death rate of AF in different SDI regions and genders. Death rate of AF per 100,000 population in different SDI regions in male and female in 2017. Graph generated by GraphPad Prism. (*Data from* GBD 2017 data visualization available from http://vizhub.healthdata.org/gbd-compare.)

of those without, which further increases to 3.23 if adjusted to the age of onset for AF less than 75 years old.[96] Familial AF has been recognized as a major risk factor for AF independent of other traditional risk factors.[97–99] In a large cohort of 4421 participants in FHS, approximately 1 in 3 developed familial AF over 8 years of follow-up.[97] Familial AF is associated with a 40% increased risk for new-onset AF after adjustment for other AF risk factors.[97]

Genetics in Familial Atrial Fibrillation

Familial clustering of early-onset AF was noted back in 1942.[100,101] Presuming Mendelian (monogenic) forms of inheritance is responsible for the familial clustering of AF, linkage analysis and candidate gene sequencing were used to identify culprit genes, occasionally whole genome or exome sequencing was used as well.

In 1997, Brugada and colleagues[102] performed the first linkage study after screening the human genome using a new strategy of pooling the DNA samples in 3 families of familial AF. They identified one of the families with autosomal-dominant inheritance of AF, and the responsible gene is located at chromosome 10q22-24. Although the exact mutation responsible is unclear, the AF-susceptible locus is noted by a genome-wide association study (GWAS) to associate with SYNPO2L and MYOZ1, both expressed on skeletal muscle and cardiomyocyte.[103] In whole-exome sequencing of AF, this locus again was highlighted as most significantly associated with AF among the variants that did not reach significance in association with AF after adjustment for multiple testing.[104]

In 2003, Chen and colleagues[105] identified the first genetic mutation in AF through linkage analysis on a 4-generation family with autosomal-dominant AF. They noted gain-of-function mutation at KCNQ1, which encodes the α-subunit of the cardiac I_{Ks} channel. This mutation in KCNQ1 causes an increase in potassium channel current, which shortens the action potential duration and effective refractory period.[105] Subsequent studies noted that gain-of-function or loss-of-function mutations in genes encoding sodium, potassium and calcium channels (such as SCN1B, SCN2B, ABCC9, HCN4, and KCNE1-5) are associated with familial AF through effects on the depolarization, repolarization, action potential duration, calcium handling, increasing cellular automaticity, and susceptibility to reentry.[105–134] To date, there are 39 genes identified in familial AF (**Table 2**) that are related to ion channels, transcription regulation (eg, GATA4 and PITX2),[135–141] cellular

junction (eg, GJA1 and JPH2),[142–146] cell structure and signaling (eg, CAV1, NPPA, and LMNA).[141,146–150]

Although familial AF studies paved the way toward the understanding of genetics in AF, they only take up a small fraction of AF in large populations, and there is a limitation to its generalization to common AF. Different disease course and traits of familial AF are noted, including earlier age of AF onset, more disabling symptoms, higher body mass index, and fewer comorbidities as compared with nonfamilial AF counterparts.[153] In a Danish twin study, a 20% higher mortality is noted in twins with AF as compared with those without an affected cotwin,[154] and the effect is even more pronounced in monozygotic twins compared with dizygotic twins, suggesting a clear genetic impact on mortality in familial AF. Overlapping cardiac phenotypes including dilated cardiomyopathy,[138] ventricular tachycardia,[150] short QT syndrome,[125] atrioventricular block,[146] and bradyarrhythmia,[129] with familial AF are also noted in the assessed families. Additionally, candidate gene studies are generally small in sample sizes and there is limited functional evaluation of genetic variants to ascertain the underlying pathophysiologic mechanism.

Genetics in Common Atrial Fibrillation

GWAS have revolutionized genetic studies in common AF. GWAS test the genome differences between AF cases and healthy controls to screen for small variations as single nucleotide polymorphisms (SNPs) to identify the association between genotype and phenotype. The SNPs identified will be mapped to gene loci in proximity. GWAS was first applied in nonfamilial common AF cases in 2007 by Gudbjartsson and colleagues[155] in 2007 in an Icelandic cohort, which identified the locus at 4q25 adjacent to PITX2 as associated with AF. PITX2 encodes paired-like homeodomain transcription factor 2, which is involved in left–right differentiation during cardiac development.[156] Functional variants at 4q25 leads to decreased expression of PITX2,[157] which subsequently modulates the atrial rhythm homeostasis causing AF susceptibility.[158] Familial AF study also noted that deleterious mutation of PITX2 is associated with AF.[140]

A part of some loci also noted from familial AF studies, GWAS revealed more novel loci that were not found in previous linkage and candidate gene analyses. One of them is PRRX1, which encodes a homeodomain transcription factor highly expressed in the developing heart.[103] PRRX1-deficient mouse model demonstrated impaired pulmonary vasculature,[159] and suppression of

Table 2
Genetic variants associated with familial AF

Gene	Gene Product	Functional Effect	Reference
Sodium Channels			
SCN1B	β-Subunit of I_{Na}	Loss of function	[106]
SCN2B	β-Subunit of I_{Na}	Loss of function	[107]
SCN3B	β-Subunit of I_{Na}	Loss of function	[108]
SCN4B	β-Subunit of I_{Na}	Loss of function	[109]
SCN5A	α-Subunit of I_{Na}	Gain and loss of function	[110,111,151]
SCN10 A	α-Subunit of I_{Na}	Gain and loss of function	[112,113]
Potassium channels			
ABCC9	K_{ATP} channel	Loss of function	[114]
HCN4	Hyperpolarization-activated and cyclic nucleotide gated potassium channel 4	Loss of function	[115]
KCNA5	Kv1.5	Gain and loss of function	[116–118]
KCND3	Kv4.3	Gain of function	[119]
KCNE1	β-Subunit of I_{ks}	Gain of function	[120]
KCNE2	β-Subunit of I_{ks}	Gain of function	[121]
KCNE3	β-Subunit of I_{ks}	Gain of function	[122]
KCNE4	β-Subunit of I_{ks}	Gain of function	[123]
KCNE5	β-Subunit of I_{ks}	Gain of function	[124]
KCNH2	α-Subunit of I_{kr}	Gain and loss of function	[125,126]
KCNJ2	Kir2.1	Gain of function	[127]
KCNJ5	Kir3.4	Gain of function	[128,129]
KCNJ8	Kir6.1	Gain of function	[130]
KCNQ1	α-subunit of I_{ks}	Gain of function	[105,131–133]
Calcium channels			
CACNB2	Cavβ2	Loss of function	[134]
CACNA2D4	Cavα2β4	Loss of function	[134]
Non-ion channel variant			
CAV1	Caveolin 1	Loss of function	[141]
GATA4	Transcription factor	Loss of function	[135]
GATA5	Transcription factor	Loss of function	[136]
GATA6	Transcription factor	Loss of function	[137,152]
GJA1	Connexin43	Loss of function	[142]
GJA5	Connexin40	Loss of function	[143,144]
GREM2	Gremlin-2	Gain of function	[147]
JPH2	Junctophilin-2	Loss of function	[145]
LMNA	Lamin A/C	N/A	[146]
NKX2-5	Transcription factor	Loss of function	[138]
NKX2-6	Transcription factor	Loss of function	[139]
NPPA	Natriuretic peptide A	Gain of function	[148]
NUP155	Nucleoporin 155	Loss of function	[149]
PITX2	Transcription factor	Loss of function	[140]
RYR2	Ryanodine receptor 2	Gain of function	[150]

(*continued on next page*)

Table 2 (continued)			
Gene	**Gene Product**	**Functional Effect**	**Reference**
SYNE2	Nesprin-2	N/A	141
ZFHX3	Transcription factor	Loss of function	141

Abbreviation: N/A, not applicable.

PRRX1 results in shortening of atrial action potential duration in human stem cell derived cardiomyocytes, which could induce AF.[160]

A locus in 1q21, which is intronic to KCCN3, is identified as being associated with lone AF by GWAS.[161] KCCN3 encodes calcium activated potassium channel SK3,[161] which carries an important role regulating repolarization of action potential in atrial myocyte.[162] In an animal study, modulation of SK3 levels causes shortening of action potential duration, and subsequently predisposes animal to inducible atrial arrythmia.[162]

Thus far, approximately 260 SNPs (Supplementary Table 1) in 166 new genetic loci have been identified as associated with AF in multiple ethnic populations in multiple GWAS, which is significantly boosted after 2 large-scale GWAS by Roselli and colleagues[163] and Nielsen and colleagues[164] in 2018 (**Table 3**). A large whole-exome analysis in 2016 showed that no coding variants are associated with common AF, suggesting that large-effect coding variants are not the predominant hereditary mechanism of AF.[104]

The majority of these identified genetic loci by GWAS are in noncoding regions. Gene enrichment tests suggest that these functional candidates are likely involved in fetal cardiac development, cell structure and function, ion channels and calcium handling inside cardiomyocytes, angiogenesis and hormone signaling[163,164] (**Fig. 7**).

A recent study by van Ouwerkerk and colleagues[174] further elucidates the translational significance of functional noncoding variants by cross-referencing transcriptional, epigenomic and chromatin conformation datasets and short-listing the candidate variant regulatory element target genes involved in AF. They note top ranked functional involvement of these genes include regulation of heart rate, muscle and cardiomyocyte contraction, heart development, sarcomere organization, repolarization of cardiomyocytes, calcium handling, and mitochondrial translation.[174] At tissue-specific transcriptional level in left atrium, persistent AF is associated with reduced expression of genes encoding potassium and calcium channels such as KCCN2, KCNJ4&5, CACNA1C, and CACNB2, whereas the expression of KCNJ2 and KCNJ4 is increased, which leads to a shortening of the atrial refractory period.[175] The susceptibility to AF is associated with decreased transcriptional response to cellular stress, inflammation, and oxidation.[175]

Risk Stratification of Incident Atrial Fibrillation Using Polygenic Risk Scores

The timely diagnosis and management of AF is vital given the huge public health burden and the availability of effective treatment options; however, 40% of AF are clinically asymptomatic and undiagnosed, leaving these patients at risk of developing cryptogenic stroke, heart failure, and coronary artery disease.[176,177] Therefore, risk stratification of target populations using clinical and genetic risk factors has become increasingly important with more genetic loci revealed through large-scale studies. Given that no coding region has been found through a whole genome sequencing study to be directly related to AF,[104] although both polygenic and monogenic factors contribute to pathogenesis of AF in general population,[178] polygenic risk score recruiting numerous AF-related SNPs could maximize the effect size and predictive value compared with single SNP. Lubitz and associatesv[179] noted a significant association of comprehensive polygenic risk score with incident AF and cardioembolic stroke; however, there was only a small discriminative effect with incremental polygenic risk scores. Weng and colleagues[180] found both clinical risk factors and polygenic risk scores derived from approximately 1000 SNPs to be associated with the lifetime risk of AF after age of 55 years. Participants in low polygenic and clinical risk tertiles have a lifetime risk for AF less than half of the those at high risk tertiles (22.3% vs 48.2%).[180] The study also found that lower clinical risk factors is associated with reduced chances of developing AF, however, for those with few clinical risk factors but high genetic predisposition, the lifetime risk for AF remains high at 43.6%, suggestive of substantial determinant role of genetics in the development of AF independent of clinical risks.[180] More studies are required to evaluate the reproducibility and cost-effectiveness of combined polygenic risk score

Table 3
Overview of GWAS for AF

Study	Ancestry	AF Cohort Studies Included	No. of AF Cases	No. of Referents	No. of New Locus
Gudbjartsson et al,[155] 2007	European	Iceland cohort	550	4476	1 (PITX2)
Benjamin et al,[165] 2009	European	AGES, ARIC, CHS, FHS, RS	3413	37,105	1 (ZFHX3)
Ellinor et al,[161] 2010	European	AFNET and KORA S4, HVH and CHS, MGH and FHS	1335	12,844	1 (KCNN3)
Ellinor et al,[103] 2012	European	AFNET, AGES, ARIC, CC, CHS, FHS, HVH, KORA, MGH, MIGEN, RS-I, SHIP, Vanderbilt, WGHS	6707	52,426	6 (PRRX1, CAV1, SYNE2, C9orf3, HCN4, SYNPO2L)
Lubitz et al,[166] 2014	European	AFNET/KORA, AGES, ARIC, CC, CHS, FHS, LURIC, MGH, PHASE/PROSPER, RS, SHIP, WGHS	7171	57,512	0 (PITX2)
Sinner et al,[167] 2014	European and Japanese	AFNET/KORA, AGES, ARIC, Biobank Japan, DANFIB, CC, CHS, FHS, Health ABC, HVH, MAC, METASTROKE, MGH, Ottawa, PROSPER, RS, SHIP, WGH	European: 6707; Japanese: 843	European: 52,426; Japanese: 3350	4 in European (NEURL, GJA1, TBX5, CAND2); 2 in Japanese (NEURL, CUX2)
Tsai et al,[168] 2016	Asian	Taiwanese cohort	275	546	1 (KCHIP1)
Christophersen et al,[169] 2017	European, African American, Asian	31 studies in GWAS, 17 studies in ExWAS	18,398 in GWAS; 22,806 in ExWAS and RVAS	91,536 in GWAS; 132,612 in ExWAS and RVAS	12 (METTL11 B/KIFAP3, ANXA4/GMCL1, CEP68, TTN/TTN-AS1, KCNN2, KLHL3/WNT8A/FAM13 B, SLC35F1/PLN, ASAH1/PCM1, SH3PXD2A, KCNJ5, SCN10 A, SOX5)

Low et al,[170] 2017	Asian	Biobank Japan	8180	28,612	6 (HAND2, KCND3, NEBL, PPFIA4, SH3PXD2A, SLC1A-CEP68)
Lee et al,[171] 2017	Asian	Yonsei AF cohort, KoGES-HEXA control	672	3700	2 (HAND2, PPFIA4) concomitantly reported by Low et al. 2017
Thorolfsdottir et al,[172] 2017	European	ICELANDIC AF	14,255	374,939	2 (LINC01142, METTL11 B)
Nielsen et al,[173] 2018	European	HUNT biobank (Norway)	6337	61,607	1 (1p32–DMRTA2/FAF1/CDKN2C/RNF11)
Roselli et al,[163] 2018	European, Japanese, African American, Brazilian and Hispanic	AFGen Consortium, Broad AF Study, UK Biobank, Biobank Japan	65,446	522,774	70
Nielsen et al,[164] 2018	European	AFGen Consortium, deCODE, DiscovEHR, HUNT, MGI, UK Biobank	60,620	970,216	80

Abbreviations: AFNET, the German Competence Network on Atrial Fibrillation; AGES, Age, Gene/Environment Susceptibility study; ARIC, Atherosclerosis Risk in Community study; CC, Cleveland Clinic; CHS, Cardiovascular Healthy Study; DANFIB, Danish National Research Foundation Center for Cardiac Arrhythmia; ExWAS, Exome-Wide Association Analysis; FHS, Framingham Heart Study; HVH, Heart and Vascular Health Study; KoGES, Korean Genome Epidemiology Study; KORA, Cooperative Research in the Region of Augsburg; LURIC, Ludwigshafen Risk and Cardiovascular Health Study; MAC, Malmö Diet and Cancer study; MGH, Massachusetts General Hospital Atrial Fibrillation Study; MGI, Michigan Genomics Initiative; MIGEN, Myocardial Infarction Genetics Consortium; PHASE/PROSPER, PHArmacogenetic study of Statins in the Elderly at risk/PROspective Study of Pravastatin in the Elderly at Risk for vascular disease; RS, Rotterdam Study; RS-I, Rotterdam Study-I; RVAS, rare variant association studies; SHIP, Study of Health in Pomerania; WGHS, Women's Genome Health Study.

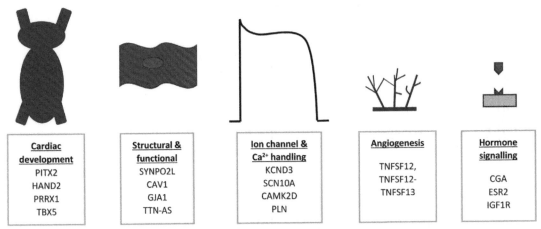

Fig. 7. Functional groups of AF-associated genetic loci. Diagram demonstrating the 5 major functional groups (fetal cardiac development, cellular structural and functional, ion channel and intracellular calcium handling, angiogenesis, and hormone signaling) of genetic loci identified as associated with AF by genome-wide association study (GWAS). Examples of genetic loci are listed in the boxes below each functional group. (*Data* Roselli C, Chaffin MD, Weng LC, et al. Multi-ethnic genome-wide association study for atrial fibrillation. *Nat Genet.* 2018;50(9):1225-1233; and Nielsen JB, Thorolfsdottir RB, Fritsche LG, et al. Biobank-driven genomic discovery yields new insight into atrial fibrillation biology. *Nat Genet.* 2018;50(9):1234-1239.)

and clinical risk factors in different populations before it could become widely implemented for risk stratification of AF.

SUMMARY

AF is the most common arrhythmia with major public health burden. In FHS, there is a 4-fold increase in prevalence and a 3 times increase in incidence over 50 years.[2] The geographic distribution of AF is in keeping with SDI, with sub-Saharan countries generally having the lowest disease burden as compared with North America.[26] However, there are concerns of under-reporting of the epidemiology in Africa, where patients with AF tend to be younger with a higher percentage of rheumatic valvular disease.[28,29] Advancing age, male sex, and Caucasian race are predisposing factors to AF[2,26,51]; however, female sex is associated with higher AF mortality, likely owing to their high thromboembolism risk.[43,49] African American, Hispanic, and Asian ethnicities are associated with lower prevalence and incidence of AF compared with Caucasians.[58,60,61] Indeed, there is major ethnic variation but limited studies regarding indigenous populations.[34,62–64]

AF may be a heritable disease, and familial AF is recognized as a major risk factor for AF. Familial AF provides unique opportunity for research into the genetics of AF.[96,97] Using linkage study and candidate gene sequencing, 39 genes have been identified in familial AF which are associated with ion channels, transcription, cellular junction, structure, and signaling (see **Table 2**). However, there is a barrier for the genetic findings from familial AF to be directly extrapolated into the general population where AF is influenced by multiple risk factors and shares different clinical features with diverse presentation.[153,154] Using GWAS, small variations as SNPs are identified in large-scale common AF population against healthy controls to link with AF. The technique revolutionized the discovery of genetics of AF in large population and has identified more than 160 genetic loci as associated in AF across multiple ethnic groups (see **Table 3**). Whole-exome sequencing identified no direct coding variant is associated with common AF, suggesting that majority of these loci are related to AF through regulatory effect.[104] Using a gene enrichment test, there are a few functional groups involved the genetic loci of AF, including fetal cardiac development, cellular structure and function, ion channels and intracellular calcium handling, angiogenesis, and hormone signaling (see **Fig. 7**).[163,164] Using numerous genetic variants, a polygenic risk score has proven to be effective and feasible in combination with clinical risk factors of AF in risk stratifying the target population,[179,180] although further studies are still required to test its reproducibility and validity in larger population with more diverse ethnic background.

CLINICS CARE POINTS

- The prevalence of atrial fibrillation (AF) is positively correlated with the sociodemographic level globally.

- Elderly patients with AF have longer hospital stay, higher in-patient mortality, and associate with chronic kidney disease compared to younger patients.
- Male sex associates with higher prevalence of AF, although female sex correlates with higher mortality in AF.
- Caucasians have almost two-fold risk for AF compared to African Americans, Hispanics, and Asians.
- AF has strong hereditary characteristics. Most of the genetic loci discovered in common AF population are in non-coding domains. Polygenic risk score has shown potential in risk stratification for AF.

DISCLOSURE

Professor G.Y.H. Lip discloses serving as a consultant for Bayer/Janssen, BMS/Pfizer, Medtronic, Boehringer Ingelheim, Novartis, Verseon, and Daiichi Sankyo and serving as a speaker for Bayer, BMS/Pfizer, Medtronic, Boehringer Ingelheim, and Daiichi Sankyo. No fees are directly received personally.

REFERENCES

1. Kirchhof P, Benussi S, Kotecha D, et al. 2016 ESC Guidelines for the management of atrial fibrillation developed in collaboration with EACTS. Europace 2016;18(11):1609–78.
2. Schnabel RB, Yin X, Gona P, et al. 50 year trends in atrial fibrillation prevalence, incidence, risk factors, and mortality in the Framingham Heart Study: a cohort study. Lancet 2015;386(9989):154–62.
3. Turakhia MP, Shafrin J, Bognar K, et al. Estimated prevalence of undiagnosed atrial fibrillation in the United States. PLoS One 2018;13(4):e0195088.
4. Krijthe BP, Kunst A, Benjamin EJ, et al. Projections on the number of individuals with atrial fibrillation in the European Union, from 2000 to 2060. Eur Heart J 2013;34(35):2746–51.
5. Lippi G, Sanchis-Gomar F, Cervellin G. Global epidemiology of atrial fibrillation: an increasing epidemic and public health challenge. Int J Stroke 2020. https://doi.org/10.1177/1747493019897870. 1747493019897870.
6. Patel NJ, Deshmukh A, Pant S, et al. Contemporary trends of hospitalization for atrial fibrillation in the United States, 2000 through 2010: implications for healthcare planning. Circulation 2014;129(23): 2371–9.
7. Johnsen SP, Dalby LW, Tackstrom T, et al. Cost of illness of atrial fibrillation: a nationwide study of societal impact. BMC Health Serv Res 2017;17(1): 714.
8. Odutayo A, Wong CX, Hsiao AJ, et al. Atrial fibrillation and risks of cardiovascular disease, renal disease, and death: systematic review and meta-analysis. BMJ 2016;354:i4482.
9. Centers for disease control and prevention NCfHS. Underlying causes of death, 1999-2008. Available at: https://wonder.cdc.gov/ucd-icd10.html. Accessed June 2, 2020.
10. Muthalaly RG, Koplan BA, Albano A, et al. Low population prevalence of atrial fibrillation in rural Uganda: a community-based cross-sectional study. Int J Cardiol 2018;271:87–91.
11. Tegene E, Tadesse I, Markos Y, et al. Prevalence and risk factors for atrial fibrillation and its anticoagulant requirement in adults aged ≥40 in Jimma Town, Southwest Ethiopia: a community based cross-sectional study. Int J Cardiol Heart Vasc 2019;22:199–204.
12. Wang X, Fu Q, Song F, et al. Prevalence of atrial fibrillation in different socioeconomic regions of China and its association with stroke: results from a national stroke screening survey. Int J Cardiol 2018;271:92–7.
13. c L, Lin M, Du Z, et al. Epidemiology of atrial fibrillation in northeast China: a cross-sectional study, 2017-2019. Heart 2020;106(8):590–5.
14. Lip GYH, Brechin CM, Lane DA. The global burden of atrial fibrillation and stroke: a systematic review of the epidemiology of atrial fibrillation in regions outside North America and Europe. Chest 2012; 142(6):1489–98.
15. Kodani E, Kaneko T, Fujii H, et al. Prevalence and incidence of atrial fibrillation in the general population based on national health insurance special health checkups - TAMA MED Project-AF. Circ J 2019;83(3):524–31.
16. Narita N, Okumura K, Kinjo T, et al. Trends in prevalence of non-valvular atrial fibrillation and anticoagulation therapy in a Japanese region - analysis using the national health insurance database. Circ J 2020;84(5):706–13.
17. Proietti M, Mairesse GH, Goethals P, et al. A population screening programme for atrial fibrillation: a report from the Belgian heart rhythm week screening programme. Europace 2016; 18(12):1779–86.
18. Marzona I, Proietti M, Vannini T, et al. Sex-related differences in prevalence, treatment and outcomes in patients with atrial fibrillation. Intern Emerg Med 2020;15(2):231–40.
19. Friberg L, Bergfeldt L. Atrial fibrillation prevalence revisited. J Intern Med 2013;274(5):461–8.
20. Diouf I, Magliano DJ, Carrington MJ, et al. Prevalence, incidence, risk factors and treatment of atrial fibrillation in Australia: the Australian Diabetes, Obesity and Lifestyle (AusDiab) longitudinal, population cohort study. Int J Cardiol 2016;205:127–32.

21. Naccarelli GV, Varker H, Lin J, et al. Increasing prevalence of atrial fibrillation and flutter in the United States. Am J Cardiol 2009;104(11): 1534–9.

22. de Moraes ERFL, Cirenza C, Lopes RD, et al. Prevalence of atrial fibrillation and stroke risk assessment based on telemedicine screening tools in a primary healthcare setting. Eur J Intern Med 2019;67:36–41.

23. Marcolino MS, Palhares DM, Benjamin EJ, et al. Atrial fibrillation: prevalence in a large database of primary care patients in Brazil. Europace 2015; 17(12):1787–90.

24. Lee SR, Choi EK, Han K, et al. Prevalence of non-valvular atrial fibrillation based on geographical distribution and socioeconomic status in the entire Korean population. Korean Circ J 2018;48(7):622–34.

25. Mou L, Norby FL, Chen LY, et al. Lifetime risk of atrial fibrillation by race and socioeconomic status: ARIC study (atherosclerosis risk in communities). Circ Arrhythm Electrophysiol 2018;11(7):e006350.

26. Institute for Health Metrics and Evaluation (IHME). GBD compare data visualization. Seattle (WA): IHME, University of Washington; 2018. Available at: http://vizhub.healthdata.org/gbd-compare. Accessed June 3, 2020.

27. Guhl E, Althouse A, Sharbaugh M, et al. Association of income and health-related quality of life in atrial fibrillation. Open Heart 2019;6(1):e000974.

28. Jacobs MS, van Hulst M, Adeoye AM, et al. Atrial fibrillation in Africa-an under-reported and unrecognized risk factor for stroke: a systematic review. Glob Heart 2019;14(3):269–79.

29. Stambler BS, Ngunga LM. Atrial fibrillation in Sub-Saharan Africa: epidemiology, unmet needs, and treatment options. Int J Gen Med 2015;8:231–42.

30. Magnussen C, Niiranen TJ, Ojeda FM, et al. Sex differences and similarities in atrial fibrillation epidemiology, risk factors, and mortality in community cohorts: results from the BiomarCaRE consortium (biomarker for cardiovascular risk assessment in Europe). Circulation 2017;136(17): 1588–97.

31. Dewhurst MJ, Adams PC, Gray WK, et al. Strikingly low prevalence of atrial fibrillation in elderly Tanzanians. J Am Geriatr Soc 2012;60(6):1135–40.

32. Huang G, Xu RH, Xu JB, et al. Hyperuricemia is associated with atrial fibrillation prevalence in very elderly - a community based study in Chengdu, China. Sci Rep 2018;8(1):12403.

33. Chan NY, Choy CC. Screening for atrial fibrillation in 13 122 Hong Kong citizens with smartphone electrocardiogram. Heart 2017;103(1):24–31.

34. Wong CX, Brooks AG, Cheng YH, et al. Atrial fibrillation in Indigenous and non-Indigenous Australians: a cross-sectional study. BMJ Open 2014; 4(10):e006242.

35. Go AS, Hylek EM, Phillips KA, et al. Prevalence of diagnosed atrial fibrillation in adults: national implications for rhythm management and stroke prevention: the AnTicoagulation and risk factors in atrial fibrillation (ATRIA) Study. JAMA 2001;285(18): 2370–5.

36. Marinigh R, Lip GY, Fiotti N, et al. Age as a risk factor for stroke in atrial fibrillation patients: implications for thromboprophylaxis. J Am Coll Cardiol 2010;56(11):827–37.

37. Soo Y, Chan N, Leung KT, et al. Age-specific trends of atrial fibrillation-related ischaemic stroke and transient ischaemic attack, anticoagulant use and risk factor profile in Chinese population: a 15-year study. J Neurol Neurosurg Psychiatr 2017;88(9): 744–8.

38. Inoue H, Atarashi H, Therapy RGfAD. Risk factors for thromboembolism in patients with paroxysmal atrial fibrillation. Am J Cardiol 2000;86(8):852–5.

39. Moulton AW, Singer DE, Haas JS. Risk factors for stroke in patients with nonrheumatic atrial fibrillation: a case-control study. Am J Med 1991;91(2): 156–61.

40. Naderi S, Wang Y, Miller AL, et al. The impact of age on the epidemiology of atrial fibrillation hospitalizations. Am J Med 2014;127(2). 158.e151-157.

41. O'Neal WT, Nazarian S, Alonso A, et al. Sex hormones and the risk of atrial fibrillation: the Multi-Ethnic Study of Atherosclerosis (MESA). Endocrine 2017;58(1):91–6.

42. Bose A, O'Neal WT, Wu C, et al. Sex differences in risk factors for incident atrial fibrillation (from the reasons for geographic and racial differences in stroke [REGARDS] study). Am J Cardiol 2019; 123(9):1453–7.

43. Benjamin EJ, Wolf PA, D'Agostino RB, et al. Impact of atrial fibrillation on the risk of death: the Framingham Heart Study. Circulation 1998;98(10):946–52.

44. Lee E, Choi EK, Han KD, et al. Mortality and causes of death in patients with atrial fibrillation: a nationwide population-based study. PLoS One 2018; 13(12):e0209687.

45. Emdin CA, Wong CX, Hsiao AJ, et al. Atrial fibrillation as risk factor for cardiovascular disease and death in women compared with men: systematic review and meta-analysis of cohort studies. BMJ 2016;532:h7013.

46. Humphries KH, Kerr CR, Connolly SJ, et al. New-onset atrial fibrillation: sex differences in presentation, treatment, and outcome. Circulation 2001; 103(19):2365–70.

47. Murphy NF, Simpson CR, Jhund PS, et al. A national survey of the prevalence, incidence, primary care burden and treatment of atrial fibrillation in Scotland. Heart 2007;93(5):606–12.

48. Mazurek M, Huisman MV, Rothman KJ, et al. Gender differences in antithrombotic treatment for

newly diagnosed atrial fibrillation: the GLORIA-AF registry program. Am J Med 2018;131(8):945–55. e943.

49. Fang MC, Singer DE, Chang Y, et al. Gender differences in the risk of ischemic stroke and peripheral embolism in atrial fibrillation: the AnTicoagulation and risk factors in atrial fibrillation (ATRIA) study. Circulation 2005;112(12):1687–91.

50. Lip GY, Nieuwlaat R, Pisters R, et al. Refining clinical risk stratification for predicting stroke and thromboembolism in atrial fibrillation using a novel risk factor-based approach: the euro heart survey on atrial fibrillation. Chest 2010;137(2):263–72.

51. Marcus GM, Alonso A, Peralta CA, et al. European ancestry as a risk factor for atrial fibrillation in African Americans. Circulation 2010;122(20):2009–15.

52. Ruo B, Capra AM, Jensvold NG, et al. Racial variation in the prevalence of atrial fibrillation among patients with heart failure: the Epidemiology, Practice, Outcomes, and Costs of Heart Failure (EPOCH) study. J Am Coll Cardiol 2004;43(3):429–35.

53. Upshaw CB. Reduced prevalence of atrial fibrillation in black patients compared with white patients attending an urban hospital: an electrocardiographic study. J Natl Med Assoc 2002;94(4):204–8.

54. Michael Smith J, Soneson EA, Woods SE, et al. Coronary artery bypass graft surgery outcomes among African-Americans and Caucasian patients. Int J Surg 2006;4(4):212–6.

55. Shen AY, Contreras R, Sobnosky S, et al. Racial/ethnic differences in the prevalence of atrial fibrillation among older adults–a cross-sectional study. J Natl Med Assoc 2010;102(10):906–13.

56. Hernandez MB, Asher CR, Hernandez AV, et al. African American race and prevalence of atrial fibrillation: a meta-analysis. Cardiol Res Pract 2012;2012:275624.

57. Guo Y, Tian Y, Wang H, et al. Prevalence, incidence, and lifetime risk of atrial fibrillation in China: new insights into the global burden of atrial fibrillation. Chest 2015;147(1):109–19.

58. Rodriguez CJ, Soliman EZ, Alonso A, et al. Atrial fibrillation incidence and risk factors in relation to race-ethnicity and the population attributable fraction of atrial fibrillation risk factors: the Multi-Ethnic Study of Atherosclerosis. Ann Epidemiol 2015;25(2):71–55.e943.

59. Dewland TA, Olgin JE, Vittinghoff E, et al. Incident atrial fibrillation among Asians, Hispanics, blacks, and whites. Circulation 2013;128(23):2470–7.

60. Perez MV, Hoffmann TJ, Tang H, et al. African American race but not genome-wide ancestry is negatively associated with atrial fibrillation among postmenopausal women in the Women's Health Initiative. Am Heart J 2013;166(3):566–72.

61. Perez MV, Wang PJ, Larson JC, et al. Risk factors for atrial fibrillation and their population burden in postmenopausal women: the Women's health initiative observational study. Heart 2013;99(16):1173–8.

62. Borzecki AM, Bridgers DK, Liebschutz JM, et al. Racial differences in the prevalence of atrial fibrillation among males. J Natl Med Assoc 2008;100(2):237–45.

63. Atzema CL, Khan S, Lu H, et al. Cardiovascular disease rates, outcomes, and quality of care in Ontario Metis: a population-based cohort study. PLoS One 2015;10(3):e0121779.

64. Teh R, Martin A, Kerse N, et al. The burden of atrial fibrillation in octogenarians. Heart Lung Circ 2013;22(7):580–1.

65. Koopman JJ, van Bodegom D, Westendorp RG, et al. Scarcity of atrial fibrillation in a traditional African population: a community-based study. BMC Cardiovasc Disord 2014;14:87.

66. Li LH, Sheng CS, Hu BC, et al. The prevalence, incidence, management and risks of atrial fibrillation in an elderly Chinese population: a prospective study. BMC Cardiovasc Disord 2015;15:31.

67. Chao T, Chen S. P1693 the results of screen of atrial fibrillation event in Taiwan: the SAFE-Taiwan study. Europace 2017;19:iii363-iii.

68. Soni A, Karna S, Fahey N, et al. Age-and-sex stratified prevalence of atrial fibrillation in rural Western India: results of SMART-India, a population-based screening study. Int J Cardiol 2019;280:84–8.

69. Lim CW, Kasim S, Ismail JR, et al. Prevalence of atrial fibrillation in the Malaysian communities. Heart Asia 2016;8(2):62–6.

70. Kim D, Yang PS, Jang E, et al. 10-year nationwide trends of the incidence, prevalence, and adverse outcomes of non-valvular atrial fibrillation nationwide health insurance data covering the entire Korean population. Am Heart J 2018;202:20–6.

71. Phrommintikul A, Detnuntarat P, Prasertwitayakij N, et al. Prevalence of atrial fibrillation in Thai elderly. J Geriatr Cardiol 2016;13(3):270–3.

72. Kvist TV, Lindholt JS, Rasmussen LM, et al. The DanCavas pilot study of multifaceted screening for subclinical cardiovascular disease in men and women aged 65-74 years. Eur J Vasc Endovasc Surg 2017;53(1):123–31.

73. Schnabel RB, Wilde S, Wild PS, et al. Atrial fibrillation: its prevalence and risk factor profile in the German general population. Dtsch Arztebl Int 2012;109(16):293–9.

74. Smyth B, Marsden P, Corcoran R, et al. Opportunistic screening for atrial fibrillation in a rural area. QJM 2016;109(8):539–43.

75. Di Carlo A, Bellino L, Consoli D, et al. Prevalence of atrial fibrillation in the Italian elderly population and

projections from 2020 to 2060 for Italy and the European Union: the FAI Project. Europace 2019; 21(10):1468–75.

76. Kaasenbrood F, Hollander M, Rutten FH, et al. Yield of screening for atrial fibrillation in primary care with a hand-held, single-lead electrocardiogram device during influenza vaccination. Europace 2016; 18(10):1514–20.

77. Berge T, Lyngbakken MN, Ihle-Hansen H, et al. Prevalence of atrial fibrillation and cardiovascular risk factors in a 63-65 years old general population cohort: the Akershus Cardiac Examination (ACE) 1950 Study. BMJ Open 2018;8(7):e021704.

78. Rodriguez-Manero M, Lopez-Pardo E, Cordero-Fort A, et al. Prevalence and outcomes of atrial fibrillation in a European healthcare area gained through the processing of a health information technology system. Rev Port Cardiol 2019;38(1): 21–9.

79. Monteiro P, endide Safira. The SAFIRA study: a reflection on the prevalence and treatment patterns of atrial fibrillation and cardiovascular risk factors in 7500 elderly subjects. Rev Port Cardiol 2018;37(4): 307–13.

80. Shkolnikova MA, Jdanov DA, Ildarova RA, et al. Atrial fibrillation among Russian men and women aged 55 years and older: prevalence, mortality, and associations with biomarkers in a population-based study. J Geriatr Cardiol 2020;17(2):74–84.

81. Gomez-Doblas JJ, Muniz J, Martin JJ, et al. Prevalence of atrial fibrillation in Spain. OFRECE study results. Rev Esp Cardiol (Engl Ed) 2014;67(4): 259–69.

82. Lahoz C, Cardenas J, Salinero-Fort M, et al. Prevalence of atrial fibrillation and associated anticoagulant therapy in the nonagenarian population of the Community of Madrid, Spain. Geriatr Gerontol Int 2019;19(3):203–7.

83. González Blanco V, Pérula de Torres L, Martín Rioboó E, et al. Opportunistic screening for atrial fibrillation versus detecting symptomatic patients aged 65 years and older: a cluster-controlled clinical trial. Med Clin (Barc) 2017;148(1):8–15.

84. Lindberg T, Wimo A, Elmståhl S, et al. Prevalence and incidence of atrial fibrillation and other arrhythmias in the general older population: findings from the Swedish national study on aging and care. Gerontol Geriatr Med 2019;5. 2333721419859687.

85. Adderley NJ, Ryan R, Nirantharakumar K, et al. Prevalence and treatment of atrial fibrillation in UK general practice from 2000 to 2016. Heart 2019;105(1):27–33.

86. Fitzmaurice DA, Hobbs FD, Jowett S, et al. Screening versus routine practice in detection of atrial fibrillation in patients aged 65 or over: cluster randomised controlled trial. BMJ 2007; 335(7616):383.

87. Lowres N, Neubeck L, Salkeld G, et al. Feasibility and cost-effectiveness of stroke prevention through community screening for atrial fibrillation using iPhone ECG in pharmacies. The SEARCH-AF study. Thromb Haemost 2014;111(6):1167–76.

88. Tomlin AM, Lloyd HS, Tilyard MW. Atrial fibrillation in New Zealand primary care: prevalence, risk factors for stroke and the management of thromboembolic risk. Eur J Prev Cardiol 2017;24(3): 311–9.

89. Sandhu RK, Dolovich L, Deif B, et al. High prevalence of modifiable stroke risk factors identified in a pharmacy-based screening programme. Open Heart 2016;3(2):e000515.

90. Quinn FR, Gladstone DJ, Ivers NM, et al. Diagnostic accuracy and yield of screening tests for atrial fibrillation in the family practice setting: a multicentre cohort study. CMAJ Open 2018;6(3):E308–15.

91. Linares JD, Jackson LR, Dawood FZ, et al. Prevalence of atrial fibrillation and association with clinical, sociocultural, and ancestral correlates among Hispanic/Latinos: the Hispanic community health study/study of Latinos. Heart Rhythm 2019; 16(5):686–93.

92. Loehr LR, Soliman EZ, Poon AK, et al. The prevalence of atrial fibrillation on 48-hour ambulatory electrocardiography in African Americans compared to Whites: the atherosclerosis risk in communities (ARIC) study. Am Heart J 2019;216:1–8.

93. Keen W, Martin J, Lopez C, et al. Abstract 18153: screening for atrial fibrillation is feasible in US managed care outpatient facilities. Circulation 2017;136(Suppl 1):A18153.

94. Rooney MR, Soliman EZ, Lutsey PL, et al. Prevalence and characteristics of subclinical atrial fibrillation in a community-dwelling elderly population: the ARIC study. Circ Arrhythm Electrophysiol 2019;12(10):e007390.

95. Del Brutto OH, Costa AF, Cano JA, et al. Low prevalence of atrial fibrillation in Amerindians: a population-based study in frequent fish consumers living in rural coastal Ecuador (The Atahualpa Project). Aging Clin Exp Res 2018;30(5):539–42.

96. Fox CS, Parise H, D'Agostino RB, et al. Parental atrial fibrillation as a risk factor for atrial fibrillation in offspring. JAMA 2004;291(23):2851–5.

97. Lubitz SA, Yin X, Fontes JD, et al. Association between familial atrial fibrillation and risk of new-onset atrial fibrillation. JAMA 2010;304(20):2263–9.

98. Gundlund A, Christiansen MN, Hansen ML, et al. Familial clustering and subsequent incidence of atrial fibrillation among first-degree relatives in Denmark. Europace 2016;18(5):658–64.

99. Christophersen IE, Ravn LS, Budtz-Joergensen E, et al. Familial aggregation of atrial fibrillation: a study in Danish twins. Circ Arrhythm Electrophysiol 2009;2(4):378–83.

100. Levy R. Paroxysmal auricular fibrillation and flutter without signs of organic cardiac disease in two brothers. J Mt Sinai Hosp N Y 1942;8:765–70.

101. Gould WL. Auricular fibrillation; report on a study of a familial tendency, 1920-1956. AMA Arch Intern Med 1957;100(6):916–26.

102. Brugada R, Tapscott T, Czernuszewicz GZ, et al. Identification of a genetic locus for familial atrial fibrillation. N Engl J Med 1997;336(13):905–11.

103. Ellinor PT, Lunetta KL, Albert CM, et al. Meta-analysis identifies six new susceptibility loci for atrial fibrillation. Nat Genet 2012;44(6):670–5.

104. Lubitz SA, Brody JA, Bihlmeyer NA, et al. Whole exome sequencing in atrial fibrillation. PLoS Genet 2016;12(9):e1006284.

105. Chen YH, Xu SJ, Bendahhou S, et al. KCNQ1 gain-of-function mutation in familial atrial fibrillation. Science 2003;299(5604):251–4.

106. Olesen MS, Holst AG, Svendsen JH, et al. SCN1Bb R214Q found in 3 patients: 1 with Brugada syndrome and 2 with lone atrial fibrillation. Heart Rhythm 2012;9(5):770–3.

107. Watanabe H, Darbar D, Kaiser DW, et al. Mutations in sodium channel β1- and β2-subunits associated with atrial fibrillation. Circ Arrhythm Electrophysiol 2009;2(3):268–75.

108. Olesen MS, Jespersen T, Nielsen JB, et al. Mutations in sodium channel β-subunit SCN3B are associated with early-onset lone atrial fibrillation. Cardiovasc Res 2011;89(4):786–93.

109. Li RG, Wang Q, Xu YJ, et al. Mutations of the SCN4B-encoded sodium channel β4 subunit in familial atrial fibrillation. Int J Mol Med 2013;32(1):144–50.

110. Darbar D, Kannankeril PJ, Donahue BS, et al. Cardiac sodium channel (SCN5A) variants associated with atrial fibrillation. Circulation 2008;117(15):1927–35.

111. Makiyama T, Akao M, Shizuta S, et al. A novel SCN5A gain-of-function mutation M1875T associated with familial atrial fibrillation. J Am Coll Cardiol 2008;52(16):1326–34.

112. Jabbari J, Olesen MS, Yuan L, et al. Common and rare variants in SCN10A modulate the risk of atrial fibrillation. Circ Cardiovasc Genet 2015;8(1):64–73.

113. Savio-Galimberti E, Weeke P, Muhammad R, et al. SCN10A/Nav1.8 modulation of peak and late sodium currents in patients with early onset atrial fibrillation. Cardiovasc Res 2014;104(2):355–63.

114. Olson TM, Alekseev AE, Moreau C, et al. KATP channel mutation confers risk for vein of Marshall adrenergic atrial fibrillation. Nat Clin Pract Cardiovasc Med 2007;4(2):110–6.

115. Macri V, Mahida SN, Zhang ML, et al. A novel trafficking-defective HCN4 mutation is associated with early-onset atrial fibrillation. Heart Rhythm 2014;11(6):1055–62.

116. Christophersen IE, Olesen MS, Liang B, et al. Genetic variation in KCNA5: impact on the atrial-specific potassium current IKur in patients with lone atrial fibrillation. Eur Heart J 2013;34(20):1517–25.

117. Olson TM, Alekseev AE, Liu XK, et al. Kv1.5 channelopathy due to KCNA5 loss-of-function mutation causes human atrial fibrillation. Hum Mol Genet 2006;15(14):2185–91.

118. Yang Y, Li J, Lin X, et al. Novel KCNA5 loss-of-function mutations responsible for atrial fibrillation. J Hum Genet 2009;54(5):277–83.

119. Olesen MS, Refsgaard L, Holst AG, et al. A novel KCND3 gain-of-function mutation associated with early-onset of persistent lone atrial fibrillation. Cardiovasc Res 2013;98(3):488–95.

120. Olesen MS, Bentzen BH, Nielsen JB, et al. Mutations in the potassium channel subunit KCNE1 are associated with early-onset familial atrial fibrillation. BMC Med Genet 2012;13:24.

121. Yang Y, Xia M, Jin Q, et al. Identification of a KCNE2 gain-of-function mutation in patients with familial atrial fibrillation. Am J Hum Genet 2004;75(5):899–905.

122. Lundby A, Ravn LS, Svendsen JH, et al. KCNE3 mutation V17M identified in a patient with lone atrial fibrillation. Cell Physiol Biochem 2008;21(1–3):47–54.

123. Mann SA, Otway R, Guo G, et al. Epistatic effects of potassium channel variation on cardiac repolarization and atrial fibrillation risk. J Am Coll Cardiol 2012;59(11):1017–25.

124. Ravn LS, Aizawa Y, Pollevick GD, et al. Gain of function in IKs secondary to a mutation in KCNE5 associated with atrial fibrillation. Heart Rhythm 2008;5(3):427–35.

125. Hong K, Bjerregaard P, Gussak I, et al. Short QT syndrome and atrial fibrillation caused by mutation in KCNH2. J Cardiovasc Electrophysiol 2005;16(4):394–6.

126. Sinner MF, Pfeufer A, Akyol M, et al. The nonsynonymous coding IKr-channel variant KCNH2-K897T is associated with atrial fibrillation: results from a systematic candidate gene-based analysis of KCNH2 (HERG). Eur Heart J 2008;29(7):907–14.

127. Xia M, Jin Q, Bendahhou S, et al. A Kir2.1 gain-of-function mutation underlies familial atrial fibrillation. Biochem Biophys Res Commun 2005;332(4):1012–9.

128. Calloe K, Ravn LS, Schmitt N, et al. Characterizations of a loss-of-function mutation in the Kir3.4 channel subunit. Biochem Biophys Res Commun 2007;364(4):889–95.

129. Yamada N, Asano Y, Fujita M, et al. Mutant KCNJ3 and KCNJ5 Potassium channels as novel molecular targets in bradyarrhythmias and atrial fibrillation. Circulation 2019;139(18):2157–69.

130. Delaney JT, Muhammad R, Blair MA, et al. A KCNJ8 mutation associated with early repolarization and atrial fibrillation. Europace 2012;14(10):1428–32.

131. Bartos DC, Anderson JB, Bastiaenen R, et al. A KCNQ1 mutation causes a high penetrance for familial atrial fibrillation. J Cardiovasc Electrophysiol 2013;24(5):562–9.

132. Das S, Makino S, Melman YF, et al. Mutation in the S3 segment of KCNQ1 results in familial lone atrial fibrillation. Heart Rhythm 2009;6(8):1146–53.

133. Otway R, Vandenberg JI, Guo G, et al. Stretch-sensitive KCNQ1 mutation A link between genetic and environmental factors in the pathogenesis of atrial fibrillation? J Am Coll Cardiol 2007;49(5):578–86.

134. Weeke P, Muhammad R, Delaney JT, et al. Whole-exome sequencing in familial atrial fibrillation. Eur Heart J 2014;35(36):2477–83.

135. Yang YQ, Wang MY, Zhang XL, et al. GATA4 loss-of-function mutations in familial atrial fibrillation. Clin Chim Acta 2011;412(19–20):1825–30.

136. Gu JY, Xu JH, Yu H, et al. Novel GATA5 loss-of-function mutations underlie familial atrial fibrillation. Clinics (Sao Paulo) 2012;67(12):1393–9.

137. Li J, Liu WD, Yang ZL, et al. Novel GATA6 loss-of-function mutation responsible for familial atrial fibrillation. Int J Mol Med 2012;30(4):783–90.

138. Yuan F, Qiu XB, Li RG, et al. A novel NKX2-5 loss-of-function mutation predisposes to familial dilated cardiomyopathy and arrhythmias. Int J Mol Med 2015;35(2):478–86.

139. Wang J, Zhang DF, Sun YM, et al. NKX2-6 mutation predisposes to familial atrial fibrillation. Int J Mol Med 2014;34(6):1581–90.

140. Wang J, Zhang DF, Sun YM, et al. A novel PITX2c loss-of-function mutation associated with familial atrial fibrillation. Eur J Med Genet 2014;57(1):25–31.

141. Tsai CT, Hsieh CS, Chang SN, et al. Next-generation sequencing of nine atrial fibrillation candidate genes identified novel de novo mutations in patients with extreme trait of atrial fibrillation. J Med Genet 2015;52(1):28–36.

142. Thibodeau IL, Xu J, Li Q, et al. Paradigm of genetic mosaicism and lone atrial fibrillation: physiological characterization of a connexin 43-deletion mutant identified from atrial tissue. Circulation 2010;122(3):236–44.

143. Yang YQ, Zhang XL, Wang XH, et al. Connexin40 nonsense mutation in familial atrial fibrillation. Int J Mol Med 2010;26(4):605–10.

144. Gollob MH, Jones DL, Krahn AD, et al. Somatic mutations in the connexin 40 gene (GJA5) in atrial fibrillation. N Engl J Med 2006;354(25):2677–88.

145. Beavers DL, Wang W, Ather S, et al. Mutation E169K in junctophilin-2 causes atrial fibrillation due to impaired RyR2 stabilization. J Am Coll Cardiol 2013;62(21):2010–9.

146. Pan H, Richards AA, Zhu X, et al. A novel mutation in LAMIN A/C is associated with isolated early-onset atrial fibrillation and progressive atrioventricular block followed by cardiomyopathy and sudden cardiac death. Heart Rhythm 2009;6(5):707–10.

147. Müller II, Melville DB, Tanwar V, et al. Functional modeling in zebrafish demonstrates that the atrial-fibrillation-associated gene GREM2 regulates cardiac laterality, cardiomyocyte differentiation and atrial rhythm. Dis Model Mech 2013;6(2):332–41.

148. Ren X, Xu C, Zhan C, et al. Identification of NPPA variants associated with atrial fibrillation in a Chinese GeneID population. Clin Chim Acta 2010;411(7–8):481–5.

149. Zhang X, Chen S, Yoo S, et al. Mutation in nuclear pore component NUP155 leads to atrial fibrillation and early sudden cardiac death. Cell 2008;135(6):1017–27.

150. Zhabyeyev P, Hiess F, Wang R, et al. S4153R is a gain-of-function mutation in the cardiac Ca(2+) release channel ryanodine receptor associated with catecholaminergic polymorphic ventricular tachycardia and paroxysmal atrial fibrillation. Can J Cardiol 2013;29(8):993–6.

151. Li Q, Huang H, Liu G, et al. Gain-of-function mutation of Nav1.5 in atrial fibrillation enhances cellular excitability and lowers the threshold for action potential firing. Biochem Biophys Res Commun 2009;380(1):132–7.

152. Yang YQ, Li L, Wang J, et al. GATA6 loss-of-function mutation in atrial fibrillation. Eur J Med Genet 2012;55(10):520–6.

153. Gundlund A, Olesen JB, Peterson ED, et al. Familial clustering of atrial fibrillation and comparative longitudinal outcomes of familial and non-familial atrial fibrillation. J Comp Eff Res 2017. https://doi.org/10.2217/cer-2016-0088.

154. Christophersen IE, Budtz-Jorgensen E, Olesen MS, et al. Familial atrial fibrillation predicts increased risk of mortality: a study in Danish twins. Circ Arrhythm Electrophysiol 2013;6(1):10–5.

155. Gudbjartsson DF, Arnar DO, Helgadottir A, et al. Variants conferring risk of atrial fibrillation on chromosome 4q25. Nature 2007;448(7151):353–7.

156. Franco D, Campione M. The role of Pitx2 during cardiac development. Linking left-right signaling and congenital heart diseases. Trends Cardiovasc Med 2003;13(4):157–63.

157. Ye J, Tucker NR, Weng LC, et al. A functional variant associated with atrial fibrillation regulates PITX2c Expression through TFAP2a. Am J Hum Genet 2016;99(6):1281–91.

158. Nadadur RD, Broman MT, Boukens B, et al. Pitx2 modulates a Tbx5-dependent gene regulatory

network to maintain atrial rhythm. Sci Transl Med 2016;8(354):354ra115.

159. Ihida-Stansbury K, McKean DM, Gebb SA, et al. Paired-related homeobox gene Prx1 is required for pulmonary vascular development. Circ Res 2004;94(11):1507–14.

160. Tucker NR, Dolmatova EV, Lin H, et al. Diminished PRRX1 expression is associated with increased risk of atrial fibrillation and shortening of the cardiac action potential. Circ Cardiovasc Genet 2017;10(5):e001902.

161. Ellinor PT, Lunetta KL, Glazer NL, et al. Common variants in KCNN3 are associated with lone atrial fibrillation. Nat Genet 2010;42(3):240–4.

162. Zhang XD, Timofeyev V, Li N, et al. Critical roles of a small conductance Ca^{2+}-activated K^+ channel (SK3) in the repolarization process of atrial myocytes. Cardiovasc Res 2014;101(2):317–25.

163. Roselli C, Chaffin MD, Weng LC, et al. Multi-ethnic genome-wide association study for atrial fibrillation. Nat Genet 2018;50(9):1225–33.

164. Nielsen JB, Thorolfsdottir RB, Fritsche LG, et al. Biobank-driven genomic discovery yields new insight into atrial fibrillation biology. Nat Genet 2018;50(9):1234–9.

165. Benjamin EJ, Rice KM, Arking DE, et al. Variants in ZFHX3 are associated with atrial fibrillation in individuals of European ancestry. Nat Genet 2009; 41(8):879–81.

166. Lubitz SA, Lunetta KL, Lin H, et al. Novel genetic markers associate with atrial fibrillation risk in Europeans and Japanese. J Am Coll Cardiol 2014; 63(12):1200–10.

167. Sinner MF, Tucker NR, Lunetta KL, et al. Integrating genetic, transcriptional, and functional analyses to identify 5 novel genes for atrial fibrillation. Circulation 2014;130(15):1225–35.

168. Tsai CT, Hsieh CS, Chang SN, et al. Genome-wide screening identifies a KCNIP1 copy number variant as a genetic predictor for atrial fibrillation. Nat Commun 2016;7:10190.

169. Christophersen IE, Rienstra M, Roselli C, et al. Large-scale analyses of common and rare variants identify 12 new loci associated with atrial fibrillation. Nat Genet 2017;49(6):946–52.

170. Low SK, Takahashi A, Ebana Y, et al. Identification of six new genetic loci associated with atrial fibrillation in the Japanese population. Nat Genet 2017; 49(6):953–8.

171. Lee JY, Kim TH, Yang PS, et al. Korean atrial fibrillation network genome-wide association study for early-onset atrial fibrillation identifies novel susceptibility loci. Eur Heart J 2017;38(34):2586–94.

172. Thorolfsdottir RB, Sveinbjornsson G, Sulem P, et al. A missense variant in PLEC increases risk of atrial fibrillation. J Am Coll Cardiol 2017; 70(17):2157–68.

173. Nielsen JB, Fritsche LG, Zhou W, et al. Genome-wide study of atrial fibrillation identifies seven risk loci and highlights biological pathways and regulatory elements involved in cardiac development. Am J Hum Genet 2018;102(1):103–15.

174. van Ouwerkerk AF, Bosada FM, van Duijvenboden K, et al. Identification of atrial fibrillation associated genes and functional non-coding variants. Nat Commun 2019;10(1):4755.

175. Deshmukh A, Barnard J, Sun H, et al. Left atrial transcriptional changes associated with atrial fibrillation susceptibility and persistence. Circ Arrhythm Electrophysiol 2015;8(1):32–41.

176. Xiong Q, Proietti M, Senoo K, et al. Asymptomatic versus symptomatic atrial fibrillation: a systematic review of age/gender differences and cardiovascular outcomes. Int J Cardiol 2015;191:172–7.

177. Sanna T, Diener HC, Passman RS, et al. Cryptogenic stroke and underlying atrial fibrillation. N Engl J Med 2014;370(26):2478–86.

178. Choi SH, Jurgens SJ, Weng LC, et al. Monogenic and polygenic contributions to atrial fibrillation risk: results from a national biobank. Circ Res 2020;126(2):200–9.

179. Lubitz SA, Yin X, Lin HJ, et al. Genetic risk prediction of atrial fibrillation. Circulation 2017;135(14): 1311–20.

180. Weng LC, Preis SR, Hulme OL, et al. Genetic predisposition, clinical risk factor burden, and lifetime risk of atrial fibrillation. Circulation 2018;137(10):1027–38.

Implications of Inflammation and Fibrosis in Atrial Fibrillation Pathophysiology

Masahide Harada, MD, PhD[a],*, Stanley Nattel, MD[b]

KEYWORDS

- Atrial fibrillation • Atrial remodeling • Inflammation • Inflammasome • Fibrosis

KEY POINTS

- Inflammation and fibrosis play a critical role in the pathophysiology of atrial fibrillation.
- Atrial fibrillation induces atrial inflammatory signaling. Systemic inflammatory diseases (hypertension, heart failure, and metabolic disorders) also increase atrial fibrillation risk.
- Inflammation activates cardiac fibroblasts, developing atrial fibrotic remodeling.
- Inflammation and fibrosis increase thrombogenicity in atrial fibrillation.
- Risk factor management and life style changes that target inflammatory conditions are important for the suppression of atrial fibrosis and atrial fibrillation risk.

INTRODUCTION

Inflammation has been implicated in the pathophysiology of atrial fibrillation (AF) and mediates various pathologic processes such as oxidative stress and apoptosis. Atrial fibrosis causes conduction disturbances and contributes to the progression of atrial remodeling. Innate immune cells secrete inflammatory mediators. Recent evidence also suggests that cardiomyocytes can secrete inflammatory mediators. Cardiac fibroblasts (FBs), the cells responsible for fibrous tissue formation, are activated by cytokines, growth factors, and adipokines associated with systemic inflammatory diseases and metabolic derangements comorbid with AF. Therefore, inflammation can underlie atrial fibrosis; the complex interplay of these maladaptive components creates a vicious cycle of atrial remodeling progression, maintaining AF and increasing thrombogenicity. In addition, the inflammasome, an intracellular inflammatory platform, has been identified in atrial cardiomyocytes and inflammasome signaling also contributes to the fibroinflammatory process in AF. This review provides current knowledge about inflammation and fibrosis in the pathophysiology of AF, diagnostic modalities to assess the fibroinflammatory condition, and the potential of these conditions as therapeutic targets.

EVIDENCE OF ATRIAL FIBRILLATION RISK IN SYSTEMIC INFLAMMATORY DISEASES

Inflammation is a biological response to infection and tissue damage that protects the host.[1] Left uncontrolled, inflammation causes the overproduction of cytokines and reactive oxygen species that can lead to disease states, including AF (**Fig. 1**).[2] Inflammatory consequences induce fibrosis, cell apoptosis, and hypertrophy, which predispose to AF when these changes occur in the atria.

[a] Department of Cardiology, Fujita Health University School of Medicine, 1-98 Dengakugakubo, Kutsukake-cho, Toyoake 4701192, Japan; [b] Montreal Heart Institute, University of Montreal, Montreal, Quebec, Canada
* Corresponding author.
E-mail address: mharada@fujita-hu.ac.jp

Card Electrophysiol Clin 13 (2021) 25–35
https://doi.org/10.1016/j.ccep.2020.11.002
1877-9182/21/© 2020 Elsevier Inc. All rights reserved.

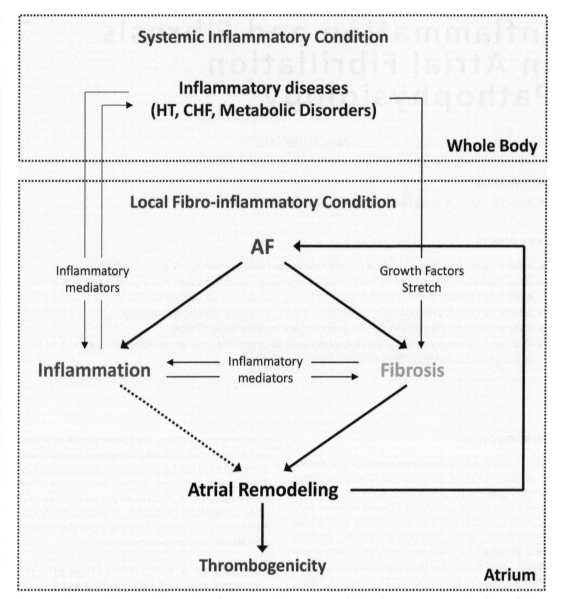

Fig. 1. Mechanistic link AF and systemic inflammatory diseases comorbid with AF. CHF, congestive heart failure; HT, hypertension.

Hypertension

Hypertension is the most attributable risk factor for AF. Hypertension activates the renin–angiotensin–aldosterone system and increases the production of angiotensin II (AT-II). The binding of AT-II to AT-II receptors (ATRs) in atrial cells increases oxidative stress by activation of nicotinamide adenine dinucleotide phosphate oxidase 2, a potential enzymatic source of reactive oxygen species production.[3]

Heart Failure

Heart failure (HF) and cardiomyopathy are associated with a 4- to 6-fold increase in the prevalence

of AF.[4] Maladaptive inflammation and oxidative stress have been implicated in the pathophysiology of HF remodeling. The serum levels of tumor necrosis factor-α were increased in patients with a history of AF in a community-based HF cohort.[5]

Metabolic Disorders

Diabetic patients exhibit a more than 40% greater risk of developing AF versus nondiabetic patients.[6] Obesity is independently associated with AF[7] and also promotes diabetes. Visceral fat accumulation transforms adipocytes from a small benign brown cell type into a large potentially pathogenic white cell type that can secrete a large number of inflammatory cytokines, promoting immune cell recruitment.[8] Glucose fluctuation stimulates the overproduction of reactive oxygen species in diabetic hearts, causing oxidative stress and inflammation.[9]

Other Inflammatory Diseases

Coronary artery disease and chronic kidney disease are chronic proinflammatory conditions that increase AF prevalence.[3] Inflammatory bowel disease, rheumatoid arthritis, and psoriasis are systemic inflammatory diseases that are accompanied by an increased AF incidence.[10–12]

EVIDENCE OF INFLAMMATION IN ATRIAL FIBRILLATION

Stagnant blood flow in AF causes the endothelial microinjury/dysfunction in the atrial endocardium, allowing immune cell migration into atrial tissue. In a histologic examination of lone patients with AF, the atrial tissue showed low-grade inflammation with immune cell infiltration.[13] Increased leukocyte infiltration and macrophage migration has been confirmed in the atrial tissue of patients with AF, but not in those with sinus rhythm, along with deposition of adhesion molecules and inflammatory cytokines.[14–16] Marcus and colleagues[17] demonstrated that a history of AF did not affect the serum levels of C-reactive protein (CRP) and IL-6, although the presence of AF at the time of the blood sample collection was associated with an elevation of CRP and IL-6. Furthermore, coronary sinus blood samples showed higher CRP levels than those from the other regions, suggesting that cardiac tissue is a source of CRP.[17]

The inflammasome, an intracellular protein complex in innate immune cells, reacts to the pathogens and triggers an inflammatory response to protect the body from infection or injury.[18] The inflammasome consists of 3 proteins: a NOD-like receptor (NLR), an adaptor protein like apoptosis-associated speck-like protein containing a CARD, and a cysteine protease such as caspase-1 or caspase-5.[18] There are several types of inflammasomes such as NLRC4, NLRP1, and NLRP3, each containing a distinct NLR protein. The inflammasome can activate the intracellular protease caspase-1 and regulate the production of IL-1β and IL-18. Inflammasomes exists both in innate immune cells and in cardiomyocytes. Yao and colleagues[19] have demonstrated that the NLRP3 inflammasome is activated in atrial cardiomyocytes from patients with AF and in a canine AF model, and inflammasome priming (increased production of the components) is correlated with the

progression of AF to persistent forms. A genetically engineered mouse model expressing constitutively active NLRP-3 shows increased inducibility of AF; NLRP3 knockdown or inhibition decreases the AF burden in this model.[19] Genetic ablation of NLRP3 protected against age-related spontaneous atrial arrhythmias, prevented PR interval prolongation, atrial conduction delay, and AF inducibility in a mouse model (CREM transgenics) of spontaneous AF.[20] Activated NLRP3 inflammasomes increase the production of IL-1β and IL-18; circulating IL-1β and IL-18 levels are positively correlated with arrhythmia progression from paroxysmal to persistent forms in patients with AF, along with the development of structural remodeling and atrial dilatation (**Fig. 2**).[21,22]

FUNDAMENTALS OF CARDIAC FIBROBLASTS AND FIBROSIS

Atrial fibrosis is central to atrial structural remodeling. Cardiac FBs are key players in the fibrotic process. FBs may account for up to 60% to 70% of cells in the heart; cardiomyocytes constitute only 30% to 40%.[23] FBs exist in the interstitial space and maintain the integrity of the extracellular matrix (ECM) to preserve the arrangement of cardiomyocytes and tissue structure. However, FBs can be activated and proliferate and differentiate into ECM-secreting cardiac myofibroblasts in response to various mediators, including neurohumoral factors (eg, AT-II), growth factors (eg, transforming growth factor-β1), and inflammatory mediators. The accumulation of interstitial ECM is associated with changes in the cardiac architecture, leading to conduction disturbance and reentry stabilization, thus facilitating AF maintenance (**Fig. 3**).[24]

EVIDENCE OF A LINK BETWEEN INFLAMMATION AND FIBROSIS IN ATRIAL FIBRILLATION

Cross talk among FBs, cardiomyocytes, and immune cells is important for the development of AF-promoting fibrotic remodeling in the atrium under inflammatory conditions. The infiltrated immune cells produce a large number of inflammatory mediators in the atrial tissue, injuring and destroying the cardiomyocytes. The injured cells release intracellular components, stimulating innate immune mechanisms and augmenting the local inflammatory response. AF also activates the NLRP3 inflammasome in atrial cardiomyocytes, producing the inflammatory cytokines (IL-1β, IL-18) that promote local inflammation. FBs can be activated by inflammatory mediators. The

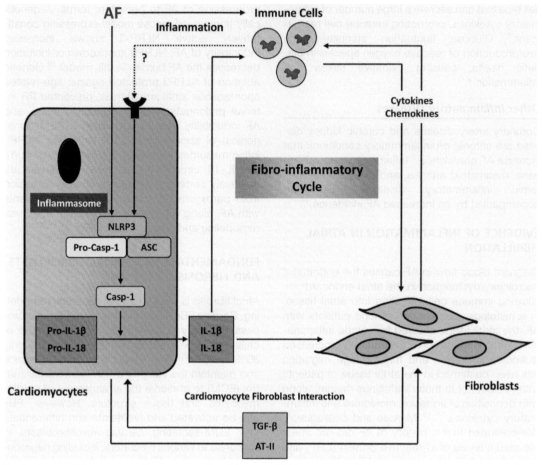

Fig. 2. Cross talk between cardiomyocytes, fibroblasts and inflammatory cells in AF. Cardiomyocyte NLRP3 inflammasome activation contribute to fibroinflammatory condition in AF. ASC, apoptosis-associated speck-like protein containing a CARD; Casp-1, caspase 1; NLRP3, nucleotide-binding oligomerization domain-like receptor family, pyrin domain-containing 3; TGF-β, transforming growth factor-β.

loss of cardiomyocytes activates the FBs to replace the affected area with fibrous tissue. Furthermore, activated FBs can release proinflammatory cytokines and attract additional immune cells to intensify the local inflammatory response.[18,23,25] The fibroinflammatory process causes a vicious cycle to develop AF-promoting fibrotic remodeling (see **Fig. 2**).

In atrial tissue from patients with AF, there were positive correlations among the inflammatory mediators (nuclear factor-κB activity, serum tumor necrosis factor-α, and IL-6 concentrations) and ECM volume.[26] The serum levels of fibroinflammatory biomarkers (matrix metalloproteinase-9, type III procollagen, and highly sensitive CRP) increased in patients with persistent AF, but not in those with sinus rhythm and were positively correlated with left atrial volume on echocardiography, an index of atrial remodeling.[27] In a

postmortem analysis, inflammatory macrophage markers and fibrosis were colocalized in subendocardial atrial tissues of patients with AF, consistent with an association between inflammation and fibrosis in AF.[28]

Epicardial adipose tissue, the visceral fat adjacent to the epicardium, also contributes to the fibroinflammatory process in the atrium. The inflammatory changes and metabolic dysfunction comorbid with AF are accompanied by an increased epicardial adipose tissue volume.[29] Epicardial adipose tissue plays a role in energy metabolism, but also produces a number of proinflammatory adipocytokines (eg, IL-1β, IL-6, IL-8, and tumor necrosis factor-α), which can diffuse into the neighboring atrial tissue, recruiting inflammatory cells and triggering FB activation.[30–32] Epicardial adipocytes can also permeate the adjacent myocardium and disrupt the myocardial

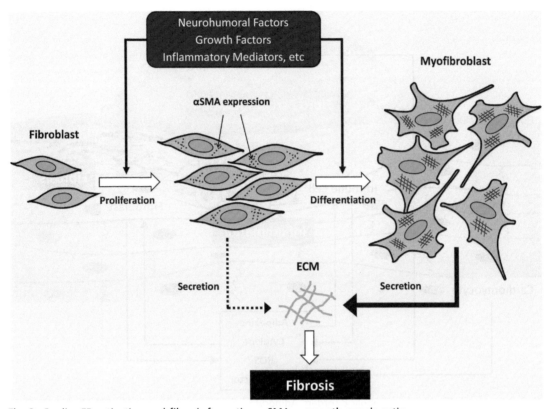

Fig. 3. Cardiac FB activation and fibrosis formation. αSMA, α smooth muscle actin.

architecture, causing fibrosis formation and conduction disturbance (via fibrofatty infiltration) that promote AF (**Fig. 4**).[31]

THROMBOGENICITY IN FIBROINFLAMMATORY CONDITIONS IN ATRIAL FIBRILLATION

AF-induced endothelial damage and dysfunction allows for the recruitment of immune cells via the injured endothelium. The loss of endothelial integrity accelerates the attachment of von Willebrand factor, an adhesion molecule, to the injured endothelium. The von Willebrand factors interact with fibrinogen and GPIIb/IIIa proteins and cause platelet aggregation. Platelet aggregation induces the expression of P-selectin, another adhesion molecule, and recruits more leukocytes and monocytes with P-selectin–binding protein (P-selectin glycoprotein ligand-1) onto the cell surface. The immune cells and injured endothelium start to express tissue factors in the atrial endocardial surface. Upon exposure to blood circulation, tissue factors trigger the extrinsic coagulation cascade and increase thrombogenicity. FBs are also activated to repair the injured endothelium

and express tissue factors, thereby enhancing thrombogenicity (**Fig. 5**).[5]

CLINICAL ASSESSMENT OF FIBROINFLAMMATORY CONDITION IN ATRIAL FIBRILLATION
Biomarkers

Recruited immune cells secrete inflammatory mediators that can be measured in the blood circulation. Inflammatory biomarker profiles can predict AF risk. Fibrosis development is favored by the activation of numerous biochemical pathways. The profibrotic mediators and end products can enter the blood circulation; thus, these molecules can be used as clinical biomarkers to assess the fibroinflammatory condition (**Table 1**).[33]

Galectin (Gal-3) is a protein that binds galactose, a monosaccharide sugar, that is used as an energy source in the body. Gal-3 also binds to various types of cells and matrix and plays a biological role in cell–cell adhesion, cell–matrix interactions, macrophage activation, angiogenesis, metastasis, apoptosis, and fibrosis. Gal-3 has been implicated in the pathophysiology of atrial fibrosis in AF. Intracardiac serum levels of Gal-3 are higher in patients with persistent AF than with

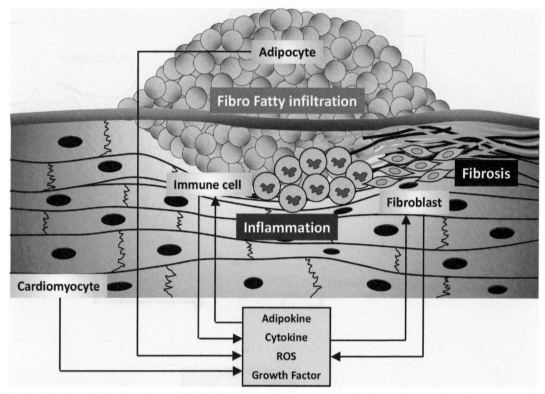

Fig. 4. Fibrofatty infiltration in metabolic disorders. Adipocytes secrete adipokines that recruit inflammatory cells and activate FBs. The epicardial adipose tissue accumulation and its infiltration into the subepicardium contribute to the progression of the AF substrate. ROS, reactive oxygen species.

paroxysmal AF. Gal-3 is an independent predictor of atrial tachyarrhythmia recurrence after a single ablation procedure.[34]

Imaging

Echocardiography (2-dimensional, pulsed-wave Doppler, speckle-tracking echo, strain and strain rate imaging) and cardiac computed tomography (CT) scans can evaluate atrial chamber size and volume in patients with AF. A large left atrium size and volume imply the progression of atrial remodeling associated with fibrosis. The left atrium size and volume also correlate with recurrence of AF after catheter ablation and risk of ischemic stroke.[35,36] The left atrium contractile and diastolic function changes are associated with atrial fibrosis and can be evaluated by speckle-tracking echocardiography.[37] Attenuation of the left atrium wall strain assessed by speckle-tracking echocardiography was an independent predictor of AF recurrence after catheter ablation.[38]

Late gadolinium enhancement MRI directly visualizes scarred and fibrotic areas in the atrium. Atrial fibrosis detected by late gadolinium enhancement MRI is associated with the success of acute peripheral vascular interventions, the chronic durability of peripheral vascular interventions, atrial function, and stroke risk. However, because the atrial walls are much thinner than the ventricular walls and because the spatial resolution of cardiac MRI is limited, the imaging of atrial fibrosis using late gadolinium enhancement MRI remains a challenge.[39,40]

PET/CT scans with 18F-fluorodeoxyglucose can detect inflammatory regions. Watanabe and colleagues[41] demonstrated the diagnostic value of PET/CT scans with 18F-fluorodeoxyglucose for the detection of inflammatory activity in the atria of patients with AF. Sinigaglia and colleagues[42] showed a significant correlation between 18F-fluorodeoxyglucose atrial uptake and AF. This pattern was associated with the risk of thromboembolism.

THERAPEUTIC OPTIONS
Anticoagulation Therapy

Inflammation and fibrosis increase thrombogenicity. Anticoagulation therapy should be considered based on the assessment of thromboembolic risk.

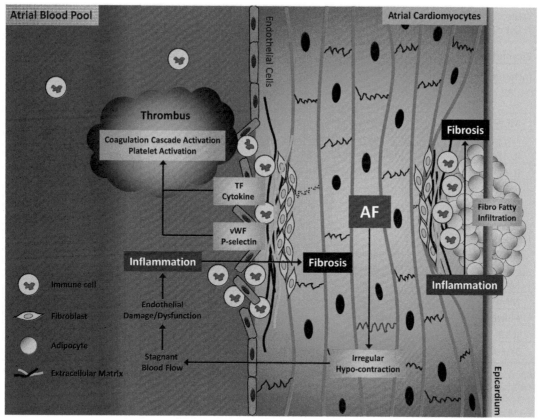

Fig. 5. Increased thrombogenicity under fibroinflammatory condition in AF. TF, tissue factor; vWF, von Willebrand factor.

In clinical practice, $CHADS_2$/CHA_2DS_2-VASc scores are used for risk stratification. These scores include factors promoting atrial inflammation and cardiomyopathy like HF, hypertension, and diabetes, along with age, and so evaluate proinflammatory conditions comorbid with AF.

Life Style Changes and Risk Factor Management

Recent studies have demonstrated that life style changes targeting obesity, physical activity, and risk factor modification decrease AF burden.[43–45] Abed and colleagues[43] demonstrated that a decrease in risk factors (obesity, hypertension, hyperglycemia, sleep apnea, and smoking/alcohol habits) decreased AF symptoms, episodes, and the burden associated with atrial remodeling in obese patients with symptomatic AF. The ARREST-AF study demonstrated that aggressive risk factor management improved AF-free survival rate after catheter ablation.[44] Uncontrolled AF comorbidities promote atrial remodeling and

increase AF risk; any underlying inflammatory conditions should be targeted.

Anti-inflammatory Drugs

Statins, corticosteroids, vitamins, polyunsaturated fatty acids, and colchicine have potent anti-inflammatory effects and have been tested for AF prevention in animal and clinical studies. However, because of potential adverse effects and/or little effect on AF, their clinical use is limited, especially as a long-term treatment.[5]

Monoclonal antibodies against IL-1β (canakinumab and gevokizumab) and human IL-1 receptor antagonist (anakinra and rilonacept) might have the potential to decreased the risk of AF via their anti-inflammatory effects. Canakinumab's ability to decrease cardiovascular events has been tested in patients with a prior myocardial infarction and elevated CRP to decrease cardiovascular events (Canakinumab Anti-inflammatory Thrombosis Outcome Study [CANTOS] trial).[46] Canakinumab decreased the plasma CRP levels and decreased cardiovascular events.[46] In addition,

Table 1
A list of fibroinflammatory biomarkers in AF

Biomarker	Blood Circulating Levels and Findings	PMID
Inflammation		
CRP	Increases in AF vs SR. Increases in PeAF/PmAF vs PAF.	11739301
	Increases in AF REC vs no AF REC after CV/CA.	24095158
MCP-1	Increases in AF vs controls	28886122
TNF-α	Increases in AF vs SR. Increases in PeAF vs PAF.	20153266
IL-1β	Increases in AF vs SR.	
IL-6	Correlates with development to PeAF/PmAF.	26839066
IL-8	Increases in PmAF vs PeAF/SR.	18523031
IL-10	Increases in PeAF/PmAF vs PAF	20153266
IL-18	Increases in AF vs controls. Increases in PeAF vs PAF	20833691
Fibrosis		
Gal-3	Increases in PeAF vs PAF.	27525318
	Increase in AF REC vs no AF REC after CA.	
MPO	Increase in AF vs SR.	20305660
MMP-9	Predictor for new onset AF	23554968
PIIINP	Predictor for new onset AF (≥8.5 µg/L)	30354407
ICTP	Predictor for new onset AF(≥7.0 µg/L)	30354407
TGF-β	Correlates with low voltage area and LA dimension	21186331

Abbreviations: CA, catheter ablation; CV, cardioversion; ICTP, pyridinoline cross-linked carboxyterminal telopeptide of type I collagen; LA, left atrium; MCP-1, monocyte chemotactic protein-1; MMP-9, matrix metalloproteinase-9; MPO, myeloperoxidase; PAF, paroxysmal AF; PeAF, persistent AF; PIIINP, procollagen III N-terminal propeptide; PmAF, permanent AF; REC, recurrence; SR, sinus rhythm; TGF-β, transforming growth factor-β; TNF-α, tumor necrosis factor-α.

cardiovascular events were correlated with the plasma CRP levels.[47] Canakinumab might also act to prevent AF.

Renin–Angiotensin–Aldosterone System Inhibitors

Renin–angiotensin–aldosterone system regulators and products (eg, AT-II and aldosterone) are profibrotic mediators. Angiotensin-converting enzyme inhibitors (ACEIs) and angiotensin receptor blockers (ARBs) have been of particular interest as an "upstream therapy" against fibrotic remodeling in AF. In retrospective studies, treatment with ACEIs and ARBs has demonstrated efficacy for primary prevention of AF in patients with HF, hypertension, and left ventricular hypertrophy. The efficacy seems to be greater in primary than secondary prevention, and greatest in conditions involving substantial renin–angiotensin–aldosterone system activation like HF and hypertension with left ventricular hypertrophy.[48,49] For the secondary prevention of AF, ACEIs and ARBs did not prevent the recurrence of AF in patients with paroxysmal and persistent AF after pharmacologic or electrical cardioversion to restore sinus rhythm.[50–52] However, Du and colleagues[53] demonstrated that treatment with an ARB (telmisartan) suppressed AF progression from paroxysmal to persistent forms, suggesting that ARBs may suppress AF maintenance.

Mineralocorticoid receptor antagonists are also expected to decrease the risk of AF by preventing fibrosis. In a subanalysis of the EMPHASIS-HF trial, patients treated with a mineralocorticoid receptor antagonist (eplerenone) showed a lower incidence of new-onset AF than those treated with placebo, suggesting its potential to prevent AF.[54] A recent randomized controlled trial demonstrated that risk factor-driven upstream therapy with ACEI, ARB, mineralocorticoid receptor antagonists, statins, and cardiac rehabilitation (physical activity, dietary restrictions, counseling) improved sinus rhythm maintenance in patients with persistent AF and HF.[55]

SUMMARY

Accumulating evidence suggests that AF is a multifactorial arrhythmia; inflammation and atrial fibrosis play critical roles in the pathophysiology. Inflammation is a physiologic response to infection and tissue damage, and fibrosis is its healing step; inflammation and fibrosis are therefore intertwined processes. However, under pathologic conditions, these components create a vicious cycle and synergistically contribute to the development of AF-promoting atrial remodeling. Although the mechanistic link between inflammation and fibrosis has yet to be fully understood, the clinical assessment and targeted intervention of underlying inflammatory conditions are promising therapeutic strategies for AF.

CLINICAL CARE POINTS

- Inflammation leads to atrial fibrosis and increases the risks of AF.
- Measuring inflammatory biomarkers helps with the assessment of inflammatory conditions in AF.
- Increased atrial size is associated with atrial fibrosis and is assessed by echocardiography, cardiac CT scan, and cardiac MRI.
- Inflammation and fibrosis increase thrombogenicity; anticoagulation therapy should be considered, based on the assessment of thromboembolic risks.
- Risk factor management and life style changes are important in the prevention of atrial remodeling and AF. Treatment with ACEI, ARB, and mineralocorticoid receptor antagonists is considered in patients with AF, especially those with underlying diseases (hypertension, left ventricular hypertrophy, and HF).

DISCLOSURE

None.

REFERENCES

1. Buckley CD, Gilroy DW, Serhan CN, et al. The resolution of inflammation. Nat Rev Immunol 2013;13(1):59–66.
2. Yeh YH, Kuo CT, Chang GJ, et al. Nicotinamide adenine dinucleotide phosphate oxidase 4 mediates the differential responsiveness of atrial versus ventricular fibroblasts to transforming growth factor-β. Circ Arrhythm Electrophysiol 2013;6(4):790–8.
3. Yagi S, Akaike M, Aihara K, et al. Endothelial nitric oxide synthase-independent protective action of statin against angiotensin II-induced atrial remodeling via reduced oxidant injury. Hypertension 2010;55(4):918–23.
4. Andrade J, Khairy P, Dobrev D, et al. The clinical profile and pathophysiology of atrial fibrillation relationship among clinical features, epidemiology, and mechanisms. Circ Res 2014;114(9):1453–68.
5. Harada M, Van Wagoner DR, Nattel S. Role of inflammation in atrial fibrillation pathophysiology and management. Circ J 2015;79(3):495–502.
6. Huxley RR, Filion KB, Konety S, et al. Meta-analysis of cohort and case-control studies of type 2 diabetes mellitus and risk of atrial fibrillation. Am J Cardiol 2011;108(1):56–62.
7. Baek YS, Yang PS, Kim TH, et al. Associations of abdominal obesity and new-onset atrial fibrillation in the general population. J Am Heart Assoc 2017;6(6):e004705.
8. Aldiss P, Davies G, Woods R, et al. 'Browning' the cardiac and peri-vascular adipose tissues to modulate cardiovascular risk. Int J Cardiol 2017;228:265–74.
9. Saito S, Teshima Y, Fukui A, et al. Glucose fluctuations increase the incidence of atrial fibrillation in diabetic rats. Cardiovasc Res 2014;104(1):5–14.
10. Lazzerini PE, Capecchi PL, Laghi-Pasini F. Systemic inflammation and arrhythmic risk: lessons from rheumatoid arthritis. Eur Heart J 2017;38(22):1717–27.
11. Ahlehoff O, Gislason GH, Jørgensen CH, et al. Psoriasis and risk of atrial fibrillation and ischaemic stroke: a Danish Nationwide Cohort Study. Eur Heart J 2012;33(16):2054–64.
12. Kristensen SL, Lindhardsen J, Ahlehoff O, et al. Increased risk of atrial fibrillation and stroke during active stage of inflammatory bowel disease: a nationwide study. Europace 2014;16(4):477–84.
13. Frustaci A, Chimenti C, Bellocci F, et al. Histological substrate of atrial biopsies in patients with lone atrial fibrillation. Circulation 1997;96(4):1180–4.
14. Chen MC, Chang JP, Liu WH, et al. Increased inflammatory cell infiltration in the atrial myocardium of patients with atrial fibrillation. Am J Cardiol 2008;102(7):861–5.
15. Rudolph V, Andrié RP, Rudolph TK, et al. Myeloperoxidase acts as a profibrotic mediator of atrial fibrillation. Nat Med 2010;16(4):470–4.
16. Yamashita T, Sekiguchi A, Iwasaki YK, et al. Recruitment of immune cells across atrial endocardium in human atrial fibrillation. Circ J 2010;74(2):262–70.
17. Marcus GM, Smith LM, Ordovas K, et al. Intra and extracardiac markers of inflammation during atrial fibrillation. Heart Rhythm 2010;7(2):149–54.
18. Chen G, Chelu MG, Dobrev D, et al. Cardiomyocyte inflammasome signaling in cardiomyopathies and atrial fibrillation: mechanisms and potential therapeutic implications. Front Physiol 2018;9:1115.
19. Yao C, Veleva T, Scott L Jr, et al. Enhanced cardiomyocyte NLRP3 inflammasome signaling promotes atrial fibrillation. Circulation 2018;138(20):2227–42.

20. Marín-Aguilar F, Lechuga-Vieco AV, Alcocer-Gómez E, et al. NLRP3 inflammasome suppression improves longevity and prevents cardiac aging in male mice. Aging Cell 2020;19(1):e13050.

21. Gungor B, Ekmekci A, Arman A, et al. Assessment of interleukin-1 gene cluster polymorphisms in lone atrial fibrillation: new insight into the role of inflammation in atrial fibrillation. Pacing Clin Electrophysiol 2013;36(10):1220–7.

22. Luan Y, Guo Y, Li S, et al. Interleukin-18 among atrial fibrillation patients in the absence of structural heart disease. Europace 2010;12(12):1713–8.

23. Van Linthout S, Miteva K, Tschöpe C. Crosstalk between fibroblasts and inflammatory cells. Cardiovasc Res 2014;102(2):258–69.

24. Nattel S. Molecular and cellular mechanisms of atrial fibrosis in atrial fibrillation. JACC Clin Electrophysiol 2017;3(5):425–35.

25. Frangogiannis NG. The inflammatory response in myocardial injury, repair and remodeling. Nat Rev Cardiol 2014;11(5):255–65.

26. Qu YC, Du YM, Wu SL, et al. Activated nuclear factor-kappaB and increased tumor necrosis factor-alpha in atrial tissue of atrial fibrillation. Scand Cardiovasc J 2009;43(5):292–7.

27. Sonmez O, Ertem FU, Vatankulu MA, et al. Novel fibro-inflammation markers in assessing left atrial remodeling in non-valvular atrial fibrillation. Med Sci Monit 2014;20:463–70.

28. Okumura Y, Watanabe I, Nakai T, et al. Impact of biomarkers of inflammation and extracellular matrix turnover on the outcome of atrial fibrillation ablation: importance of matrix metalloproteinase-2 as a predictor of atrial fibrillation recurrence. J Cardiovasc Electrophysiol 2011;22(9):987–93.

29. Packer M. Characterization, pathogenesis, and clinical implications of inflammation-related atrial myopathy as an important cause of atrial fibrillation. J Am Heart Assoc 2020;9(7):e015343.

30. Greulich S, Maxhera B, Vandenplas G, et al. Secretory products from epicardial adipose tissue of patients with type 2 diabetes mellitus induce cardiomyocyte dysfunction. Circulation 2012;126(12):2324–34.

31. Haemers P, Hamdi H, Guedj K, et al. Atrial fibrillation is associated with the fibrotic remodelling of adipose tissue in the subepicardium of human and sheep atria. Eur Heart J 2017;38(1):53–61.

32. Mazurek T, Zhang L, Zalewski A, et al. Human epicardial adipose tissue is a source of inflammatory mediators. Circulation 2003;108(20):2460–6.

33. Zhou X, Dudley SC Jr. Evidence for inflammation as a driver of atrial fibrillation. Front Cardiovasc Med 2020;7:62.

34. Takemoto Y, Ramirez RJ, Yokokawa M, et al. Galectin-3 regulates atrial fibrillation remodeling and predicts catheter ablation outcomes. JACC Basic Transl Sci 2016;1(3):143–54.

35. Njoku A, Kannabhiran M, Arora R, et al. Left atrial volume predicts atrial fibrillation recurrence after radiofrequency ablation: a meta-analysis. Europace 2018;20(1):33–42.

36. Ogata T, Matsuo R, Kiyuna F, et al. Left atrial size and long-term risk of recurrent stroke after acute ischemic stroke in patients with nonvalvular atrial fibrillation. J Am Heart Assoc 2017;6(8):e006402.

37. Pathan F, D'Elia N, Nolan MT, et al. Normal ranges of left atrial strain by speckle-tracking echocardiography: a systematic review and meta-analysis. J Am Soc Echocardiogr 2017;30(1):59–70.e8.

38. Mirza M, Caracciolo G, Khan U, et al. Left atrial reservoir function predicts atrial fibrillation recurrence after catheter ablation: a two-dimensional speckle strain study. J Interv Card Electrophysiol 2011;31(3):197–206.

39. Marrouche NF, Wilber D, Hindricks G, et al. Association of atrial tissue fibrosis identified by delayed enhancement MRI and atrial fibrillation catheter ablation: the DECAAF study. JAMA 2014;311(5):498–506.

40. Siebermair J, Kholmovski EG, Marrouche N. Assessment of left atrial fibrosis by late gadolinium enhancement magnetic resonance imaging: methodology and clinical implications. JACC Clin Electrophysiol 2017;3(8):791–802.

41. Watanabe E, Miyagawa M, Uetani T, et al. Positron emission tomography/computed tomography detection of increased (18)F-fluorodeoxyglucose uptake in the cardiac atria of patients with atrial fibrillation. Int J Cardiol 2019;283:171–7.

42. Sinigaglia M, Mahida B, Piekarski E, et al. FDG atrial uptake is associated with an increased prevalence of stroke in patients with atrial fibrillation. Eur J Nucl Med Mol Imaging 2019;46(6):1268–75.

43. Abed HS, Wittert GA, Leong DP, et al. Effect of weight reduction and cardiometabolic risk factor management on symptom burden and severity in patients with atrial fibrillation: a randomized clinical trial. JAMA 2013;310(19):2050–60.

44. Pathak RK, Middeldorp ME, Lau DH, et al. Aggressive risk factor reduction study for atrial fibrillation and implications for the outcome of ablation: the ARREST-AF cohort study. J Am Coll Cardiol 2014;64(21):2222–31.

45. Chung MK, Eckhardt LL, Chen LY, et al. Lifestyle and risk factor modification for reduction of atrial fibrillation: a scientific statement from the American Heart Association. Circulation 2020;141(16):e750–72.

46. Ridker PM, Everett BM, Thuren T, et al. Antiinflammatory therapy with canakinumab for atherosclerotic disease. N Engl J Med 2017;377(12):1119–31.

47. Ridker PM, MacFadyen JG, Everett BM, et al, CANTOS Trial Group. Relationship of C-reactive protein reduction to cardiovascular event reduction following treatment with canakinumab: a secondary

analysis from the CANTOS randomised controlled trial. Lancet 2018;391(10118):319–28.

48. Schneider MP, Hua TA, Böhm M, et al. Prevention of atrial fibrillation by Renin-Angiotensin system inhibition a meta-analysis. J Am Coll Cardiol 2010;55(21):2299–307.

49. Savelieva I, Kakouros N, Kourliouros A, et al. Upstream therapies for management of atrial fibrillation: review of clinical evidence and implications for European Society of Cardiology guidelines. Part II: secondary prevention. Europace 2011;13(5):610–25.

50. Disertori M, Latini R, Barlera S, et al. GISSI-AF Investigators. Valsartan for prevention of recurrent atrial fibrillation. N Engl J Med 2009;360(16):1606–17.

51. Goette A, Schön N, Kirchhof P, et al. Angiotensin II-antagonist inparoxysmal atrial fibrillation (ANTIPAF) trial. Circ Arrhythm Electrophysiol 2012;5(1):43–51.

52. Yusuf S, Healey JS, Pogue J, et al. Irbesartan in patients with atrial fibrillation. N Engl J Med 2011;364(10):928–38.

53. Du H, Fan J, Ling Z, et al. Effect of nifedipine versus telmisartan on prevention of atrial fibrillation recurrence in hypertensive patients. Hypertension 2013;61(4):786–92.

54. Swedberg K, Zannad F, McMurray JJ, et al. Eplerenone and atrial fibrillation in mild systolic heart failure: results from the EMPHASIS-HF study. J Am Coll Cardiol 2012;59(18):1598–603.

55. Rienstra M, Hobbelt AH, Alings M, et al. Targeted therapy of underlying conditions improves sinus rhythm maintenance in patients with persistent atrial fibrillation: results of the RACE 3 trial. Eur Heart J 2018;39(32):2987–96.

Risk Factors

Hypertension, Prehypertension, Hypertensive Heart Disease, and Atrial Fibrillation

Dennis H. Lau, MBBS, PhD[a],*, Hassan A. Shenasa, BS[b],
Mohammad Shenasa, MD[b]

KEYWORDS

- Atrial fibrillation • Hypertension • Prehypertension • Remodeling
- Renin-angiotensin aldosterone system • Risk factor management

KEY POINTS

- Hypertension (HT) is a major risk factor for atrial fibrillation (AF) development and progression.
- The pathophysiologic mechanisms underlying HT-related atrial remodeling are complex, but current evidence suggests a progressive process that also is reversible.
- Inhibition of the renin-angiotensin-aldosterone system appears to provide the best protection against AF onset and progression in patients with HT.
- HT is seldom the sole risk factor in individuals with AF. A comprehensive risk factor management approach is warranted to optimize outcomes.
- Further studies are needed to delineate targeting of aortic stiffness and HT-related structural remodeling to improve outcomes in individuals with HT, independent of blood pressure levels.

INTRODUCTION

There has been increasing focus on the role of risk factors in atrial fibrillation (AF) pathogenesis and the importance of targeting these factors as upstream noninvasive management strategy to improve outcomes.[1] Due to its high prevalence, the population-attributable risk of hypertension (HT) for AF has been shown to be highest among the risk factors studied in the Atherosclerosis Risk in Communities Study.[2] Specifically, nearly a quarter of AF burden can be attributable to HT if borderline blood pressure (BP) or pre-HT is taken into account. Elegant work examining the pulsatile component of BP has demonstrated that increased arterial stiffness as assessed by pulse pressure was associated strongly with incident AF in a large community-based Framingham Heart Study cohort over a mean 16 years' follow-up.[3] Furthermore, hypertensive men with left ventricular hypertrophy (LVH), a marker of end-organ damage, were found to have higher rate of AF progression than those without LVH.[4]

This review delves into the relationship between HT, pre-HT, and hypertensive heart disease and AF. First, the cardiovascular effects of HT are explored, with focus on atrial remodeling. Next, the clinical impact of HT, pre-HT, and LVH on AF development and sinus rhythm maintenance is delineated. Last, the clinical management of BP

Conflicts of interest: Dr D.H. Lau reports that the University of Adelaide has received on his behalf lecture and/or consulting fees from Abbott Medical, Bayer, Biotronik, Boehringer Ingelheim, Medtronic, Microport, and Pfizer.
[a] Department of Cardiology, Centre for Heart Rhythm Disorders, University of Adelaide, Royal Adelaide Hospital, Port Road, Adelaide, South Australia 5000, Australia; [b] Heart and Rhythm Medical Group, 18324 Twin Creeks Road, Monte Sereno, CA 95030, USA
* Corresponding author.
E-mail address: dennis.h.lau@adelaide.edu.au

Card Electrophysiol Clin 13 (2021) 37–45
https://doi.org/10.1016/j.ccep.2020.11.009

in AF individuals is focused on, highlighting the importance of a comprehensive approach and the many areas that require further research.

HIGH BLOOD PRESSURE AND ATRIAL REMODELING

The cardiovascular effects of high BP are well recognized and include LVH diastolic dysfunction, heart failure with reduced ejection fraction, and coronary atherosclerosis as well as cardiac arrhythmias. Specifically, the substrate for atrial arrhythmias in hypertensive heart disease can be explained by the underlying electrical, ionic and structural remodeling. The atria from both small and large animal models of HT have been found dilated with increased collagen and fibrous tissue content, increased inflammation, and reduced connexin 43 expression that contribute to conduction slowing, increased conduction heterogeneity, and increased AF vulnerability/duration despite variable changes in atrial refractoriness.[5–11] Other changes include subcellular calcium remodeling and increased propensity for arrhythmogenic calcium alternans that can contribute to AF triggers.[12] In patients with chronically treated HT and LVH, electrophysiologic changes that result in increased AF inducibility include increased areas of low atrial voltage, global conduction slowing, and regional conduction delay at the crista terminalis with increased electrogram fractionation and double potentials.[13]

The mechanisms underlying these atrial changes, however, due to HT are not understood fully. Atrial stretch is a key driver of atrial remodeling in HT where increased intra-atrial pressure, atrial dilatation, and diastolic dysfunction are well-established hemodynamic consequences. The impact of HT-induced atrial dilatation on increased AF stability has been shown elegantly in a swine study.[14] Both acute and chronic atrial stretch contribute to AF triggers as well as activation of the autonomic nervous and renin-angiotensin-aldosterone systems (RAAS) to result in electrical and structural remodeling with involvement of various signaling pathways.[15,16] Specifically, the proarrhythmic effects of angiotensin II are contributed by changes in ion channels, calcium handling, gap junction, and atrial fibrosis as well as increased oxidative stress and inflammation.[17,18] The mechanistic link between RAAS and AF is affirmed by the 7-fold higher prevalence of AF in individuals with primary aldosteronism compared with those with essential hypertension.[19] The atrial remodeling process has been shown to be progressive with significant electro-structural correlation, thereby implicating that

early and aggressive BP management may arrest the remodeling cascade to prevent AF development.[9] Early experimental data suggest that the substrate for AF due to HT is reversible, which is supported by a small data set on reverse atrial remodeling after renal denervation in hypertensive individuals.[20,21] It remains unclear, however, if there is a BP threshold when remodeling will accelerate and whether different circadian BP profiles will have a differential impact on atrial remodeling.[22]

BLOOD PRESSURE INDICES, ATRIAL FIBRILLATION RISK, AND SINUS RHYTHM MAINTENANCE

The clinical association between HT and incident AF is well established, with early data from the Framingham Heart Study showing multivariate adjusted odds ratio between 1.4 and 1.5.[23] The independent association between AF and HT is affirmed in a more recent meta-analysis showing a relative risk ratio of 1.46 in developing AF.[1] There also is ample evidence demonstrating the impact of LVH in hypertensive subjects, leading to additional risk of developing new-onset AF.[24] The regression of LVH after BP treatment has been found to lower the risk of new-onset AF independent of BP lowering and agents used.[25] More recently, there is increasing attention on the association between individual BP component and pre-HT with the risk of developing AF. Data from the Women's Health Study indicated that systolic BP was better predictor of incident AF than diastolic BP and that individuals with systolic BP between 130 mm Hg and 139 mm Hg were at 43% increased risk of incident AF compared with those with normal systolic BP of less than 120 mm Hg.[26] Most of the subsequent studies since have confirmed the relationship between pre-HT and AF from different population cohorts, with hazard ratio up to 1.8 (**Table 1**).[27–32] Furthermore, elevated pulse pressure, a surrogate measure of increased proximal aortic stiffness, has been found predictive of AF development. In the prospective community-based Framingham cohort, every 20–mm Hg increase in pulse pressure was associated with an adjusted hazard ratio of 1.23 for incident AF at a median follow-up of 12 years.[3] Other studies since have shown similar association between measures of aortic stiffness (pulse pressure and augmentation index) and AF development (see **Table 1**).[33–36]

In patients with AF, the negative impact of HT on the progression of AF is well established. Recent systematic review and meta-analysis of 47 studies with more than 27,000 patients followed for more

Table 1
Studies demonstrating association between prehypertension and aortic stiffness with atrial fibrillation

Author, Year	Study, Country	Cohort	Follow-up	Atrial Fibrillation Incidence	Risk of Atrial Fibrillation, Hazard Ratio (95% CI)
Prehypertension					
Conen et al,[26] 2009	Women's Health Study, USA	n = 34,221; 55 yo ± 7 yo; 100% women	12.4 y	1.9%	1.43 (1.09–1.87) SBP 130–139 mm Hg vs <120 mm Hg
Chamberlain et al,[27] 2011	Atherosclerosis Risk in Communities Study, USA	N = 14,546; 45–64 yo; 55.3% women	10 y	3.5%	1.42 (1.15–1.76) SBP 120–139 mm Hg vs <120 mm Hg
Grundvold et al,[28] 2012	Norwegian Cardiovascular Survey, Norway	n = 2014; 50 yo ± 5 yo; 0% women	30 y	13.4%	1.50 (1.10–2.03) SBP 128–138 mm Hg vs <128 mm Hg
O'Neal et al,[29] 2015	Multi-Ethnic Study of Atherosclerosis, USA	n = 5311; 62 yo ±10 yo; 53% women	5.3 y	3.4%	1.80 (1.004–3.2) SBP 120–139 mm Hg vs <120 mm Hg
Kokubo et al,[30] 2015	Japanese Urban Cohort (The Suita Study), Japan	n = 6906; 56 yo ±11 yo; 53% women	12.8 y	3.7%	1.29 (0.91–1.85) 1.72 (1.01–2.91) [a]overweight SBP 120–139 mm Hg vs <120 mm Hg
Lee et al,[31] 2017	Korean National Sample Cohort, Republic of Korea	n = 227,102; >20 yo; 51% women	7.7 y	0.7%	1.08 (nonsignificant) SBP 120–139 mm Hg vs <120 mm Hg
Kim et al,[32] 2019	Korean National Health Insurance Service, Republic of Korea	n = 9,797,418; 47 yo ± 14 yo; 55.3% women	8.2 y	2.0%	1.085 (1.073–1.096) SBP mm Hg 120–139 vs <120 mm Hg
Aortic stiffness					
Mitchell et al,[3] 2007	Framingham Heart Study, USA	n = 5331; median 57 yo; 55% women	12 y	13.1%	1.26 (1.12–1.43) per 20–mm Hg pulse pressure increase

(continued on next page)

Table 1
(continued)

Author, Year	Study, Country	Cohort	Follow-up	Atrial Fibrillation Incidence	Risk of Atrial Fibrillation, Hazard Ratio (95% CI)
Larstorp et al,[33] 2012	Losartan Intervention For Endpoint Reduction in Hypertension Study, USA, UK, and Scandinavia	n = 8810; 67 yo ± 7 yo; 54% women	4.9 y	4.0%	1.20 (1.11–1.30) per 10–mm Hg pulse pressure increase
Roetker et al,[34] 2014	Multi-Ethnic Study of Atherosclerosis, USA	n = 6630; 62 ± 10 yo; 53% women	7.8 y	4.6%	1.29 (1.05–1.59) per SD pulse pressure increase
Shaikh et al,[35] 2016	Framingham Heart Study, USA	n = 5797; 61 yo ± 10 yo; 55% women	7.1 y	7.0%	1.16 (1.02–1.32) per SD augmentation index increase
Chen et al,[36] 2016	Rotterdam Study, The Netherlands	N = 5220; 69 yo ± 8 yo; 57% women	7.5 y	5.7%	1.05 (0.93–1.19)[a] 1.15 (1.03–1.29)[b] Per SD pulse wave velocity increase

Abbreviations: CHARGE-AF, cohorts for heart and aging research in genomic epidemiology-AF; SBP, systolic BP; yo, years old.

[a] Fully adjusted for CHARGE-AF risk score (age, race, height, weight, systolic and diastolic BP, antihypertensive medication use, smoking, diabetes, previous myocardial infarction, and previous heart failure).

[b] Adjusted for CHARGE-AF risk score excluding systolic and diastolic BP, height, and weight.

than 100,000 patient-years showed that HT was a significant univariable predictor of AF progression.[37] Additionally, the presence of HT has been found associated with greater AF recurrence after rhythm control therapy; although the association was found weaker when adjusted for other components of the metabolic syndrome in this meta-analysis.[38] Similarly, LVH has been shown associated with progression from paroxysmal to persistent AF in a 10-year follow-up study from the Canadian registry.[39] In the post hoc analysis of the Atrial Fibrillation Follow-up Investigation of Rhythm Management trial, concentric LVH was associated with increased AF recurrences in the pharmacologic rhythm control group.[40] Although there are no data on the impact of pre-HT on sinus rhythm maintenance in patients with AF, 2 small studies have shown that increased aortic stiffness was associated with higher AF recurrences after rhythm control intervention,[41,42] whereas another failed to show any independent association between aortic stiffness indices and postablation AF recurrences, perhaps due to a relatively shorter follow-up duration of only 6 months.[43]

BLOOD PRESSURE CONTROL AND ATRIAL FIBRILLATION

Many studies in hypertensive subjects have provided insights on the impact of BP management in both primary and secondary prevention of AF, although there is a paucity of data on the atrial substrate changes with these interventions. It is not surprising that RAAS inhibition have shown the most promising evidence in this space given its strong mechanistic link with atrial remodeling. Meta-analysis of randomized controlled trials has shown superiority of RAAS inhibition compared with conventional BP therapy (β-blocker and calcium channel blocker) or placebo for primary prevention of nonvalvular AF in hypertensive individuals, with 21% lower risk of developing new-onset AF.[44] The evidence appears to favor angiotensin-II receptor blockers (ARBs) over angiotensin-converting enzyme inhibitors (ACEIs) and aldosterone antagonists, with the most benefits seen in those with concomitant heart failure.[44,45] In hypertensive patients with AF, current practice guideline recommends (class IIa recommendation, quality of evidence—level B-R) treatment with an ARB to prevent recurrence of AF.[46] This is supported by meta-analysis of randomized controlled trials data from more than 42,000 patients, where ACEIs and ARBs were superior to calcium antagonists/β-blockers in reducing AF recurrences.[47] In patients with AF and suboptimally controlled HT undergoing catheter ablation,

additional renal denervation at the time of pulmonary vein isolation procedure has been shown to improve 12-month freedom from AF in conjunction with significantly better BP control in a randomized study.[48]

Data remain scarce regarding the optimum BP target for AF prevention. Current practice guidelines recommend a target of less than 130/80 mm Hg for patients with HT and known cardiovascular disease or 10-year atherosclerotic cardiovascular event risk of 10% or higher.[46] Extrapolating this target to the AF population is not unreasonable because a large proportion of patients with AF would have coexisting cardiovascular risk factors. The randomized Substrate Modification with Aggressive Blood Pressure Control trial evaluated aggressive versus standard BP lowering (target <120/80 mm Hg vs <140/90 mm Hg) in 184 hypertensive patients from up to 6 months before and 3 months after the catheter ablation procedure for AF. Despite attainment of lower systolic BP (123 mm Hg vs 135 mm Hg) with a combination of quinapril, hydrochlorothiazide, atenolol, amlodipine, and terazosin, there was no significant difference in the primary outcome of recurrent symptomatic atrial arrhythmia beyond 3 months postablation (median follow-up of 14 months).[49] This seemingly negative study, however, has several limitations, including relatively short treatment duration, possible underpowering, small BP difference between treatment and control groups, and the lack of targeting of other coexisting risk factors.[50]

The landscape of AF management has evolved to include upstream therapy for lifestyle and comprehensive risk factor modification as the fourth pillar, beyond established pillars of appropriate oral anticoagulation, rhythm, and rate control.[1] The interventions of such an aggressive risk factor modification program consist of structured and goal-directed weight management through BP control of less than 130/80 mm Hg, dietary modification aiming for 10% weight loss initially followed by a target body mass index of less than 27 kg/m^2, tailored moderate-intensity exercise to improve cardiorespiratory fitness, screening and treating obstructive sleep apnea, glycemic and lipid management aiming for glycated hemoglobin less than 6.5% and low-density lipoprotein cholesterol less than 2.6 mmol/L, smoking cessation, and alcohol abstinence or reduction.[51–53] In individuals with AF who have a body mass index above 27 kg/m^2 and at least 1 AF risk factor (such as HT, hyperglycemia, dyslipidemia, obstructive sleep apnea, and alcohol excess) managed in the risk factor modification program, reverse cardiac remodeling (reduced left atrial dilatation and LVH) may underpin the improvement in sinus rhythm maintenance and reversal of the natural progression of AF.[54,55]

CLINICAL IMPLICATIONS

HT is a major risk factor for cardiovascular disease, including AF. The health care burden of AF is enormous, with recent data showing increasing AF hospitalizations outnumbering those for myocardial infarction and heart failure.[56] The rising burden of AF risk factors in both adolescents and adults will continue to fuel the worldwide trend of increasing AF prevalence.[57-60] Unfortunately, recent cross-sectional National Health and Nutrition Examination Survey data suggest that the proportion of US adults with controlled BP appears to have declined between 2013 to 2014 and 2017 to 2018.[61] The underdiagnosis of HT in younger adults who are receiving regular primary care is an area of concern.[62] There has been little improvement seen in each stage of the HT cascade of awareness, treatment, and control since 2010, whereas new population-based strategies are needed to improve detection of high BP and initiation of antihypertensive therapy.[63]

The close association between HT and other AF risk factors, such as obstructive sleep apnea and obesity, warrants a comprehensive management approach beyond isolated BP management. Current evidence is in favor of an integrated care approach involving a multidisciplinary team approach using e-health to provide comprehensive and patient-centered AF care toward improved hard cardiovascular endpoints.[64,65] The field is recognizing the challenges and complexities of AF care, with the Heart Rhythm Society highlighting the need for a new model of care delivery via centers of excellence to comprehensively address the 4 pillars of AF care: risk factor management, stroke prevention, rate control, and rhythm control.[1,66]

FUTURE DIRECTIONS

Well-designed, prospective studies are needed to delineate optimal BP targets in individuals with HT and AF. The association between aortic stiffness and AF presents opportunities for further research and it remains unclear if additional targeting of these novel parameters will contribute to favorable remodeling and improved sinus rhythm maintenance. Future studies may include novel therapeutics targeting HT-related electrostructural atrial remodeling to determine if there are additional benefits toward AF outcomes independent of BP control.

SUMMARY

The adverse effects of high BP on atrial remodeling and the consequent increases in incident AF, AF progression, and AF recurrence demand aggressive management of HT in individuals with AF. Further work is needed to improve HT detection and management to reduce the rising tide of AF.

DISCLOSURE

Dr D.H. Lau is supported by a Mid-career Fellowship from The Hospital Research Foundation, South Australia.

REFERENCES

1. Lau DH, Nattel S, Kalman JM, et al. Modifiable risk factors and atrial fibrillation. Circulation 2017; 136(6):583–96.
2. Huxley RR, Lopez FL, Folsom AR, et al. Absolute and attributable risks of atrial fibrillation in relation to optimal and borderline risk factors: the Atherosclerosis Risk in Communities (ARIC) study. Circulation 2011;123(14):1501–8.
3. Mitchell GF, Vasan RS, Keyes MJ, et al. Pulse pressure and risk of new-onset atrial fibrillation. JAMA 2007;297(7):709–15.
4. Erkuner O, Dudink E, Nieuwlaat R, et al. Effect of systemic hypertension with versus without left ventricular hypertrophy on the progression of atrial fibrillation (from the Euro Heart Survey). Am J Cardiol 2018;122(4):578–83.
5. Okazaki H, Minamino T, Tsukamoto O, et al. Angiotensin II type 1 receptor blocker prevents atrial structural remodeling in rats with hypertension induced by chronic nitric oxide inhibition. Hypertens Res 2006;29(4):277–84.
6. Kim SJ, Choisy SC, Barman P, et al. Atrial remodeling and the substrate for atrial fibrillation in rat hearts with elevated afterload. Circ Arrhythm Electrophysiol 2011;4(5):761–9.
7. Lau DH, Shipp NJ, Kelly DJ, et al. Atrial arrhythmia in ageing spontaneously hypertensive rats: unraveling the substrate in hypertension and ageing. PLoS One 2013;8(8):e72416.
8. Kistler PM, Sanders P, Dodic M, et al. Atrial electrical and structural abnormalities in an ovine model of chronic blood pressure elevation after prenatal corticosteroid exposure: implications for development of atrial fibrillation. Eur Heart J 2006;27(24):3045–56.
9. Lau DH, Mackenzie L, Kelly DJ, et al. Hypertension and atrial fibrillation: evidence of progressive atrial remodeling with electrostructural correlate in a conscious chronically instrumented ovine model. Heart Rhythm 2010;7(9):1282–90.
10. Lau DH, Mackenzie L, Kelly DJ, et al. Short-term hypertension is associated with the development of

atrial fibrillation substrate: a study in an ovine hypertensive model. Heart Rhythm 2010;7(3):396–404.

11. Hohl M, Lau DH, Muller A, et al. Concomitant obesity and metabolic syndrome add to the atrial arrhythmogenic phenotype in male hypertensive rats. J Am Heart Assoc 2017;6(9):e006717.

12. Pluteanu F, Hess J, Plackic J, et al. Early subcellular Ca2+ remodelling and increased propensity for Ca2+ alternans in left atrial myocytes from hypertensive rats. Cardiovasc Res 2015;106(1):87–97.

13. Medi C, Kalman JM, Spence SJ, et al. Atrial electrical and structural changes associated with long-standing hypertension in humans: implications for the substrate for atrial fibrillation. J Cardiovasc Electrophysiol 2011;22(12):1317–24.

14. Manninger M, Zweiker D, van Hunnik A, et al. Arterial hypertension drives arrhythmia progression via specific structural remodeling in a porcine model of atrial fibrillation. Heart Rhythm 2018;15(9):1328–36.

15. Thanigaimani S, McLennan E, Linz D, et al. Progression and reversibility of stretch induced atrial remodeling: characterization and clinical implications. Prog Biophys Mol Biol 2017;130(Pt B):376–86.

16. Schotten U, Verheule S, Kirchhof P, et al. Pathophysiological mechanisms of atrial fibrillation: a translational appraisal. Physiol Rev 2011;91(1):265–325.

17. Goette A, Lendeckel U. Electrophysiological effects of angiotensin II. Part I: signal transduction and basic electrophysiological mechanisms. Europace 2008;10(2):238–41.

18. Sun Y, Zhang J, Lu L, et al. Aldosterone-induced inflammation in the rat heart : role of oxidative stress. Am J Pathol 2002;161(5):1773–81.

19. Rossi GP, Cesari M, Cuspidi C, et al. Long-term control of arterial hypertension and regression of left ventricular hypertrophy with treatment of primary aldosteronism. Hypertension 2013;62(1):62–9.

20. Thanigaimani S, Brooks AG, Kuklik P, et al. Prevention and reverse atrial remodeling in hypertensive substrate: beneficial effects of Tranilast and antihypertensive therapies. Heart Lung Circ 2016;25(S2):S2.

21. McLellan AJ, Schlaich MP, Taylor AJ, et al. Reverse cardiac remodeling after renal denervation: atrial electrophysiologic and structural changes associated with blood pressure lowering. Heart Rhythm 2015;12(5):982–90.

22. Lip GYH, Coca A, Kahan T, et al. Hypertension and cardiac arrhythmias: a consensus document from the European Heart Rhythm Association (EHRA) and ESC Council on Hypertension, endorsed by the Heart Rhythm Society (HRS), Asia-Pacific Heart Rhythm Society (APHRS) and Sociedad Latinoamericana de Estimulacion Cardiaca y Electrofisiologia (SOLEACE). Europace 2017;19(6):891–911.

23. Benjamin EJ, Levy D, Vaziri SM, et al. Independent risk factors for atrial fibrillation in a population-based cohort. The Framingham Heart Study. JAMA 1994;271(11):840–4.

24. Chatterjee S, Bavishi C, Sardar P, et al. Meta-analysis of left ventricular hypertrophy and sustained arrhythmias. Am J Cardiol 2014;114(7):1049–52.

25. Okin PM, Wachtell K, Devereux RB, et al. Regression of electrocardiographic left ventricular hypertrophy and decreased incidence of new-onset atrial fibrillation in patients with hypertension. JAMA 2006;296(10):1242–8.

26. Conen D, Tedrow UB, Koplan BA, et al. Influence of systolic and diastolic blood pressure on the risk of incident atrial fibrillation in women. Circulation 2009;119(16):2146–52.

27. Chamberlain AM, Agarwal SK, Folsom AR, et al. A clinical risk score for atrial fibrillation in a biracial prospective cohort (from the Atherosclerosis Risk in Communities [ARIC] study). Am J Cardiol 2011;107(1):85–91.

28. Grundvold I, Skretteberg PT, Liestol K, et al. Upper normal blood pressures predict incident atrial fibrillation in healthy middle-aged men: a 35-year follow-up study. Hypertension 2012;59(2):198–204.

29. O'Neal WT, Soliman EZ, Qureshi W, et al. Sustained pre-hypertensive blood pressure and incident atrial fibrillation: the Multi-Ethnic Study of Atherosclerosis. J Am Soc Hypertens 2015;9(3):191–6.

30. Kokubo Y, Watanabe M, Higashiyama A, et al. Interaction of blood pressure and body mass index with risk of incident atrial fibrillation in a Japanese urban cohort: the suita study. Am J Hypertens 2015;28(11):1355–61.

31. Lee SS, Ae Kong K, Kim D, et al. Clinical implication of an impaired fasting glucose and prehypertension related to new onset atrial fibrillation in a healthy Asian population without underlying disease: a nationwide cohort study in Korea. Eur Heart J 2017;38(34):2599–607.

32. Kim YG, Han KD, Choi JI, et al. Impact of the duration and degree of hypertension and body weight on new-onset atrial fibrillation: a nationwide population-based study. Hypertension 2019;74(5):e45–51.

33. Larstorp AC, Ariansen I, Gjesdal K, et al. Association of pulse pressure with new-onset atrial fibrillation in patients with hypertension and left ventricular hypertrophy: the Losartan Intervention for Endpoint (LIFE) reduction in hypertension study. Hypertension 2012;60(2):347–53.

34. Roetker NS, Chen LY, Heckbert SR, et al. Relation of systolic, diastolic, and pulse pressures and aortic distensibility with atrial fibrillation (from the Multi-Ethnic Study of Atherosclerosis). Am J Cardiol 2014;114(4):587–92.

35. Shaikh AY, Wang N, Yin X, et al. Relations of arterial stiffness and brachial flow-mediated dilation with new-onset atrial fibrillation: the Framingham Heart Study. Hypertension 2016;68(3):590–6.

36. Chen LY, Leening MJ, Norby FL, et al. Carotid Intima-Media Thickness and arterial stiffness and the risk of atrial fibrillation: the atherosclerosis risk in Communities (ARIC) study, Multi-Ethnic study of atherosclerosis (MESA), and the Rotterdam study. J Am Heart Assoc 2016;5(5):e002907.

37. Blum S, Meyre P, Aeschbacher S, et al. Incidence and predictors of atrial fibrillation progression: a systematic review and meta-analysis. Heart Rhythm 2019;16(4):502–10.

38. Lin KJ, Cho SI, Tiwari N, et al. Impact of metabolic syndrome on the risk of atrial fibrillation recurrence after catheter ablation: systematic review and meta-analysis. J Interv Card Electrophysiol 2014; 39(3):211–23.

39. Padfield GJ, Steinberg C, Swampillai J, et al. Progression of paroxysmal to persistent atrial fibrillation: 10-year follow-up in the Canadian Registry of Atrial Fibrillation. Heart Rhythm 2017;14(6):801–7.

40. Shah N, Badheka AO, Grover PM, et al. Influence of left ventricular remodeling on atrial fibrillation recurrence and cardiovascular hospitalizations in patients undergoing rhythm-control therapy. Int J Cardiol 2014;174(2):288–92.

41. Lau DH, Middeldorp ME, Brooks AG, et al. Aortic stiffness in lone atrial fibrillation: a novel risk factor for arrhythmia recurrence. PLoS One 2013;8(10): e76776.

42. Fumagalli S, Giannini I, Pupo S, et al. Atrial fibrillation after electrical cardioversion in elderly patients: a role for arterial stiffness? Results from a preliminary study. Aging Clin Exp Res 2016;28(6):1273–7.

43. Kizilirmak F, Guler GB, Guler E, et al. Impact of aortic stiffness on the frequency of paroxysmal atrial fibrillation recurrences. Acta Cardiol 2015;70(4):414–21.

44. Khatib R, Joseph P, Briel M, et al. Blockade of the renin-angiotensin-aldosterone system (RAAS) for primary prevention of non-valvular atrial fibrillation: a systematic review and meta analysis of randomized controlled trials. Int J Cardiol 2013;165(1): 17–24.

45. Chaugai S, Meng WY, Ali Sepehry A. Effects of RAAS blockers on atrial fibrillation prophylaxis: an updated systematic review and meta-analysis of randomized controlled trials. J Cardiovasc Pharmacol Ther 2016;21(4):388–404.

46. Whelton PK, Carey RM, Aronow WS, et al. 2017 ACC/AHA/AAPA/ABC/ACPM/AGS/APhA/ASH/ASPC/NMA/PCNA guideline for the prevention, detection, evaluation, and management of high blood pressure in adults: Executive summary: a report of the American College of Cardiology/American Heart Association Task Force on Clinical Practice Guidelines. Circulation 2018;138(17):e426–83.

47. Zhao D, Wang ZM, Wang LS. Prevention of atrial fibrillation with renin-angiotensin system inhibitors on essential hypertensive patients: a meta-analysis of randomized controlled trials. J Biomed Res 2015;29(6):475–85.

48. Steinberg JS, Shabanov V, Ponomarev D, et al. Effect of renal denervation and catheter ablation vs catheter ablation alone on atrial fibrillation recurrence among patients with paroxysmal atrial fibrillation and hypertension: the ERADICATE-AF randomized clinical trial. JAMA 2020;323(3): 248–55.

49. Parkash R, Wells GA, Sapp JL, et al. Effect of aggressive blood pressure control on the recurrence of atrial fibrillation after catheter ablation: a randomized, open-label clinical trial (SMAC-AF [Substrate Modification with Aggressive Blood Pressure Control]). Circulation 2017;135(19):1788–98.

50. Lau DH, Hendriks J, Kalman JM, et al. Blood pressure control in atrial fibrillation: one of many critical components in risk factor modification. Circulation 2017;135(19):1799–801.

51. Pathak RK, Elliott A, Middeldorp ME, et al. Impact of CARDIOrespiratory FITness on arrhythmia recurrence in obese individuals with atrial fibrillation: the CARDIO-FIT Study. J Am Coll Cardiol 2015;66(9): 985–96.

52. Pathak RK, Middeldorp ME, Lau DH, et al. Aggressive risk factor reduction study for atrial fibrillation and implications for the outcome of ablation: the ARREST-AF cohort study. J Am Coll Cardiol 2014; 64(21):2222–31.

53. Pathak RK, Middeldorp ME, Meredith M, et al. Long-term effect of goal-directed weight management in an atrial fibrillation cohort: a long-term follow-up study (LEGACY). J Am Coll Cardiol 2015;65(20): 2159–69.

54. Middeldorp ME, Pathak RK, Meredith M, et al. PREVEntion and regReSsive Effect of weight-loss and risk factor modification on Atrial Fibrillation: the REVERSE-AF study. Europace 2018;20(12): 1929–35.

55. Abed HS, Wittert GA, Leong DP, et al. Effect of weight reduction and cardiometabolic risk factor management on symptom burden and severity in patients with atrial fibrillation: a randomized clinical trial. JAMA 2013;310(19):2050–60.

56. Gallagher C, Hendriks JM, Giles L, et al. Increasing trends in hospitalisations due to atrial fibrillation in Australia from 1993 to 2013. Heart 2019;105(17): 1358–63.

57. Choi YS, Beltran TA, Klaric JS. Prevalence of optimal metabolic health in U.S. Adolescents, NHANES 2007-2016. Metab Syndr Relat Disord 2020. https://doi.org/10.1089/met.2020.0099.

58. Gu JK, Charles LE, Fekedulegn D, et al. Temporal trends in prevalence of cardiovascular disease (CVD) and CVD risk factors among U.S. older workers: NHIS 2004-2018. Ann Epidemiol 2020. https://doi.org/10.1016/j.annepidem.2020.10.002.

59. Chugh SS, Havmoeller R, Narayanan K, et al. World-wide epidemiology of atrial fibrillation: a global burden of disease 2010 study. Circulation 2014; 129(8):837–47.

60. Wong CX, Brown A, Tse HF, et al. Epidemiology of atrial fibrillation: the Australian and Asia-Pacific perspective. Heart Lung Circ 2017;26(9):870–9.

61. Muntner P, Hardy ST, Fine LJ, et al. Trends in blood pressure control among US adults with hypertension, 1999-2000 to 2017-2018. JAMA 2020; 324(12):1190–200.

62. Johnson HM, Thorpe CT, Bartels CM, et al. Undiagnosed hypertension among young adults with regular primary care use. J Hypertens 2014;32(1):65–74.

63. Foti K, Wang D, Appel LJ, et al. Hypertension awareness, treatment, and control in US adults: trends in the hypertension control cascade by population Subgroup (National health and Nutrition Examination Survey, 1999-2016). Am J Epidemiol 2019;188(12): 2165–74.

64. Gallagher C, Elliott AD, Wong CX, et al. Integrated care in atrial fibrillation: a systematic review and meta-analysis. Heart 2017;103(24):1947–53.

65. Gallagher C, Hendriks JM, Nyfort-Hansen K, et al. Integrated care for atrial fibrillation: the heart of the matter. Eur J Prev Cardiol 2020. https://doi.org/10.1093/eurjpc/zwaa065.

66. Piccini JP Sr, Allred J, Bunch TJ, et al. Rationale, considerations, and goals for atrial fibrillation centers of excellence: a Heart Rhythm Society perspective. Heart Rhythm 2020;17(10): 1804–32.

Atrial Fibrillation and Heart Failure
Epidemiology, Pathophysiology, Prognosis, and Management

Jonathan P. Ariyaratnam, MB BChir[a], Dennis H. Lau, MBBS, PhD[a],
Prashanthan Sanders, MBBS, PhD[a], Jonathan M. Kalman, MBBS, PhD[b],*

KEYWORDS

- Atrial fibrillation • Heart failure (HF) • Heart failure with reduced ejection fraction (HFrEF)
- Heart failure with preserved ejection fraction (HFpEF)

KEY POINTS

- Atrial fibrillation (AF) and heart failure (HF) share similar risk factors and frequently coexist.
- The risk of developing AF is higher in patients with HF (both HFrEF and HFpEF). The association between HFpEF and AF appears to be particularly strong.
- Mortality rates are increased when AF coexists with HF. Incident AF confers a particularly increased risk of mortality in patients with HF.
- Management of AF-HFrEF should focus on anticoagulation, rhythm or rate control and risk factor management. There is some evidence that catheter ablation may be effective in AF-HFrEF.
- Strong data to guide management of AF-HFpEF remains lacking. Robust new studies in this area are required.

INTRODUCTION

Atrial fibrillation (AF) and heart failure (HF) are chronic cardiovascular conditions that continue to increase in prevalence worldwide and have been described as global epidemics.[1,2] AF and HF each independently worsen quality of life and increase risk of hospitalization and mortality. In addition, AF and HF commonly coexist (AF-HF), sharing common risk factors and physiologically potentiating the effect of each other. In combination, these conditions appear to have a synergistic effect on outcomes including mortality, emphasizing the need for improved strategies for management of these two conditions in combination.

A significant challenge in HF management is the vast heterogeneity in phenotype. In recent years, HF has been broadly classified into HF with reduced ejection fraction (HFrEF) and HF with preserved ejection fraction (HFpEF), based on left ventricular ejection fraction (LVEF) identified on cardiac imaging. Although HFrEF and HFpEF exhibit the same symptoms and signs, they are increasingly seen as entirely different entities with diverging etiologies, prognostic implications, and management strategies. Furthermore, their interactions with AF (AF-HFrEF and AF-HFpEF) are distinctive. In this review article, we discuss the pathophysiology, epidemiology, prognosis, and evidence-based management of AF-HF, highlighting the significant differences between AF-HFrEF and AF-HFpEF.

[a] Centre for Heart Rhythm Disorders, University of Adelaide and Royal Adelaide Hospital, Adelaide, Australia;
[b] Department of Cardiology, Royal Melbourne Hospital, Department of Medicine, University of Melbourne, Melbourne, Australia
* Corresponding author. Department of Cardiology, Royal Melbourne Hospital, Parkville, Victoria 3050, Australia.
E-mail address: jon.kalman@mh.org.au

Card Electrophysiol Clin 13 (2021) 47–62
https://doi.org/10.1016/j.ccep.2020.11.004
1877-9182/21/© 2020 Elsevier Inc. All rights reserved.

HEART FAILURE WITH REDUCED EJECTION FRACTION AND HEART FAILURE WITH PRESERVED EJECTION FRACTION

HFrEF and HFpEF have been shown to contribute equally to the global burden of HF.[3] Simplistically, HFrEF is HF due to impaired left ventricular systolic function, whereas HFpEF is HF due to impaired left ventricular diastolic function. Diagnosis of HFrEF requires symptoms of HF in association with impaired systolic function identified on cardiac imaging. On the other hand, diagnosis of HFpEF is rather more challenging and recently published guidelines highlight the complexities of the diagnosis.[4] Diagnosis of HFpEF is made even more difficult by the presence of AF, as the symptoms of AF and HFpEF commonly overlap (**Fig. 1**). In addition, the echocardiographic and natriuretic peptide measurements used to diagnose diastolic failure are altered by the presence of AF.[5] Many of the studies investigating AF-HFpEF are therefore limited by overly simplistic definitions of HFpEF. Conclusions drawn regarding the prevalence and incidence of AF-HFpEF, the mortality associated with AF-HFpEF, and the optimal management of AF-HFpEF should therefore be tempered by the knowledge that HFpEF may have been overdiagnosed in these studies.

EPIDEMIOLOGY OF ATRIAL FIBRILLATION– HEART FAILURE

The prevalence of HF worldwide is 2% with up to 26 million people affected.[6] Similarly, it is estimated that approximately 33.5 million people have AF.[1] The prevalence of both conditions is increased in men and older age; the prevalence of HF in those older than 75 is 8.4%,[7] whereas the prevalence of AF in those older than 80 is 9%.[8] With aging populations around the world, the burden of both diseases is expected to continue to climb.

The prevalence of each condition is increased in the presence of the other. Patients with AF have a high prevalence of underlying HF, whereas, conversely, patients with HF have a marked association with prevalent AF.[9,10] **Fig. 2** shows the prevalence of AF in major HF registries, highlighting the consistently higher prevalence of AF in HFpEF compared with HFrEF.

The Framingham Heart Study (FHS), in which healthy adults were biennially monitored over their lifetimes for the development of cardiovascular disease, has been particularly useful in monitoring the temporal relationships between AF and HF. In total, 382 participants developed both AF and HF between 1948 and 1995.[11] Of these participants, 38% developed AF first, 41% developed HF first, and 21% were diagnosed with both on the same day. A new diagnosis of HF was associated with incident AF at a rate of 5.4% per year, whereas a new diagnosis of AF was associated with incident HF at a rate of 3.3% per year.[11] In a more contemporary analysis of the FHS, AF and HF subtypes were specifically evaluated.[12] This study demonstrated that patients with HFpEF were more likely to have prevalent AF preceding their HF diagnosis than patients with HFrEF, and patients with a new diagnosis of AF were more likely to develop incident HFpEF than incident HFrEF. Furthermore, prevalent AF predicted the development of incident HFpEF but not incident HFrEF. These data suggest that AF may have a particularly close role to play in the pathophysiology of HFpEF.

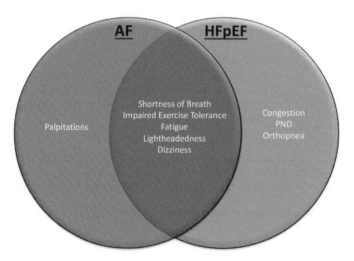

Fig. 1. Overlapping symptoms of AF and HFpEF.

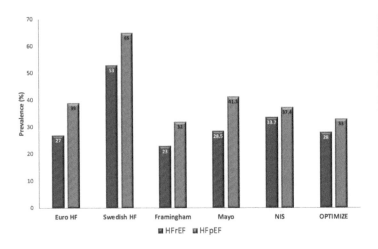

Fig. 2. Prevalence of AF in HFpEF and HFrEF. Prevalence of AF in HFrEF and HFpEF in major HF registries. There is increased prevalence of AF associated with HFpEF in comparison with HFrEF. NIS, National Inpatient Sample; OPTIMIZE, Organized Program to Initiate Life Saving Treatment in Hospitalized Patients with Heart Failure.

PATHOPHYSIOLOGY OF ATRIAL FIBRILLATION–HEART FAILURE

Fig. 3 shows the inextricable pathophysiological relationship between HF and AF. The development of the 2 conditions is driven by several common risk factors. Once developed, the 2 conditions have the potential to interact with each other in a vicious cycle.

SHARED RISK FACTORS

Many of the risk factors underlying the development of AF and HF (both HFrEF and HFpEF) are shared (**Fig. 4**). As the general population around the world becomes increasingly older, sedentary, and obese, the prevalence of AF and HF continues to rise. These risk factors cause significant hemodynamic shifts,

cardiac inflammation, atrial and ventricular fibrosis, macrovascular and microvascular ischemia, and arterial stiffening, leading to important changes in atrial and ventricular function.

Substantial research has shown the effect of untreated risk factors on the development of atrial disease and AF.[13-16] The importance of these risk factors, and in particular obesity, has been further highlighted by evidence showing that atrial disease can be reversed by aggressive treatment of risk factors through lifestyle modifications as well as by medical and surgical therapies.[17,18]

Similarly, risk factors for the development of both HFrEF and HFpEF also include aging, obesity, sedentary lifestyles, and hypertension. In HFrEF, obesity has been shown to result in a twofold increase in risk of HF development,[19]

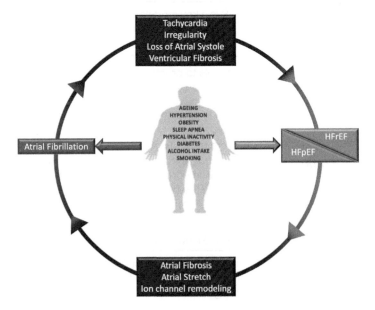

Fig. 3. AF interacts with HFrEF and HFpEF in a vicious cycle. Both AF and HF share common risk factors that lead to their development. AF and HF are then able to induce and perpetuate each other in a vicious cycle.

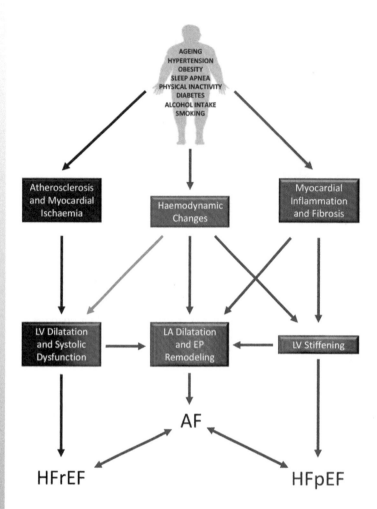

Fig. 4. Similar risk factors underlie the development of AF, HFrEF, and HFpEF. Shared risk factors cause significant alterations in cardiac hemodynamics, myocardial ischemia, and myocardial inflammation. These important changes lead to structural changes of the myocardium that can lead to HFrEF, HFpEF, or AF. AF, atrial fibrillation; EP, electrophysiological; LA, left atrium; LV, left ventricle; HFpEF, heart failure with preserved ejection fraction; HFrEF, heart failure with reduced ejection fraction.

whereas the overweight/obese phenotype is present in 80% of patients with HFpEF.[20] Further evidence from long-term follow-up registry data has shown that obesity is a comparable risk factor for the development of both incident HFrEF and HFpEF.[10] Interestingly, although obesity increases risk of HF development, substantial evidence exists to suggest that the presence of obesity actually reduces the long-term mortality of these conditions; the so-called "obesity paradox."[21]

HEART FAILURE PROMOTES INCIDENT ATRIAL FIBRILLATION

Both animal and human studies have provided evidence for the mechanistic links between prevalent HF and incident AF. These mechanisms include (1) activation of the renin-angiotensin-aldosterone system (RAAS), (2) mechanical stretch of the left atrium, and (3) electrophysiological remodeling of the atria.

Neurohormonal Activation and Atrial Fibrosis

The RAAS is a key modulator of the electrophysiological properties of the atria. HF results in activation of the RAAS in response to underperfusion of the kidneys. Activation of RAAS has been shown in animal models to promote fibrosis within the atria, partly mediated by the proinflammatory cytokine transforming growth factor-β.[22] Evidence for this association is strengthened by the fact that interstitial fibrosis appears to be significantly reduced by inhibitors of the RAAS, such as enalapril, candesartan, and spironolactone.[23–25] The pathophysiological importance of this atrial fibrosis is highlighted by the fact that its presence correlates directly with AF recurrence after AF ablation.[26]

Mechanical Stretch of the Atria

Both HFpEF and HFrEF result in significant hemodynamic alterations within the heart. One of the key changes is increased end-systolic left ventricular pressures. This increases left atrial pressures leading to left atrial stretch, activating stretch-dependent ion channels within the atria.[27] Left atrial stretch has been shown to be important in the initiation and maintenance of AF through changes in electrical conduction and cellular refractoriness.[28] Furthermore, blockade of stretch-activated channels with gadolinium has been shown to reduce propensity for AF despite increased atrial pressures and volumes.[29]

Ion Channel Dysregulation

Ion channel dysregulation and resulting alterations in atrial conduction properties have also been shown to be important in HF. Atrial mapping in sinus rhythm of patients with HFrEF identified significant changes within the atria with reduced atrial voltages, slowed conduction, and increased susceptibility to AF.[30] Underlying these electrophysiological changes is widespread ion channel remodeling, including dysregulation of voltage-dependent potassium channels, inward rectifying potassium channels, calcium handling proteins, and changes in connexin function.[31]

ATRIAL FIBRILLATION PROMOTES INCIDENT HEART FAILURE
Tachycardia-Mediated Cardiomyopathy

AF commonly presents with rapid ventricular rates. Sustained rapid ventricular rates in response to AF has the potential to impair both systolic and/or diastolic left ventricular (LV) function, inducing and worsening the effects of both HFrEF and HFpEF.

Tachycardia-mediated cardiomyopathy (TMC) specifically refers to the reversible systolic dysfunction seen following weeks of sustained and untreated elevated heart rates. Prolonged tachycardia results in a number of cellular changes that contribute to this LV systolic dysfunction.[32] These changes include impaired myocardial contractile function, upregulation of the RAAS[33,34] leading to a proinflammatory response,[35] fluid accumulation and dysfunctional hypertrophy of ventricular myocytes,[36] dysregulation of cellular calcium handling,[37] and alterations in the extracellular matrix.[38] In addition, significant hemodynamic changes further contribute to LV dysfunction with tachycardia causing increased LV wall stress, raised LV filling pressures, and increased afterload due to increased systemic vascular resistance.[39–41]

Importantly, these changes appear to be temporary, with restoration of sinus rhythm associated with normalization of hemodynamics and with normalization of LV function occurring within

weeks. However, there is evidence to suggest that chronic changes within the ventricular myocardium may persist following TMC; increased collagen deposition, LV stiffness, and impaired diastolic function have been noted in animal studies of TMC,[38,42] whereas long-term follow-up of patients with previous TMC suggests an increased propensity for these patients to develop recurrent HF and even sudden death.[43,44]

Irregular Ventricular Rhythm

There is growing evidence to suggest that irregular R-R intervals in AF also impair LV function irrespective of tachycardia. In patients with persistent AF in whom the heart rate is adequately controlled, regularization of the heart rhythm with either restoration of sinus rhythm or atrioventricular (AV) node ablation and pacing has been shown to improve ejection fraction in selected patients with HFrEF.[45,46] On a cellular level, animal studies have demonstrated that irregular cycle lengths result in abnormal calcium handling and therefore impaired cardiac myocyte function.[47]

Loss of Atrial Systole

In sinus rhythm, coordinated atrial systole contributes to approximately 20% of cardiac output by increasing ventricular filling during ventricular diastole. Loss of atrial systole caused by AF consequently results in impaired systolic function due to reduced stroke volume according to the Frank-Starling mechanism.[48] Furthermore, impaired LV filling during diastole results in diastolic dysfunction, raised left atrial pressures, and resultant symptoms of HFpEF.[49]

Ventricular Fibrosis

Cardiac MRI studies have identified diffuse ventricular fibrosis in patients with AF in the absence of any other cause.[50] This ventricular fibrosis has a dose-dependent relationship with AF; the greater the burden of AF, the greater the degree of fibrosis.[50] Ventricular fibrosis has a detrimental effect on both systolic and diastolic function and therefore has a potential impact in both HFrEF and HFpEF.[51]

PROGNOSTIC IMPLICATIONS OF ATRIAL FIBRILLATION–HEART FAILURE
Mortality

Although individual studies have demonstrated conflicting results regarding the impact of prevalent AF on all-cause mortality in HFrEF, a number of meta-analyses have now been performed confirming an overall increased long-term risk of between

17-40%.[52–54] **Table 1** shows that the pattern is similar with HFpEF, with most, but not all, randomized controlled trials (RCTs) and registries demonstrating a statistically significant increased risk of long-term all-cause mortality. In addition, there are conflicting data regarding whether AF is more dangerous in HFrEF or HFpEF; a meta-analysis pooling comparative risk estimates for all-cause mortality in AF-HFrEF and AF-HFpEF suggested that AF-HFrEF carried greater risk.[55] However, this study was limited by variable definitions of HFpEF with some studies defining patients with ejection fractions of 40% as HFpEF. On the other hand, a number of other studies have suggested that risk of all-cause mortality may rise with increasing ejection fractions in HF.[56,57]

Interestingly, developing incident AF after a diagnosis of either HFrEF or HFpEF appears to confer a much greater risk of long-term all-cause mortality than prevalent AF (AF before HF diagnosis).[54] The reasons for this remain unclear, although several mechanisms have been postulated: (1) new AF is more likely to be poorly rate-controlled than established AF, (2) risks associated with potent antiarrhythmic medications may be highest during the initiation phase, (3) over-anticoagulation or under-anticoagulation is more likely when newly prescribed compared with established regimens, and (4) a sudden change from sinus rhythm to AF is less likely to be hemodynamically tolerated in the failing heart when compared with ongoing long-standing AF.[58]

Stroke

AF is associated with a fivefold increase in risk of cerebral thromboembolism, independent of hypertension and age.[59] Studies from the pre-anticoagulation era show that congestive cardiac failure may elevate this risk of stroke,[60] although other studies demonstrate no significant association.[61,62] These conflicting data likely expose a lack of uniformity in the definition of HF in these studies. Indeed, when HF is defined purely as a moderate-to-severe reduction in LVEF, the risk of stroke is more than doubled (2.5x higher).[63] On the other hand, when the HF definition includes clinician-judged symptoms or previously documented history, the association with stroke often disappears.[64]

Data on the risk of stroke in AF-HFpEF from the pre-anticoagulation era are limited. However, recent studies have attempted to define the risk in patients with AF-HFpEF, albeit in largely anticoagulated populations. The CODE-AF registry of 10,697 Korean patients with AF showed that patients with AF-HFpEF were at significantly increased risk of stroke compared with patients with AF in the absence of HF.[65] On the other hand, the similarly sized US-based ORBIT-AF registry identified that there was no independent increased stroke risk in patients with HFpEF, albeit in a cohort with lower overall stroke rates.[66] Other studies have identified that there is no significant difference in risk of stroke between AF-HFrEF and AF-HFpEF.[55,67,68]

Overall, the data therefore suggest that the presence of HFrEF may increase the risk of stroke in patients with AF, depending on the definition of HFrEF used. Data in HFpEF are limited and more studies are required to further define this risk.

ATRIAL FIBRILLATION AND HEART FAILURE WITH MIDRANGE EJECTION FRACTION

In 2016, the European Society of Cardiology introduced the concept of HF with midrange ejection fraction (HFmrEF). These are patients with symptoms and signs of HF, ejection fraction between 40% and 49%, and elevated natriuretic peptides with evidence of structural heart disease or diastolic dysfunction. This additional classification of HF was an acknowledgment that a gray zone existed between HFrEF and HFpEF. Interestingly, studies have since shown that this group of patients demonstrate characteristics and prognoses that are intermediate between HFrEF and HFpEF. Indeed, the prevalence of AF in HFmrEF, and the risk of all-cause mortality of AF-HFmrEF, appears to lie somewhere between the prevalence and mortality in HFrEF and HFpEF.[68,69]

MANAGEMENT OF ATRIAL FIBRILLATION–HEART FAILURE

Optimal management of AF-HF mirrors the management of AF alone with 4 key principles; anticoagulation, rhythm control, rate control, and risk factor management (RFM). However, HFrEF and HFpEF differ entirely in pathophysiology and responses to treatment and must, therefore, be considered as separate entities when considering management. Although the evidence supporting various management options is significantly more advanced in AF-HFrEF, the evidence-base for AF-HFpEF continues to grow.

MANAGEMENT OF ATRIAL FIBRILLATION–HEART FAILURE WITH REDUCED EJECTION FRACTION
Anticoagulation

Anticoagulation has been extensively shown to effectively reduce the risk of stroke in patients with AF by up to 68%.[61] Current clinical

Table 1
Association of prevalent and incident AF in HFpEF with all-cause mortality

Study	Study Type	Population	Number of HFpEF Participants	Average Follow-up, y	Effect of Prevalent AF on Risk of All-Cause Mortality (Adjusted HR)	Effect of Incident AF on Risk of All-Cause Mortality (Adjusted HR)
TOPCAT 2018[97]	RCT	• At least 1 sign/ symptom of HF • LVEF >45% • >50 y • Controlled systolic BP • K <5 • GFR >30	1765	2.9	• 1.34 (1.09–1.65)	• 2.53 (1.80–3.55)
CHARM 2006[56]	RCT	• Symptomatic HF • NYHA II-IV • LVEF >40%	7599	3.1	• 1.37 (1.06–1.79)	• Odds ratio (unadjusted) – 2.57 (1.70–3.90)
I-PRESERVE 2014[98]	RCT	• Symptomatic HF (NYHA II-IV) • LVEF >45% • >1 hospitalization previous 6 mo	4128	4.4	• 1.23 (0.99–1.54)	• Not reported
PRESERVE 2012[99]	RCT	• >1 HF hospitalization OR >3 ambulatory HF visits • LVEF >50%	14,295	1.8	• 1.11 (1.03–1.20)	• 1.62 (1.42–1.84)
Zakeri et al,[100] 2013	Registry	• Olmstead County HF surveillance study cohort • LVEF >50%	939	4.3	• 1.27 (1.06–1.51)	• 2.22 (1.73–2.84)
Sartipy et al,[68] 2017	Registry	• Swedish HF • Registry • Clinician-judged HF • EF >50%	9595	2.2	• 1.11 (1.02–1.21)	• Not reported
Zafrir et al,[69] 2018	Registry	• HF Long-Term Registry of the ESC • LVEF >50%	3879	1	• 1.20 (0.95–1.50)	• Not reported
Santhana-krishnan et al,[12] 2016	Registry	• Framingham Heart Study participants 1980–2012 • LVEF >45%	309	3.6 (+/−3.4)	• 1.33 (0.97–1.83)	• 1.58 (1.08–2.3)
Rusinaru et al,[101] 2008	Registry	• HF admissions in Somme region • LVEF >50%	368	5	• 1.19 (0.89–1.6)	• Not reported

Large RCTs and HF registries providing risk estimates for all-cause mortality in patients with AF and HFpEF. Most studies suggest that prevalent AF increases risk of all-cause mortality in HFpEF but risk is significantly higher in incident AF than prevalent AF.

Abbreviations: AF, atrial fibrillation; BP, blood pressure; EF, ejection fraction; ESC, European Society of Cardiology; GFR, glomerular filtration rate; HF, heart failure; HFpEF, heart failure with preserved ejection fraction; HR, hazard ratio; LVEF, left ventricular ejection fraction; NYHA, New York Heart Association; RCT, randomized controlled trial.

guidelines propose anticoagulation according to the presence of risk factors. The CHADS2Vasc risk score is in widespread use to assist in anticoagulation decision-making.[70] Congestive cardiac failure, defined loosely as "signs/symptoms of HF or objective evidence of reduced LVEF," forms part of this risk stratification tool. Given that anticoagulation is generally recommended for patients with a CHADS2Vasc score of 1 or more, any patient with a diagnosis of AF-HFrEF would, by definition, warrant anticoagulation according to clinical guidelines. Adequately anticoagulated patients with AF-HFrEF have reduced incidence of ischemic stroke compared with non-anticoagulated patients with AF-HFrEF.[64] In addition, anticoagulated patients with AF-HFrEF have equivalent adjusted stroke risks to adequately anticoagulated patients with AF-only, with no significant difference in bleeding.[64,71–74] Therefore, although strong evidence for an increased adjusted stroke risk with AF-HFrEF compared with AF-only may be lacking, anticoagulation of these cohorts reduces overall stroke incidence and does not appear to cause significant harm.

In terms of choice of anticoagulant to use in patients with AF-HFrEF, substudies of the major direct oral anticoagulant (DOAC) RCTs have shown that each DOAC (Apixaban, Dabigatran, Rivaroxaban, and Edoxaban) is at least as safe as warfarin in this population, with some showing superiority in terms of reduced risk of stroke[71,72] and major bleeding.[71,72,74]

Pharmacological Rhythm Versus Rate Control

Although anticoagulation in AF-HFrEF is universally expected in the absence of contraindications, the choice between rate control or rhythm control remains guided by patient symptoms and physician preferences. The reason for this is the absence of clear data supporting one strategy above the other. The AF-CHF trial randomized patients with AF and either symptomatic HF (New York Heart Association class II-IV) with LVEF less than 35% or asymptomatic HF with recent decompensation or LVEF less than 25% to a strategy of rate control or rhythm control.[75] Rhythm control strategies included electrical cardioversion and/or pharmacologic rhythm control (mainly involving amiodarone) whereas rate control involved beta-blockers and/or digoxin and/or device implantation with AV node ablation. The study showed that there was no benefit of rhythm control over rate control in terms of the risk of cardiovascular mortality, all-cause mortality, stroke, and worsening HF after 3 years of follow-up.

A cautious approach should be taken in interpreting this study, however. First, 21% of the patients starting in the rhythm control group crossed-over to the rate control group because of a failure to maintain sinus rhythm. Second, 82% of the patients in the rhythm control group were treated with amiodarone compared with just 7% in the rate control group. Amiodarone has been shown in observational studies to increase risk of all-cause mortality and noncardiac mortality and may have neutralized any potential benefits associated with rhythm control.[76,77] Therefore, although the AF-CHF trial showed that pharmacologic rhythm control was not superior to rate control strategies in the AF-HFrEF population, these findings should not be generalized to include nonpharmacological methods for rhythm control, such as catheter ablation.

Catheter Ablation

Two of the main advantages of catheter ablation over pharmacologic rhythm control for treatment of AF are the lower long-term AF recurrence rates and the reduced need for toxic antiarrhythmic drugs such as amiodarone. Catheter ablation is now established as first-line therapy for patients with symptomatic AF in the absence of structural heart disease, and in recent years there has been growing interest in its potential utility for patients with AF-HFrEF. A number of RCTs have been published investigating the effect of catheter ablation on patients with AF-HFrEF (**Table 2**). In general, these studies provide consistent evidence that catheter ablation is more effective than medical rate control in improving LVEF, quality of life, and exercise tolerance. Whether this translates to long-term prognostic benefits remains unclear, with previous evidence suggesting that long-term maintenance of sinus rhythm is poor after catheter ablation for AF-HFrEF. However, the CASTLE-AF trial did show cardiovascular mortality benefits of ablation at 36 months.[78] On the other hand, these trials also suggest that patients with HFrEF are at higher risk of peri-procedural complications compared with non-HFrEF patients, perhaps highlighting the increased fragility of this population. Further evidence is required to assess the balance between efficacy and safety of catheter ablation in this population.

A major difficulty in the design and interpretation of these trials involving AF-HFrEF is the heterogeneity in underlying HF etiology. Many of these studies recruited a mix of ischemic and nonischemic patients with HF, and interpreted the results to reflect HF as an entirety. However, there is evidence to suggest that efficacy rates of catheter ablation may

Table 2
Major RCTs investigating outcomes of catheter ablation in patients with HFrEF

Study, Year	Population	Intervention	Comparator	Follow-up, mo	Outcomes
Khan et al,[82] 2008	• Symptomatic AF • NYHA II-III • EF <40% • OMT	PVI (n = 41)	AV node ablation and BiV pacing (n = 40)	6	With PVI: • Improved MLHF score • Longer 6MWT • Improved EF
MacDonald et al,[102] 2011	• Persistent AF • NYHA II-IV • EF <35% • OMT	RFA PVI ± Linear ± CFAEs (n = 22)	Medical rate control (n = 19)	9.7 (RFA group), 6.9 (control group)	With RFA • Radionuclide EF improved • CMR EF not improved • MLHF and 6MWT not improved
Jones et al,[103] 2013	• Persistent AF • NYHA II-IV • EF <35% • OMT	RFA PVI ± Linear ± CFAEs (n = 26)	Medical rate control (n = 26)	12	With RFA • Improved peak oxygen consumption • Improved MLHF • Nonsignificant trend to improved LVEF • Nonsignificant trend to improved 6MWT
Hunter et al,[104] 2014	• Persistent AF • NYHA II-IV • EF <50% • Adequate ventricular rate control	RFA PVI ± CFAEs ± Linear (n = 26)	Medical rate control (n = 24)	6	With RFA • Improved LVEF • Improved peak oxygen consumption • Improved MLHF
Di Biase et al,[105] 2016	• Persistent AF • Dual chamber ICD/CRT-D • NYHA II-IV • EF <40% • OMT	RFA PVI +/ PW + CS ± SVC ± CFAE (n = 102)	Amiodarone (n = 101)	24	With RFA • Improved freedom from AF • Reduced unplanned hospitalization • Lower all-cause mortality • Improved LVEF • Improved MLHF • Improved 6MWT

(continued on next page)

Table 2
(continued)

Study, Year	Population	Intervention	Comparator	Follow-up, mo	Outcomes
Prabhu et al,[46] 2017	• Persistent AF • NYHA II-IV • EF <45% (on CMR) • Absence of CAD • Absence of any other cause of HF	RFA PVI +/PW (n = 33)	Ongoing medical rate control (n = 33)	6	With RFA • Improved LVEF • Improved NYHA class
Marrouche et al,[78] 2018	• Paroxysmal or persistent AF • NYHA II-IV • LVEF <35% • ICD or CRT-D	RFA PVI ± additional at operator discretion	Medical therapy (rate or rhythm control)	37.8	With RFA • Reduced composite all-cause mortality and HF hospitalization • Reduced all-cause mortality • Reduced cardiovascular mortality • Reduced HF hospitalization • Improved LVEF

Abbreviations: 6MWT, 6-min walk test; AF, atrial fibrillation; AV, atrioventricular; BiV, biventricular; CAD, coronary artery disease; CFAE, complex fractionated atrial electrograms; CMR, cardiac MRI; CRT-D, cardiac resynchronization therapy and defibrillator; CS, coronary sinus; EF, ejection fraction; HF, heart failure; ICD, implantable cardiac defibrillator; MLHFQ, Minnesota Living with Heart Failure Questionnaire; NYHA, New York Heart Association; OMT, optimal medical treatment; PVI, pulmonary vein isolation; PW, posterior wall; RCT, randomized controlled trial; RFA, radiofrequency ablation; SVC, superior vena cava.

diverge according to etiology. The CAMERA-MRI RCT recruited patients with nonischemic cardiomyopathy only and used cardiac MRI to establish the presence of ventricular fibrosis before intervention (catheter ablation or continued medical rate control).[46] Absence of ventricular fibrosis implicated arrhythmia-induced cardiomyopathy as the underlying etiology. The results showed that an absence of ventricular fibrosis predicted greater improvements in LVEF in the catheter ablation arm and ventricular fibrosis volume inversely correlated with absolute improvement in LVEF. This study therefore emphasizes the need for further stratification of the HFrEF population, both in the design of future trials as well as considering management for individual patients.

Rate Control

The AF-CHF trial showed that, for patients with AF-HFrEF, controlling heart rate to less than 80 beats per minute at rest or less than 110 beats per minute during exertion was equal to restoration of sinus rhythm in terms of long-term mortality.[75] On the other hand, the RACE II trial showed that there was no significant mortality or morbidity benefit associated with a strict rate control strategy (resting heart rate [HR] <80 beats per minute) compared with a lenient strategy (resting HR <110 beats per minute).[79] Rate control is therefore an appropriate strategy for patients with AF-HFrEF but target HR remains unclear.

Strategies for rate control in the HFrEF population include medications such as beta-blockers and digoxin or pacemaker implantation and AV node ablation. The Swedish HF Registry provides evidence for the efficacy of beta-blockers in this population with the associated reduction in HR linked to a significant reduction in mortality.[80] Digoxin, on the other hand, has not been shown to be efficacious in the AF-HFrEF population but is often used empirically on the basis that it has proven benefit in patients with HFrEF and sinus rhythm.[81]

AV node ablation is established as an option for rate control in AF-HFrEF, albeit an inferior option to AF ablation as seen in the PABA-CHF trial.[82] In general, it is a strategy that is used as a last resort when attempts at rhythm control and medical rate control have failed. This is because it necessitates prior implantation of a pacemaker, on which the patient will be dependent. In patients with HFrEF and heart block, the BLOCK-HF study showed that biventricular pacing was superior to right ventricular pacing, regardless of baseline QRS duration.[83] A number of observational studies have shown the significant mortality and symptomatic benefits of AV node ablation and biventricular

pacemaker implantation compared with medical rate control, and this has been confirmed in meta-analyses.[83,84] However, HF etiology remains an important factor with evidence to suggest that patients with ischemic cardiomyopathy may respond less well compared with those with nonischemic cardiomyopathy.[85]

Risk Factor Management

RFM is an essential component of the management of AF. Numerous studies provide evidence that aggressive monitoring and treatment of the risk factors described previously improve sinus rhythm maintenance, AF-related symptoms, and quality of life.[14–16,18,86,87] Particular benefits have been seen with simple lifestyle modifications resulting in significant weight loss. However, data in the AF-HFrEF population are lacking. Cardiac rehabilitation has proven beneficial in the overall HF population, in terms of reducing hospitalizations and improving quality of life, albeit in the absence of proven benefit on mortality.[88] However, significant barriers to lifestyle modifications in the HFrEF cohort exist, with patients more likely to be elderly and frail and resistant to change because of psychosocial and behavioral issues.[88] Furthermore, there is evidence to suggest that being overweight or obese may confer a survival benefit to patients with HFrEF compared with normal-weight patients with HFrEF.[21] Further studies are required to investigate the association between aggressive RFM and outcomes in the AF-HFrEF population.

MANAGEMENT OF ATRIAL FIBRILLATION–HEART FAILURE WITH PRESERVED EJECTION FRACTION
Anticoagulation

Patients with AF-HFpEF generally have higher CHADS2Vasc scores because they are more likely to be women, elderly, and have associated comorbidities such as hypertension and diabetes.[89] Therefore, regardless of the diagnosis of AF-HFpEF, these patients often warrant anticoagulation. Despite this, the AF-HFpEF cohort has been found to be under-anticoagulated compared with patients with HFrEF, with the difference most pronounced in those with CHADS2Vasc scores of 1 or 2.[89] This perhaps reflects the difficulty in diagnosis of HFpEF and the lack of clarity on its contribution to the CHADS2Vasc scoring system. As with AF-HFrEF, the major DOAC trials showed that anticoagulated patients with AF-HFpEF had adjusted stroke rates similar to patients with AF-only without a significantly increased risk of bleeding.[71]

Rate Versus Rhythm Control

Unlike AF-HFrEF, there are no RCTs available to compare the efficacy of rhythm control versus rate control in the AF-HFpEF population. Clinical guidelines do not specifically propose one strategy over the other. A recently published retrospective analysis of the Get With the Guidelines HF Registry suggested that rhythm control may confer a modest mortality benefit in comparison with rate control.[90] However, this study was significantly limited by a weak definition of HFpEF using EF alone, weak definition of rate control based purely on documented use of beta-blockers or calcium-channel blockers, and an inability to monitor the success or failure of each strategy with follow-up electrocardiogram or Holter.

Catheter Ablation

Currently, only observational studies investigating the efficacy of catheter ablation in AF-HFpEF have been published.[91–96] Most of these studies defined HFpEF simply as HF symptoms and signs in the absence of depressed LV function, thereby likely including a substantial proportion of patients without true HFpEF. Overall, these studies have shown that long-term freedom from AF after catheter ablation is lower in patients with AF-HFpEF compared with patients with AF-only, and is similar to rates in AF-HFrEF populations.[91,92,95,96] One study specified echocardiographic evidence of LV diastolic failure as an inclusion criterion for the HFpEF group, and this showed that freedom from AF rates were intermediate between the AF-only group and the AF-HFrEF group.[92] A further single-arm observational study demonstrated that diastolic function may improve following catheter ablation in HFpEF; however, at this stage there is insufficient evidence to support catheter ablation for AF-HFpEF. Well-designed RCTs with clearly defined patients with HFpEF are required to further understand the importance of catheter ablation treatment in this population.

SUMMARY

AF and HF have similar risk factors, frequently coexist, and potentiate each other in a vicious cycle. AF appears to play a particularly important role in the pathophysiology of HFpEF. Evidence suggests that the presence of AF in both HFrEF and HFpEF increases the risk of all-cause mortality as well as stroke in these conditions, and is particularly problematic when AF is incident. Growing evidence suggests that catheter ablation may be an effective strategy in controlling symptoms and improving quality of life in patients with AF-HFrEF, although further evidence to help stratify the patients most likely to respond is needed. Evidence for mortality benefits remains tenuous at this stage. Strong data guiding management of AF-HFpEF are also lacking largely due to its challenging diagnosis. Therefore, although the dangers of these coexistent conditions are clear, improving outcomes associated with them requires further careful investigation.

CLINICS CARE POINTS

- Patients with HF are 10 times more likely to develop AF than those without HF.
- HF patients who develop AF have 17-40% increased risk of all-cause mortality compared to those without AF.
- Catheter ablation for AF-HFrEF improves symptoms and quality of life and may have mortality benefits.
- Optimal management to improve long-term prognosis in patients with AF-HFpEF has yet to be established.

FINANCIAL DISCLOSURES

Dr. J. Ariyaratnam is supported by the Australian Government Research Training Program Scholarship from the University of Adelaide. Dr D. Lau is supported by the Robert J. Craig Lectureship from the University of Adelaide. Dr P. Sanders is supported by a Practitioner Fellowships from the National Health and Medical Research Council of Australia and by the National Heart Foundation of Australia. Dr Kalman is supported by a Practitioner Fellowship from the National Health and Medical Research Council of Australia.

CONFLICT OF INTEREST DISCLOSURES

Dr P. Sanders reports having served on the advisory board of Medtronic, Abbott Medical, Boston Scientific, CathRx, and PaceMate. Dr P. Sanders reports that the University of Adelaide has received on his behalf lecture and/or consulting fees from Medtronic, Abbott Medical, and Boston Scientific. Dr P. Sanders reports that the University of Adelaide has received on his behalf research funding from Medtronic, Abbott Medical, Boston Scientific, and MicroPort.

REFERENCES

1. Chugh SS, Havmoeller R, Narayanan K, et al. Worldwide epidemiology of atrial fibrillation: a global burden of disease 2010 study. Circulation 2014;129(8):837–47.

2. Savarese G, Lund LH. Global public health burden of heart failure. Card Fail Rev 2017;3(1):7–11.
3. Bursi F, Weston SA, Redfield MM, et al. Systolic and diastolic heart failure in the community. JAMA 2006;296(18):2209–16.
4. Pieske B, Tschöpe C, de Boer RA, et al. How to diagnose heart failure with preserved ejection fraction: the HFA-PEFF diagnostic algorithm: a consensus recommendation from the Heart Failure Association (HFA) of the European Society of Cardiology (ESC). Eur J Heart Fail 2020;22(3):391–412.
5. Lam CS, Rienstra M, Tay WT, et al. Atrial fibrillation in heart failure with preserved ejection fraction: association with exercise capacity, left ventricular filling pressures, natriuretic peptides, and left atrial volume. JACC Heart Fail 2017;5(2):92–8.
6. Ponikowski P, Anker SD, AlHabib KF, et al. Heart failure: preventing disease and death worldwide. ESC Heart Fail 2014;1(1):4–25.
7. Redfield MM, Jacobsen SJ, Burnett JC Jr, et al. Burden of systolic and diastolic ventricular dysfunction in the community: appreciating the scope of the heart failure epidemic. JAMA 2003; 289(2):194–202.
8. Go AS, Hylek EM, Phillips KA, et al. Prevalence of diagnosed atrial fibrillation in adults: national implications for rhythm management and stroke prevention: the AnTicoagulation and Risk Factors in Atrial Fibrillation (ATRIA) Study. JAMA 2001;285(18): 2370–5.
9. Ling LH, Kistler PM, Kalman JM, et al. Comorbidity of atrial fibrillation and heart failure. Nat Rev Cardiol 2016;13(3):131–47.
10. Brouwers FP, de Boer RA, van der Harst P, et al. Incidence and epidemiology of new onset heart failure with preserved vs. reduced ejection fraction in a community-based cohort: 11-year follow-up of PREVEND. Eur Heart J 2013;34(19): 1424–31.
11. Wang TJ, Larson MG, Levy D, et al. Temporal relations of atrial fibrillation and congestive heart failure and their joint influence on mortality: the Framingham Heart Study. Circulation 2003; 107(23):2920–5.
12. Santhanakrishnan R, Wang N, Larson MG, et al. Atrial fibrillation begets heart failure and vice versa: temporal associations and differences in preserved versus reduced ejection fraction. Circulation 2016;133(5):484–92.
13. Abed HS, Wittert GA, Leong DP, et al. Effect of weight reduction and cardiometabolic risk factor management on symptom burden and severity in patients with atrial fibrillation: a randomized clinical trial. JAMA 2013;310(19):2050–60.
14. Pathak RK, Elliott A, Middeldorp ME, et al. Impact of CARDIOrespiratory FITness on arrhythmia recurrence in obese individuals with atrial fibrillation: the CARDIO-FIT Study. J Am Coll Cardiol 2015;66(9): 985–96.
15. Pathak RK, Middeldorp ME, Lau DH, et al. Aggressive risk factor reduction study for atrial fibrillation and implications for the outcome of ablation: the ARREST-AF cohort study. J Am Coll Cardiol 2014; 64(21):2222–31.
16. Pathak RK, Middeldorp ME, Meredith M, et al. Long-term effect of goal-directed weight management in an atrial fibrillation cohort: a long-term follow-up study (LEGACY). J Am Coll Cardiol 2015;65(20):2159–69.
17. Donnellan E, Wazni OM, Elshazly M, et al. Impact of bariatric surgery on atrial fibrillation type. Circ Arrhythm Electrophysiol 2020;13(2):e007626.
18. Middeldorp ME, Pathak RK, Meredith M, et al. PREVEntion and regReSsive Effect of weight-loss and risk factor modification on Atrial Fibrillation: the REVERSE-AF study. Europace 2018;20(12):1929–35.
19. Kenchaiah S, Evans JC, Levy D, et al. Obesity and the risk of heart failure. N Engl J Med 2002;347(5): 305–13.
20. Haass M, Kitzman DW, Anand IS, et al. Body mass index and adverse cardiovascular outcomes in heart failure patients with preserved ejection fraction: results from the Irbesartan in Heart Failure with Preserved Ejection Fraction (I-PRESERVE) trial. Circ Heart Fail 2011;4(3):324–31.
21. Oreopoulos A, Padwal R, Kalantar-Zadeh K, et al. Body mass index and mortality in heart failure: a meta-analysis. Am Heart J 2008;156(1):13–22.
22. Li D, Shinagawa K, Pang L, et al. Effects of angiotensin-converting enzyme inhibition on the development of the atrial fibrillation substrate in dogs with ventricular tachypacing-induced congestive heart failure. Circulation 2001;104(21):2608–14.
23. Kumagai K, Nakashima H, Urata H, et al. Effects of angiotensin II type 1 receptor antagonist on electrical and structural remodeling in atrial fibrillation. J Am Coll Cardiol 2003;41(12):2197–204.
24. Milliez P, Deangelis N, Rucker-Martin C, et al. Spironolactone reduces fibrosis of dilated atria during heart failure in rats with myocardial infarction. Eur Heart J 2005;26(20):2193–9.
25. Sakabe M, Fujiki A, Nishida K, et al. Enalapril prevents perpetuation of atrial fibrillation by suppressing atrial fibrosis and over-expression of connexin43 in a canine model of atrial pacing-induced left ventricular dysfunction. J Cardiovasc Pharmacol 2004;43(6):851–9.
26. Marrouche NF, Wilber D, Hindricks G, et al. Association of atrial tissue fibrosis identified by delayed enhancement MRI and atrial fibrillation catheter ablation: the DECAAF study. JAMA 2014;311(5): 498–506.
27. Sachs F. Stretch-activated ion channels: what are they? Physiology (Bethesda) 2010;25(1):50–6.

28. Solti F, Vecsey T, Kekesi V, et al. The effect of atrial dilatation on the genesis of atrial arrhythmias. Cardiovasc Res 1989;23(10):882–6.

29. Bode F, Katchman A, Woosley RL, et al. Gadolinium decreases stretch-induced vulnerability to atrial fibrillation. Circulation 2000;101(18):2200–5.

30. Sanders P, Morton JB, Davidson NC, et al. Electrical remodeling of the atria in congestive heart failure: electrophysiological and electroanatomic mapping in humans. Circulation 2003;108(12):1461–8.

31. Nattel S, Maguy A, Le Bouter S, et al. Arrhythmogenic ion-channel remodeling in the heart: heart failure, myocardial infarction, and atrial fibrillation. Physiol Rev 2007;87(2):425–56.

32. Gopinathannair R, Etheridge SP, Marchlinski FE, et al. Arrhythmia-induced cardiomyopathies: mechanisms, recognition, and management. J Am Coll Cardiol 2015;66(15):1714–28.

33. Spinale FG, de Gasparo M, Whitebread S, et al. Modulation of the renin-angiotensin pathway through enzyme inhibition and specific receptor blockade in pacing-induced heart failure: I. Effects on left ventricular performance and neurohormonal systems. Circulation 1997;96(7):2385–96.

34. Travill CM, Williams TD, Pate P, et al. Haemodynamic and neurohumoral response in heart failure produced by rapid ventricular pacing. Cardiovasc Res 1992;26(8):783–90.

35. Bradham WS, Bozkurt B, Gunasinghe H, et al. Tumor necrosis factor-alpha and myocardial remodeling in progression of heart failure: a current perspective. Cardiovasc Res 2002;53(4):822–30.

36. Spinale FG, Holzgrefe HH, Mukherjee R, et al. Angiotensin-converting enzyme inhibition and the progression of congestive cardiomyopathy. Effects on left ventricular and myocyte structure and function. Circulation 1995;92(3):562–78.

37. Cory CR, McCutcheon LJ, O'Grady M, et al. Compensatory downregulation of myocardial Ca channel in SR from dogs with heart failure. Am J Physiol 1993;264(3 Pt 2):H926–37.

38. Spinale FG, Tomita M, Zellner JL, et al. Collagen remodeling and changes in LV function during development and recovery from supraventricular tachycardia. Am J Physiol 1991;261(2 Pt 2):H308–18.

39. O'Brien PJ, Ianuzzo CD, Moe GW, et al. Rapid ventricular pacing of dogs to heart failure: biochemical and physiological studies. Can J Physiol Pharmacol 1990;68(1):34–9.

40. Ohno M, Cheng CP, Little WC. Mechanism of altered patterns of left ventricular filling during the development of congestive heart failure. Circulation 1994;89(5):2241–50.

41. Seymour AA, Burkett DE, Asaad MM, et al. Hemodynamic, renal, and hormonal effects of rapid ventricular pacing in conscious dogs. Lab Anim Sci 1994;44(5):443–52.

42. Spinale FG, Zellner JL, Johnson WS, et al. Cellular and extracellular remodeling with the development and recovery from tachycardia-induced cardiomyopathy: changes in fibrillar collagen, myocyte adhesion capacity and proteoglycans. J Mol Cell Cardiol 1996;28(8):1591–608.

43. Nerheim P, Birger-Botkin S, Piracha L, et al. Heart failure and sudden death in patients with tachycardia-induced cardiomyopathy and recurrent tachycardia. Circulation 2004;110(3):247–52.

44. Watanabe H, Okamura K, Chinushi M, et al. Clinical characteristics, treatment, and outcome of tachycardia induced cardiomyopathy. Int Heart J 2008; 49(1):39–47.

45. Natale A, Zimerman L, Tomassoni G, et al. Impact on ventricular function and quality of life of transcatheter ablation of the atrioventricular junction in chronic atrial fibrillation with a normal ventricular response. Am J Cardiol 1996;78(12):1431–3.

46. Prabhu S, Taylor AJ, Costello BT, et al. Catheter ablation versus medical rate control in atrial fibrillation and systolic dysfunction: the CAMERA-MRI study. J Am Coll Cardiol 2017;70(16):1949–61.

47. Ling LH, Khammy O, Byrne M, et al. Irregular rhythm adversely influences calcium handling in ventricular myocardium: implications for the interaction between heart failure and atrial fibrillation. Circ Heart Fail 2012;5(6):786–93.

48. Mitchell JH, Gupta DN, Payne RM. Influence of atrial systole on effective ventricular stroke volume. Circ Res 1965;17:11–8.

49. White CW, Kerber RE, Weiss HR, et al. The effects of atrial fibrillation on atrial pressure-volume and flow relationships. Circ Res 1982;51(2):205–15.

50. Ling LH, Kistler PM, Ellims AH, et al. Diffuse ventricular fibrosis in atrial fibrillation: noninvasive evaluation and relationships with aging and systolic dysfunction. J Am Coll Cardiol 2012;60(23):2402–8.

51. Liu T, Song D, Dong J, et al. Current understanding of the pathophysiology of myocardial fibrosis and its quantitative assessment in heart failure. Front Physiol 2017;8:238.

52. Cheng M, Lu X, Huang J, et al. The prognostic significance of atrial fibrillation in heart failure with a preserved and reduced left ventricular function: insights from a meta-analysis. Eur J Heart Fail 2014; 16(12):1317–22.

53. Mamas MA, Caldwell JC, Chacko S, et al. A meta-analysis of the prognostic significance of atrial fibrillation in chronic heart failure. Eur J Heart Fail 2009;11(7):676–83.

54. Odutayo A, Wong CX, Williams R, et al. Prognostic importance of atrial fibrillation timing and pattern in adults with congestive heart failure: a systematic review and meta-analysis. J Card Fail 2017;23(1):56–62.

55. Kotecha D, Chudasama R, Lane DA, et al. Atrial fibrillation and heart failure due to reduced versus

preserved ejection fraction: a systematic review and meta-analysis of death and adverse outcomes. Int J Cardiol 2016;203:660–6.

56. Olsson LG, Swedberg K, Ducharme A, et al. Atrial fibrillation and risk of clinical events in chronic heart failure with and without left ventricular systolic dysfunction: results from the Candesartan in Heart failure-Assessment of Reduction in Mortality and morbidity (CHARM) program. J Am Coll Cardiol 2006;47(10):1997–2004.

57. Pai RG, Varadarajan P. Prognostic significance of atrial fibrillation is a function of left ventricular ejection fraction. Clin Cardiol 2007;30(7):349–54.

58. Anter E, Jessup M, Callans DJ. Atrial fibrillation and heart failure: treatment considerations for a dual epidemic. Circulation 2009;119(18):2516–25.

59. Wolf PA, Dawber TR, Thomas HE Jr, et al. Epidemiologic assessment of chronic atrial fibrillation and risk of stroke: the Framingham study. Neurology 1978;28(10):973–7.

60. Benjamin EJ, Levy D, Vaziri SM, et al. Independent risk factors for atrial fibrillation in a population-based cohort. The Framingham Heart Study. JAMA 1994; 271(11):840–4.

61. Risk factors for stroke and efficacy of antithrombotic therapy in atrial fibrillation. Analysis of pooled data from five randomized controlled trials. Arch Intern Med 1994;154(13):1449–57.

62. Hart RG, Pearce LA, McBride R, et al. Factors associated with ischemic stroke during aspirin therapy in atrial fibrillation: analysis of 2012 participants in the SPAF I-III clinical trials. The Stroke Prevention in Atrial Fibrillation (SPAF) Investigators. Stroke 1999;30(6):1223–9.

63. Echocardiographic predictors of stroke in patients with atrial fibrillation: a prospective study of 1066 patients from 3 clinical trials. Arch Intern Med 1998;158(12):1316–20.

64. Friberg L, Lund LH. Heart failure: a weak link in CHA2 DS2 -VASc. ESC Heart Fail 2018;5(3): 231–9.

65. Chung S, Kim TH, Uhm JS, et al. Stroke and systemic embolism and other adverse outcomes of heart failure with preserved and reduced ejection fraction in patients with atrial fibrillation (from the COmparison study of Drugs for symptom control and complication prEvention of Atrial Fibrillation [CODE-AF]). Am J Cardiol 2020;125(1):68–75.

66. Cherian TS, Shrader P, Fonarow GC, et al. Effect of atrial fibrillation on mortality, stroke risk, and quality-of-life scores in patients with heart failure (from the outcomes registry for better informed treatment of atrial fibrillation [ORBIT-AF]). Am J Cardiol 2017;119(11):1763–9.

67. Sobue Y, Watanabe E, Lip GYH, et al. Thromboembolisms in atrial fibrillation and heart failure patients with a preserved ejection fraction (HFpEF) compared to those with a reduced ejection fraction (HFrEF). Heart Vessels 2018;33(4):403–12.

68. Sartipy U, Dahlstrom U, Fu M, et al. Atrial fibrillation in heart failure with preserved, mid-range, and reduced ejection fraction. JACC Heart Fail 2017; 5(8):565–74.

69. Zafrir B, Lund LH, Laroche C, et al. Prognostic implications of atrial fibrillation in heart failure with reduced, mid-range, and preserved ejection fraction: a report from 14 964 patients in the European Society of Cardiology Heart Failure Long-Term Registry. Eur Heart J 2018;39(48):4277–84.

70. Lip GY, Nieuwlaat R, Pisters R, et al. Refining clinical risk stratification for predicting stroke and thromboembolism in atrial fibrillation using a novel risk factor-based approach: the euro heart survey on atrial fibrillation. Chest 2010;137(2):263–72.

71. McMurray JJ, Ezekowitz JA, Lewis BS, et al. Left ventricular systolic dysfunction, heart failure, and the risk of stroke and systemic embolism in patients with atrial fibrillation: insights from the ARISTOTLE trial. Circ Heart Fail 2013;6(3):451–60.

72. Ferreira J, Ezekowitz MD, Connolly SJ, et al. Dabigatran compared with warfarin in patients with atrial fibrillation and symptomatic heart failure: a subgroup analysis of the RE-LY trial. Eur J Heart Fail 2013;15(9):1053–61.

73. van Diepen S, Hellkamp AS, Patel MR, et al. Efficacy and safety of rivaroxaban in patients with heart failure and nonvalvular atrial fibrillation: insights from ROCKET AF. Circ Heart Fail 2013;6(4): 740–7.

74. Magnani G, Giugliano RP, Ruff CT, et al. Efficacy and safety of edoxaban compared with warfarin in patients with atrial fibrillation and heart failure: insights from ENGAGE AF-TIMI 48. Eur J Heart Fail 2016;18(9):1153–61.

75. Roy D, Talajic M, Nattel S, et al. Rhythm control versus rate control for atrial fibrillation and heart failure. N Engl J Med 2008;358(25):2667–77.

76. Qin D, Leef G, Alam MB, et al. Mortality risk of long-term amiodarone therapy for atrial fibrillation patients without structural heart disease. Cardiol J 2015;22(6):622–9.

77. Steinberg JS, Sadaniantz A, Kron J, et al. Analysis of cause-specific mortality in the atrial fibrillation follow-up investigation of rhythm management (AFFIRM) study. Circulation 2004;109(16):1973–80.

78. Marrouche NF, Brachmann J, Andresen D, et al. Catheter ablation for atrial fibrillation with heart failure. N Engl J Med 2018;378(5):417–27.

79. Van Gelder IC, Groenveld HF, Crijns HJ, et al. Lenient versus strict rate control in patients with atrial fibrillation. N Engl J Med 2010;362(15): 1363–73.

80. Li SJ, Sartipy U, Lund LH, et al. Prognostic significance of resting heart rate and use of β-blockers in

atrial fibrillation and sinus rhythm in patients with heart failure and reduced ejection fraction: findings from the Swedish heart failure registry. Circ Heart Fail 2015;8(5):871–9.

81. The effect of digoxin on mortality and morbidity in patients with heart failure. N Engl J Med 1997; 336(8):525–33.

82. Khan MN, Jaïs P, Cummings J, et al. Pulmonary-vein isolation for atrial fibrillation in patients with heart failure. N Engl J Med 2008;359(17):1778–85.

83. Mustafa U, Atkins J, Mina G, et al. Outcomes of cardiac resynchronisation therapy in patients with heart failure with atrial fibrillation: a systematic review and meta-analysis of observational studies. Open Heart 2019;6(1):e000937.

84. Ganesan AN, Brooks AG, Roberts-Thomson KC, et al. Role of AV nodal ablation in cardiac resynchronization in patients with coexistent atrial fibrillation and heart failure a systematic review. J Am Coll Cardiol 2012;59(8):719–26.

85. Sohinki D, Ho J, Srinivasan N, et al. Outcomes after atrioventricular node ablation and biventricular pacing in patients with refractory atrial fibrillation and heart failure: a comparison between non-ischaemic and ischaemic cardiomyopathy. Europace 2014;16(6):880–6.

86. Pathak RK, Evans M, Middeldorp ME, et al. Cost-effectiveness and clinical effectiveness of the risk factor management clinic in atrial fibrillation: the CENT study. JACC Clin Electrophysiol 2017;3(5):436–47.

87. Middeldorp ME, Ariyaratnam J, Lau D, et al. Lifestyle modifications for treatment of atrial fibrillation. Heart 2020;106(5):325–32.

88. Long L, Mordi IR, Bridges C, et al. Exercise-based cardiac rehabilitation for adults with heart failure. Cochrane Database Syst Rev 2019;1(1):Cd003331.

89. Contreras JP, Hong KN, Castillo J, et al. Anticoagulation in patients with atrial fibrillation and heart failure: insights from the NCDR PINNACLE-AF registry. Clin Cardiol 2019;42(3):339–45.

90. Kelly JP, DeVore AD, Wu J, et al. Rhythm control versus rate control in patients with atrial fibrillation and heart failure with preserved ejection fraction: insights from Get with the guidelines-heart failure. J Am Heart Assoc 2019;8(24):e011560.

91. Black-Maier E, Ren X, Steinberg BA, et al. Catheter ablation of atrial fibrillation in patients with heart failure and preserved ejection fraction. Heart Rhythm 2018;15(5):651–7.

92. Cha YM, Wokhlu A, Asirvatham SJ, et al. Success of ablation for atrial fibrillation in isolated left ventricular diastolic dysfunction: a comparison to systolic dysfunction and normal ventricular function. Circ Arrhythm Electrophysiol 2011;4(5):724–32.

93. Elkaryoni A, Al Badarin F, Spertus JA, et al. Comparison of the effect of catheter ablation for atrial fibrillation on all-cause hospitalization in patients

with versus without heart failure (from the nationwide readmission database). Am J Cardiol 2020; 125(3):392–8.

94. Ichijo S, Miyazaki S, Kusa S, et al. Impact of catheter ablation of atrial fibrillation on long-term clinical outcomes in patients with heart failure. J Cardiol 2018;72(3):240–6.

95. Jayanna MB, Mohsen A, Inampudi C, et al. Procedural outcomes of patients with heart failure undergoing catheter ablation of atrial fibrillation. Am J Ther 2019;26(3):e333–8.

96. Vecchio N, Ripa L, Orosco A, et al. Atrial fibrillation in heart failure patients with preserved or reduced ejection fraction. prognostic significance of rhythm control strategy with catheter ablation. J Atr Fibrillation 2019;11(5):2128.

97. Cikes M, Claggett B, Shah AM, et al. Atrial fibrillation in heart failure with preserved ejection fraction: the TOPCAT trial. JACC Heart Fail 2018;6(8):689–97.

98. Oluleye OW, Rector TS, Win S, et al. History of atrial fibrillation as a risk factor in patients with heart failure and preserved ejection fraction. Circ Heart Fail 2014;7(6):960–6.

99. McManus DD, Hsu G, Sung SH, et al. Atrial fibrillation and outcomes in heart failure with preserved versus reduced left ventricular ejection fraction. J Am Heart Assoc 2013;2(1):e005694.

100. Zakeri R, Chamberlain AM, Roger VL, et al. Temporal relationship and prognostic significance of atrial fibrillation in heart failure patients with preserved ejection fraction: a community-based study. Circulation 2013;128(10):1085–93.

101. Rusinaru D, Leborgne L, Peltier M, et al. Effect of atrial fibrillation on long-term survival in patients hospitalised for heart failure with preserved ejection fraction. Eur J Heart Fail 2008;10(6):566–72.

102. MacDonald MR, Connelly DT, Hawkins NM, et al. Radiofrequency ablation for persistent atrial fibrillation in patients with advanced heart failure and severe left ventricular systolic dysfunction: a randomised controlled trial. Heart 2011;97(9):740–7.

103. Jones DG, Haldar SK, Hussain W, et al. A randomized trial to assess catheter ablation versus rate control in the management of persistent atrial fibrillation in heart failure. J Am Coll Cardiol 2013;61(18):1894–903.

104. Hunter RJ, Berriman TJ, Diab I, et al. A randomized controlled trial of catheter ablation versus medical treatment of atrial fibrillation in heart failure (the CAMTAF trial). Circ Arrhythm Electrophysiol 2014; 7(1):31–8.

105. Di Biase L, Mohanty P, Mohanty S, et al. Ablation versus amiodarone for treatment of persistent atrial fibrillation in patients with congestive heart failure and an implanted device: results from the AATAC Multicenter randomized trial. Circulation 2016; 133(17):1637–44.

Diabetes and Endocrine Disorders (Hyperthyroidism/ Hypothyroidism) as Risk Factors for Atrial Fibrillation

Satoshi Higa, MD, PhD[a],*, Akira Maesato, MD, PhD[a], Sugako Ishigaki, MD[a], Kazuyoshi Suenari, MD, PhD[b], Yi-Jen Chen, MD, PhD[c], Shih-Ann Chen, MD[d]

KEYWORDS

- Atrial fibrillation • Risk factors • Diabetes mellitus • Thyroid disease

KEY POINTS

- Diabetes mellitus and hyperthyroidism are strong independent risk factors for AF.
- Glycemic control and achieving euthyroid status can affect the pathophysiology of AF and improve the outcomes of pharmacologic and/or electrical cardioversion and catheter ablation.
- Controlling thromboembolism is an important aspect of DM and the early period of uncontrolled hyperthyroidism.

INTRODUCTION

Atrial fibrillation (AF) is a diversified disease resulting from electrophysiologic disorders, and its adverse events significantly impact health care costs. Pulmonary vein (PV) isolation is a cornerstone of AF ablation strategies.[1] However, multiple procedures because of recurrence have become problematic. The management of risk factors may have a significant impact on atrial remodeling and clinical outcomes.[2] Therefore, treatment strategies combined with rhythm control and risk factor management may improve the overall clinical outcomes. This article highlights the current state of knowledge about AF risk factors diabetes mellitus (DM) and thyroid diseases, and discusses the impact of managing these risk factors on primary and secondary prevention of AF.

DIABETES MELLITUS
Prevalence of Atrial Fibrillation Associated with Diabetes Mellitus

DM has been reported to have a higher risk of AF (**Table 1**).[3–9] A longer duration with poor glycemic control has been independently associated with an increased incidence of AF.[5] The NAVIGATOR Trial reported that the fasting plasma glucose level could be a predictor of AF.[8] Furthermore, DM independently increased the overall risk of AF onset more in females.[4] The younger DM population has a significantly higher relative risk of AF than the elderly DM population.[9]

[a] Cardiac Electrophysiology and Pacing Laboratory, Division of Cardiovascular Medicine, Makiminato Central Hospital, 1199 Makiminato, Urasoe City, Okinawa 901-2131, Japan; [b] Department of Cardiology, Hiroshima City Hiroshima Citizens Hospital, 7-33 Motomachi, Naka-ku, Hiroshima City, Hiroshima 703-8518, Japan; [c] Division of Cardiovascular Medicine, Department of Internal Medicine, Wan Fang Hospital, Taipei Medical University, 111 Hsin-Lung Road, Section 3, Taipei 116, Taiwan; [d] Division of Cardiology and Cardiovascular Research Center, Taipei Veterans General Hospital, 201, Sec. 2, Shih-Pai Road, Taipei, Taiwan
* Corresponding author.
E-mail address: sa_higa@yahoo.co.jp

Card Electrophysiol Clin 13 (2021) 63–75
https://doi.org/10.1016/j.ccep.2020.11.005
1877-9182/21/© 2020 Elsevier Inc. All rights reserved.

Table 1
Association between DM and the risk of the onset of AF

Publication Year (Ref.)	Study Design	Study Period (y)	Characteristics of Sample Population (n)	AF Patients (n)	Mean Follow-Up (mo)	Risk of New Onset of AF
Nichols et al,[4] 2009	Observational cohort	1999–2008	50% DM (+)/50% DM (−) (total 34,744)	3.6% in DM (+) 2.5% in DM (−)	86	AF was significantly greater among DM patients (9.1 per 1000 person/year in DM [+] and 6.6 per 1000 person/year in DM [-]; $P<.0001$). DM was associated with a 26% increased risk of AF among females (HR, 1.26; 95% CI, 1.08–1.46; $P = .003$) but was not statistically significant factor among males (HR, 1.09; 95% CI, 0.96–1.24; $P = .17$) after a full adjustment of the other risk factors.
Dublin et al,[5] 2010	Population-based case control	2001–2004	Newly diagnosed AF/control (total 3613)	1410	NA	Among patients treated for DM, the risk of developing AF was 3% higher for each additional year of the DM duration (95% CI, 1%–6%). AF risk was higher with poor glycemic control (HR, 1.06; 95% CI, 0.74–1.51, in HbA_{1c} <7), (HR, 1.48; 95% CI, 1.09–2.01, in HbA_{1c} 7–8), (HR, 1.46; 95% CI, 1.02–2.08, in HbA_{1c} 8–9), (HR, 1.96; 95% CI, 1.22–3.14, in HbA_{1c} >9) per an additional 1 y.

Study	Study type	Years	Population			Results
Huxley et al,[6] 2012	Prospective cohort[a]	1990–2007	Pre-DM (51.4%)/DM (14.9%)/non-DM (33.7%) (total 13,025)	1311	174	Type II DM was associated with a significant increase in the risk of AF (HR, 1.35; 95% CI, 1.14–1.60) after an adjustment for cofounders (HR, 1.13; 95% CI, 1.07–1.20) in DM (+) and (HR, 1.05; 95% CI, 0.96–1.15) in DM (−) patients per a 1% increment increase in the HbA$_{1c}$.
Schoen et al,[7] 2012	Randomized[b]	1993–2011	Females without CVD (total 34,720)	1079	197	A significant relationship between baseline DM and the onset of AF (HR, 1.95; 95% CI, 1.49–2.56; $P<.0001$ [age adjusted]), (HR, 1.37; 95% CI, 1.03–1.83; $P = .03$ [multivariate adjusted]), (HR, 1.14; 95% CI, 0.93–1.40; $P = .02$ [time updated model adjusted]) for changes in the risk factors and cardiovascular events.
Latini et al,[8] 2013	Double-blinded randomized[c]	NA	IGT (total 8943)	613	78	IGT could predicted the risk of AF (HR, 1.33; 95% CI, 1.11–1.59; $P = .018$) (per 1 mmol/L increment increase in fasting plasma glucose).
Pallisgaard et al,[9] 2016	Danish nationwide cohort	1996–2012	DM (5%)/non-DM (95%) (total 5,081,087)	d	216	DM is an independent predictor of AF, particularly in young DM patients.

Abbreviations: CI, confidence interval; CVD, cardiovascular disease; HbA$_{1c}$, hemoglobin A$_{1c}$; HR, hazard ratio; IGT, impaired glucose tolerance; NA, data not available.

[a] These study results were based on the data from the Atherosclerosis Risk in Communities Study (ARIC).
[b] This study population included health professional women who were free of cardiovascular disease at baseline and participated in the Women's Health Study (WHS).
[c] These study results were based on the data from the Nateglinide and Valsaltan in Impaired Glucose Tolerance Outcomes Research Trial (NAVIGATOR).
[d] This study showed that the adjusted incidence rate ratios in those with DM and with non-DM as a reference were 2.34 (95% CI, 1.52–3.60; 18–39 y/o), 1.52 (95% CI, 1.47–1.56; 40–64 y/o), 1.20 (95% CI, 1.18–1.23; 65–74 y/o), and 0.99 (95% CI, 0.97–1.01; 75–100 y/o), respectively, for AF per 1000 person/years in the four age groups.

Pathophysiology of Atrial Fibrillation Associated with Diabetes Mellitus

Electrical, structural, and electromechanical remodeling, and cardiac autonomic neuropathy

Several important concepts regarding the pathophysiologic association between AF and DM have been reported. Basic studies have demonstrated that DM is associated with proarrhythmic conditions including a decrease in sodium currents and increase in L-type calcium currents, prolonged interatrial conduction time and action potential duration, and increased expression of connexin-43 and suppressed expression of connexin-40.[10,11] Exposure to a hyperglycemic state enhances oxidative stress and inflammation, and causes excessive production of advanced glycation end products and reactive oxygen species, and activation of the renin angiotensin-aldosterone system can cause fibrosis.[10,12–14] Animals with DM have been shown to have an impaired atrial electromechanical function, which is associated with fibrotic changes and conduction slowing.[15] In clinical studies, DM had a higher interatrial electromechanical delay,[16] which is an independent predictor of the onset and recurrence of AF.[16,17] A clinical study also showed a significantly longer atrial activation time and lower bipolar voltage with DM suggesting advanced electrical remodeling.[18] Cardiac autonomic neuropathy in DM encompasses parasympathetic denervation and subsequent sympathetic denervation. AF is caused by an imbalance in the sympathetic and parasympathetic nerve activity.[19]

Blood glucose fluctuations

High blood glucose levels with larger fluctuations may have a significant impact on the risk of cardiovascular complications. A previous study reported the correlation between larger blood glucose fluctuations and the onset of AF.[20] In basic studies, glucose fluctuations are associated with enhanced oxidative stress, fibrosis, and AF inducibility.[21] Therefore, glucose fluctuations are more harmful because of increased oxidative stress[22] and abnormal sympathetic nerve stimulation[23] rather than a hyperglycemic state. Considering those issues, care must be given to the importance of glucose fluctuations, rather than hyperglycemia alone, in AF genesis.

Previous Reports Regarding Primary and Secondary Prevention of Atrial Fibrillation Associated with Diabetes Mellitus

Regarding primary prevention, controversial results of the efficacy of antidiabetic agents for the prevention of AF have been reported (**Table 2**).[24–30]

The use of metformin or thiazolidinediones is independently associated with a reduction in the incidence of AF.[24,25] These favorable results may be caused by the anti-inflammatory action of those agents.[31] However, sulfonylureas have not shown any favorable outcome.[27] Furthermore, there was no significant benefit of an intensive glycemic control on the incidence of AF.[26] Therefore, larger glucose fluctuations during glycemic control are harmful.[32,33] Elderly patients with DM have a higher incidence of AF among insulin users but a lower incidence among dipeptidyl peptidase-4 (DPP-4) inhibitors users.[27] However, controversial efficacy results of DPP-4 inhibitors on AF have been reported.[34] Although, glucagon-like peptide-1 (GLP-1) receptor agonists and sodium-glucose cotransporter-2 (SGLT2) inhibitors have been associated with a lower risk of major cardiovascular events, those agents have not shown any significant impact on the incidence of AF.[35,36] Recently, Zelniker and colleagues[30] demonstrated that dapagliflozin reduced the risk of the onset of AF/atrial flutter. Considering the safety profile of that without severe hypoglycemia or cardiovascular benefits from GLP-1 receptor agonists and SGLT2 inhibitors, further research to confirm the efficacy of AF suppression needs to be conducted.

According to secondary prevention, DM could be a risk factor of a poor cardioversion efficacy in patients with or without AF ablation.[37,38] Because of the poor efficacy and adverse events of antiarrhythmic drugs, there may be less benefit of antiarrhythmic drugs for DM.[39,40] Although, a meta-analysis showed the association between the hemoglobin A_{1c} level and risk of late AF recurrences with DM,[41] there have been controversial results of the impact of DM on catheter ablation outcomes (**Table 3**).[41–49] According to those reports, preoperative pioglitazone use and better glycemic control may improve ablation outcomes.

THYROID DISEASE

Prevalence of Atrial Fibrillation Associated with Thyroid Disease

Hyperthyroidism has been reported to have a three- to six-fold risk of AF as compared with euthyroid.[50,51] Furthermore, AF is reported in 10% to 15% of those with hyperthyroidism and the prevalence increases with age. Twenty-five percent of elderly patients with hyperthyroidism (>60 years old) had AF as compared with 5% in younger patients (<60 years old).[52] Currently, there are little data about the relationship between hypothyroidism and AF. Although a few previous studies suggested that hypothyroidism might be

Table 2
Efficacy of antidiabetic agents for primary prevention of AF in type II DM

Publication Year (Ref.)	Study Design	Population (n)	Age y/o (SD)	User Group (n, %)	Nonuser Group (n, %)	Mean Follow-Up (mo)	Risk of New Onset of AF
Chao et al,[24] 2012	NHIRD Cohort[a] 2000–2007	12,065	54 (12)	TZD (4137)	Nonusers (7928)	63	TZD reduced the AF onset (HR, 0.69; 95% CI, 0.49–0.91; P = .028)
Chang et al,[25] 2014	NHIRD Cohort[a] 1999–2010	645,710	59 (17)	Metformin (85,198)	Nonusers (560,512)	156	Metformin reduced the AF onset (HR, 0.81; 95% CI, 0.76–0.86; P<.001)
Fatemi et al,[26] 2014	Multicenter, randomized, double-blind, prospective	10,082	62 (7)	Intensive control (HbA$_{1c}$ <6.0%) (5040)	Standard control (HbA$_{1c}$ 7.0%–7.9%) (5042)	56	Intensive (5.9/1000) and standard (6.37/1000) control did not show any statistical significance for the AF onset (P = .52)
Chen et al,[27] 2017[d]	NHIRD Cohort[ac] 2005–2012	9790[b]	>65	Insulin (805; 8.2%) DPP4 inhibitors (312; 3.2%)	Nonsers	84	Higher risk of an AF onset among insulin users (HR, 1.58; 95% CI, 1.37–1.82; P<.05) Lower risk among DPP4 inhibitor users (HR, 0.65; 95% CI, 0.45–0.93; P<.05)
Chang et al,[28] 2017[e]	NHIRD Cohort[a] 2009–2012	90,880	55 (12)	Metformin plus DPP4 inhibitors (16,017; 17.6%)	Metformin plus other hypoglycemic agents-users (74,863; 82.4%)	24	Lower risk of AF onset among DPP4 inhibitor users (HR, 0.69; 95% CI, 0.59–0.81; P<.0001)
Liou et al,[29] 2018[f]	NHIRD Cohort[ac] 2002–2013	14,410	69	Insulin (2739; 19.0%) Biguanide (7756; 53.8%) TDZs (3009; 20.9%)	Nonusers	120	Higher risk of AF onset among insulin users (HR, 1.19; 95% CI, 1.06–1.35; P<.05) Lower among biguanide users (HR, 0.81; 95% CI, 0.71–0.95; P<.05) and TZDs (OR, 0.72; 95% CI, 0.63–0.83; P<.05)

(continued on next page)

Table 2
(continued)

Publication Year (Ref.)	Study Design	Population (n)	Age y/o (SD)	User Group (n, %)	Nonuser Group (n, %)	Mean Follow-Up (mo)	Risk of New Onset of AF
Zelniker et al,[30] 2020	DECRELARE-TIMI 58[9]	17,160	NA	SGLT2 inhibitor (dapagliflozin)	Placebo	NA	Dapagliflozin reduced the risk of an AF/AFL onset (HR, 0.81; 95% CI, 0.68–0.95; P = .009)

Abbreviations: AFL, atrial flutter; CI, confidence interval; HbA$_{1c}$, hemoglobin A$_{1c}$; HR, hazard ratio; NA, data not available; NHIRD, Taiwan's National Health Insurance Research Database; SGLT2 inhibitor, sodium-glucose cotransporter 2 inhibitor; TDZs, thiazolidinediones.

a These studies were nationwide, population-based, retrospective, observational studies using the Taiwan's National Health Insurance Research Database.

b Study population was newly diagnosed DM.

c This study was a nested case control study.

d This study also showed the comparison data of metformin (n = 5055; 51.6%; HR, 1.01; 95% CI, 0.88–1.15), acarbose (n = 1198; 12.2%; HR, 0.91; 95% CI, 0.76–1.10), glinides (n = 798; 8.2%; HR, 1.11; 95% CI, 0.90–1.37), sulfonylurea (n = 5474; 55.9%; HR, 1.07; 95% CI, 0.94–1.22), and TDZs (n = 1396; 14.3%; HR, 0.93; 95% CI, 0.77–1.13).

e Most patients were prescribed sitagliptin (n = 12,180; 76%) among the DPP4 inhibitors users and sulfonylureas (n = 60,606; 81%) among the non-DPP4 inhibitors users.

f This study also showed the comparison data of sulfonylurea (n = 7443; 51.7%; HR, 1.13; 95% CI, 0.99–1.30), alfa-glucosidase inhibitor (n = 3308; 23.0%; HR, 1.03; 95% CI, 0.92–1.16), and DPP4 inhibitors (n = 2598; 18.0%; HR, 1.06; 95% CI, 0.94–1.19; P>.05). Those were not associated with an increased risk of new-onset AF.

g These study results were based on the data from the Trials of Dapagliflozin Effect on Cardiovascular Events-Thrombolysis in Myocardial Infarction 58. In this study, the reduction in AF/AFL events was consistent regardless of presence (HR, 0.79; 95% CI, 0.58–1.09) or absence (HR, 0.81; 95% CI, 0.67–0.98) of a previous history of AF/AFL at baseline, P for interaction 0.89.

Table 3
Effects of antidiabetic agents and glycemic control on secondary prevention of AF after catheter ablation in DM

Publication Year (Ref.)	Study Design	Characteristics of Sample Population n (%)	Age y/o (SD)	Intervention Group (n)	Control Group (n)	Mean Follow-Up (mo)	Risk of an AF/AT Recurrence
Gu et al,[42] 2011[a]	Prospective/ observational	Type II DM/ paroxysmal (100%) (total 150)	59 (9)	TZD (pioglitazone) (51)	Nonusers (99)	23	TZD was associated with reduced recurrences (HR, 0.32; 95% CI, 0.12–0.86; $P = .024$)
Lu et al,[43] 2015[b]	Retrospective/ observational	Type II DM/ paroxysmal (100%) (total 149)	62 (9)	Basal HbA$_{1c}$ (<6.9%)	Basal HbA$_{1c}$ ($\geq$6.9%)	12	Basal HbA$_{1c}$ was an independent predictor of a recurrence (after the first ablation (HR, 1.22; 95% CI, 1.02–1.47; $P = .034$)
Anselmino et al,[41] 2015[c]	Meta-analysis of 15 randomized control trials	Type I/II DM (2.2%/ 97.8%), paroxysmal/ persistent/long-lasting persistent (65%/21%/14%) (total 1464)	62	—	—	27	Basal HbA$_{1c}$ level was related to a higher incidence of recurrences after first ablation ($P<.001$)
Yang et al,[44] 2016[d]	Retrospective/ observational	DM/non-DM (28.6%/ 71.4%)/ paroxysmal/ nonparoxysmal (64.1%/35.9%) (total 496)	62 (9)	—	—	25	Preprocedural high sRAGE ($\geq$418 pg/ mL) in DM patients was related to lower recurrences (HR, 0.40; 95% CI, 0.18–0.89; $P = .026$)

(continued on next page)

Table 3
(continued)

Publication Year (Ref.)	Study Design	Characteristics of Sample Population n (%)	Age y/o (SD)	Intervention Group (n)	Control Group (n)	Mean Follow-Up (mo)	Risk of an AF/AT Recurrence
Providencia et al,[45] 2019[e]	Multicenter/ retrospective/ observational	DM/non-DM (9.4%/ 90.6%)/ paroxysmal nonparoxysmal/ LAAT (57.6%/ 36.3%/6.1%) (total 2497)	61 (10)	—	—	19	DM was an independent predictor of recurrences (HR, 1.36; 95% CI, 1.03–1.78)
Donnellan et al,[46] 2019[f]	Retrospective/ observational	Type I/II DM (12.1%/ 87.9%) (total 298)	67 (8)	Preprocedural HbA1c (<7%) (12 mo before)	Preprocedural HbA1c (>9%) (12 mo before)	26	Preprocedural HbA1c level was independently associated with recurrences (P<.0001)
Creta et al,[47] 2020[g]	Multicenter/ retrospective/ observational	DM/non-DM (9.3%/ 90.7%)/ paroxysmal nonparoxysmal (57.5%/42.5%) (total 2504)	61 (10)	Type II DM (+) 234	Type II DM (−) 2270	17	DM was an independent predictor of recurrences (HR, 1.39; 95% CI, 1.07–1.82; P = .016)

Abbreviations: AF/AT, atrial fibrillation/atrial tachycardia; CI, confidence interval; HbA1c, hemoglobin A1c; HR, hazard ratio; sRAGE, soluble receptor for advanced glycation end products; TDZ, thiazolidinedione.

[a] In this study, TZD users had a higher single ablation success rate (86.3% vs 70.7%; $P = .034$) and lower redo ablation rate (9.8% vs 24.2%; $P = .034$) compared with nonusers. The left atrial diameter was associated with increased recurrences (HR, 1.18; 95% CI, 1.06–1.31; $P = .002$) and the use of ACEIs/ARBs was associated with reduced recurrences (HR, 0.37; 95% CI, 0.16–0.87; $P = .023$).

[b] In this study, the HbA1c <6.9% group had a higher AF-free survival rate as compared with those with ≥6.9% (69.0% vs 46.8%; $P = .004$). A multivariate Cox regression analysis also demonstrated that the left atrial size (HR, 1.11; 95% CI, 1.05–1.17; $P<.001$) was an independent predictor of arrhythmia recurrences after first ablation.

[c] A metaregression analysis also demonstrated that an advanced age ($P<.001$) and higher body mass index ($P<.001$) was related to a higher incidence of arrhythmia recurrences.

[d] A multivariate Cox regression analysis also demonstrated that paroxysmal AF (HR, 0.39; 95% CI, 0.18–0.84; $P = .016$) was an independent predictor of favorable outcomes of rhythm control after ablation.

[e] A multivariate Cox regression analysis also demonstrated that the AF duration (HR, 1.02; 95% CI, 1.01–1.03; $P = .001$), paroxysmal AF (HR, 0.54; 95% CI, 0.45–0.66; $P<.001$), BMI (HR, 1.03; 95% CI, 1.01–1.05; $P = .001$), and indexed left atrial volume (HR, 1.01; 95% CI, 1.00–1.01; $P = .002$) were independent predictors of arrhythmia recurrences.

[f] A higher AF-free survival rate among those with an HbA1c <7% as compared with those with greater than 9% (32.4% vs 68.8%).

[g] A multivariate Cox regression analysis also demonstrated that the total AF duration (HR, 1.02; 95% CI, 1.01–1.04; $P<.001$), paroxysmal AF (HR, 0.55; 95%CI, 0.46–0.65; $P<.001$), BMI (HR, 1.03; 95% CI, 1.02–1.05, $P<.001$), and indexed left atrial volume (HR, 1.01; 95% CI, 1.00–1.01, $P<.001$) were independent predictor of arrhythmia recurrences.

Table 4
Previous publications regarding catheter ablation outcomes related to thyroid disease

Publication Year (Ref.)	Study Design	Population n (%)	Age y/o (SD)	History of Hyperthyroidism (+) n (%)	History of Hyperthyroidism (−) n (%)	Mean Follow-Up (mo)	Risk of AF/AT Recurrence
Ma et al,[69] 2007	Retrospective/ observational	16, paroxysmal/ persistent (62%/38%)	60 (11)	16 (100%)	—	16	9 (56%) were AF free (off drug) 7 (44%) recurred, and 4 (25%) responded to AADs
Machino et al,[70] 2012	Retrospective/ observational	337, paroxysmal/ persistent (57%/43%)	61 (9)	16 (4.7%)	321 (95.3%)	48	No significant difference between the 2 groups (HR, 0.87; 95% CI, 0.40–1.88; P = .73)
Mikhaylov et al,[71] 2013[a]	Retrospective/ observational/ case-control	704, paroxysmal (100%)	58 (5)	AIH (+) 20 (33%)	AIH (−) 40 (67%)	12	AIH (+) was an independent predictor of a recurrence
Sousa et al,[72] 2015[b]	Retrospective/ observational	1095, paroxysmal/ persistent/LAAT (59.7%/ 32.3%/8%)	60 (10)	FT4 (ng/L): 10.6–14.6, ≥14.6 824 (75%)	FT4 (ng/L): <10.6 271 (25%)	13	FT4 level could predict recurrence with a 15% increase per quartile (interquartile range, 10.6–14.6; HR, 1.15; 95% CI, 1.03–1.29; P = .014)
Wongcharoen et al,[73] 2015[c]	Retrospective/ observational	717, paroxysmal/ persistent (75%/25%)	55 (10)	84 (12%)	633 (88%)	32	History of hyperthyroidism could be an independent predictor of a recurrence after a single procedure (HR, 2.07; 95% CI, 1.27–3.38; P = .014)
Wang et al,[74] 2016	Retrospective/ observational/ case-control	146, paroxysmal (100%)	61 (9)	20 AIH (+)	30 AIH (−)	<3, 3–12	AIH (+) exhibited a significantly higher early recurrence within the blanking period but not beyond 3–12 mo

Abbreviations: AAD, antiarrhythmic drug; AF/AT, atrial fibrillation/atrial tachycardia; AIH (+/-), with or without a history of amiodarone induced hyperthyroidism; CI, confidence interval; HR, hazard ratio; TSH, thyroid-stimulating hormone.

[a] In the AIH (+) group, only 6 (30%) were arrhythmia free (vs AIH [-]; P = .01), 7 (35%) had AT recurrences (vs AIH [-]; P = .01), and 10 (50%) had AF recurrence (vs AIH [-]; P = .2) in the first session. Seven patients (35%) in the AIH (+) group received a redo procedure (vs AIH [-]; P = .01) and 5 (25%) had a higher incidence of non-PV arrhythmias (vs AIH [-]; P = .003). The final arrhythmia-free rate after multiple procedures was similar between the two groups (12 [60%] with AIH [+] vs 28 [70%] with AIH [-] group; P = .56).

[b] This study showed that 71.1% of the total population was arrhythmia free and TSH could not predict recurrence.

[c] In this study, a euthyroid status was achieved for >3 months before the ablation in hyperthyroid patients. A higher number and prevalence of non-PV foci were observed with hyperthyroidism (vs nonhyperthyroidism; P<.01). Ectopic foci from the ligament of Marshall were demonstrated more often in hyperthyroid patients (7.1% vs 1.6%; P<.01) in whom ethanol ablations were applied. After multiple procedures, the AF recurrence rates were similar between the two groups.

associated with AF,[53,54] a population cohort from Denmark demonstrated that there is a low risk of AF in overt hypothyroidism.[51]

Pathophysiology of Atrial Fibrillation Associated with Thyroid Disease

Both genomic and nongenomic actions of thyroid hormones on ionic currents and their mRNA expression, myosin heavy chain (alfa isoforms) expression, sarcoplasmic reticulum calcium-activated ATPase, β_1-adrenergic receptors, and phospholamban all contribute to AF genesis.[55–61] Chen and colleagues[62] first demonstrated that thyroid hormone increased the automaticity and enhanced triggered activity of PV cardiomyocytes. These findings were followed by a clinical study showing increased ectopic activity in hyperthyroidism.[63] Recently, genome-wide association studies have highlighted PITX2 as a major player causing AF. Lozano-Valasco and coworkers[64] report that hyperthyroidism impairs PITX2 expression leading to Wnt-microRNA-ion channel remodeling.

There are few studies regarding the association between hypothyroidism and AF. An increased AF susceptibility in hypothyroidism has been reported.[55] Chen and colleagues[65] reported that hypothyroidism accelerates myocardial fibrosis. Therefore, increased myocardial fibrosis may lead to prolongation of the effective refractory period and slow conduction with anisotropy promoting reentry formation causing AF arrhythmogenesis. Because hyperthyroid and hypothyroid animals show different anatomic and electrophysiologic remodeling, different mechanisms may be involved in AF genesis in hyperthyroidism and hypothyroidism.

Previous Reports Regarding Managements of Atrial Fibrillation Associated with Thyroid Disease

If either clinical or subclinical forms of thyroid dysfunction occur, appropriate treatments (anti-thyroid agents, radioiodine, surgical resections, and β-blockers) should be applied if they exhibit AF.[50] Fortunately, AF spontaneously converts to sinus rhythm in 62% of patients once a euthyroid state is achieved,[66] but a higher age and longer AF duration can predict persistent AF.[67] In amiodarone-induced hypothyroidism, Huang and colleagues[68] reported that thyroxine monotherapy without amiodarone enhanced AF recurrences and might be an unfavorable treatment. Ablation outcomes in patients with a previous history of hyperthyroidism have been reported (**Table 4**).[69–74] Machino and colleagues[70] reported that hyperthyroidism was not associated with a higher risk of AF

recurrences. Sousa and colleagues[72] showed that the F-T3 level influenced ablation outcomes. Although PV isolation alone has a lower efficacy for hyperthyroidism, the final overall outcomes after repeat procedures are similar to control subjects.[71,73,74] A higher prevalence of non-PV ectopy is demonstrated in hyperthyroidism.[71,73] These results reinforced that ablation strategies to eliminate all AF-initiating ectopic foci are essential to achieve favorable outcomes.

MANAGEMENTS OF STROKES

DM is a risk factor for thromboembolisms, especially that requiring insulin and a longer DM history.[75] Regarding the safety and efficacy of direct oral anticoagulants in DM,[76] even without any other major thromboembolic risk factors, patients with insulin use and a longer DM history may benefit from direct oral anticoagulants. Previous studies suggested a higher incidence of thromboembolisms in the early period of an uncontrolled hyperthyroid state and recommend anticoagulants.[77] In contrast, Bruere and colleagues[78] reported that hyperthyroidism was not an independent risk factor for thromboembolisms, but hypothyroidism was associated with a bleeding risk. Therefore, the stroke risk in thyroid disease–related AF is still controversial.

SUMMARY AND FUTURE DIRECTIONS

DM and thyroid diseases are associated with not only an increased risk of AF but also recurrence after interventions. Glycemic control and achieving a euthyroid state may improve the overall clinical outcomes. To maximize primary and secondary prevention, innovative approaches to stratify patient-specific risks and to clarify the mechanisms responsible for AF are needed.

CLINICS CARE PERSPECTIVE

- For AF prevention, an appropriate glycemic control without larger glucose fluctuations is essential.
- Controlling thromboembolisms is an important aspect of DM and the early period of uncontrolled hyperthyroidism.
- Further investigations are required to establish risk stratification and patient-specific long-term rhythm control strategies for AF.

DISCLOSURE

Dr S. Higa is a consultant to Japan Life Line and Johnson & Johnson; and received speaker's honoraria from Japan Life Line, Medtronic, Abbott, Bayer, Biotronik, Boehringer-Ingelheim, Bristol-Myers, Daiichi-Sankyo Pharmaceutical Company, and Pfizer. The other authors have nothing to declare.

REFERENCES

1. Calkins H, Hindricks G, Cappato R, et al. 2017 HRS/EHRA/ECAS/APHRS/SOLAECE expert consensus statement on catheter and surgical ablation of atrial fibrillation: executive summary. Heart Rhythm 2017;14:e445–94.
2. Ariyaratnam JP, Middeldorp M, Thomas G, et al. Risk factor management before and after atrial fibrillation ablation. Card Electrophysiol Clin 2020;12:141–54.
3. Huxley RR, Filion KB, Konety S, et al. Meta-analysis of cohort and case-control studies of type 2 diabetes mellitus and risk of atrial fibrillation. Am J Cardiol 2011;108:56–62.
4. Nichols GA, Reinier K, Chugh SS. Independent contribution of diabetes to increased prevalence and incidence of atrial fibrillation. Diabetes Care 2009;32:1851–6.
5. Dublin S, Glazer NL, Smith NL, et al. Diabetes mellitus, glycemic control, and risk of atrial fibrillation. J Gen Intern Med 2010;25:853–8.
6. Huxley RR, Alonso A, Lopez FL, et al. Type 2 diabetes, glucose homeostasis and incident atrial fibrillation: the atherosclerosis risk in communities study. Heart 2012;98:133–8.
7. Schoen T, Pradhan AD, Albert CM, et al. Type 2 diabetes mellitus and risk of incident atrial fibrillation in women. J Am Coll Cardiol 2012;60:1421–8.
8. Latini R, Staszewsky L, Sun JL, et al. Incidence of atrial fibrillation in a population with impaired glucose tolerance: the contribution of glucose metabolism and other risk factors. A post hoc analysis of the nateglinide and valsartan in impaired glucose tolerance outcomes research trial. Am Heart J 2013;166:935–40.
9. Pallisgaard JL, Schjerning AM, Lindhardt TB, et al. Risk of atrial fibrillation in diabetes mellitus: a nationwide cohort study. Eur J Prev Cardiol 2016;23:621–7.
10. Liu C, Fu H, Li J, et al. Hyperglycemia aggravates atrial interstitial fibrosis, ionic remodeling and vulnerability to atrial fibrillation in diabetic rabbits. Anadolu Kardiyol Derg 2012;12:543–50.
11. Watanabe M, Yokoshiki H, Mitsuyama H, et al. Conduction and refractory disorders in the diabetic atrium. Am J Physiol Heart Circ Physiol 2012;303:86–95.
12. Russo I, Frangogiannis NG. Diabetes-associated cardiac fibrosis: cellular effectors, molecular mechanisms and therapeutic opportunities. J Mol Cell Cardiol 2016;90:84–93.
13. Kato T, Yamashita T, Sekiguchi A, et al. AGEs-RAGE system mediates atrial structural remodeling in the diabetic rat. J Cardiovasc Electrophysiol 2008;19:415–20.
14. Anderson EJ, Kypson AP, Rodriguez E, et al. Substrate-specific derangements in mitochondrial metabolism and redox balance in the atrium of the type 2 diabetic human heart. J Am Coll Cardiol 2009;54:1891–8.
15. Fu H, Liu C, Li J, et al. Impaired atrial electromechanical function and atrial fibrillation promotion in alloxan-induced diabetic rabbits. Cardiol J 2013;20:59–67.
16. Demir K, Avci A, Kaya Z, et al. Assessment of atrial electromechanical delay and P-wave dispersion in patients with type 2 diabetes mellitus. J Cardiol 2016;67:378–83.
17. De Vos CB, Weijs B, Crijns HJ, et al. Atrial tissue Doppler imaging for prediction of new-onset atrial fibrillation. Heart 2009;95:835–40.
18. Chao TF, Suenari K, Chang SL, et al. Atrial substrate properties and outcome of catheter ablation in patients with paroxysmal atrial fibrillation associated with diabetes mellitus or impaired fasting glucose. Am J Cardiol 2010;106:1615–20.
19. Otake H, Suzuki H, Honda T, et al. Influences of autonomic nervous system on atrial arrhythmogenic substrates and the incidence of atrial fibrillation in diabetic heart. Int Heart J 2009;50:627–41.
20. Gu J, Fan YQ, Zhang JF, et al. Impact of long-term glycemic variability on development of atrial fibrillation in type 2 diabetic patients. Anatol J Cardiol 2017;18:410–6.
21. Saito S, Teshima Y, Fukui A, et al. Glucose fluctuations increase the incidence of atrial fibrillation in diabetic rats. Cardiovasc Res 2014;104:5–14.
22. Monnier L, Mas E, Ginet C, et al. Activation of oxidative stress by acute glucose fluctuations compared with sustained chronic hyperglycemia in patients with type 2 diabetes. JAMA 2006;295:1681–7.
23. Ko SH, Park YM, Yun JS, et al. Severe hypoglycemia is a risk factor for atrial fibrillation in type 2 diabetes mellitus: nationwide population-based cohort study. J Diabet Complications 2018;32:157–63.
24. Chao TF, Leu HB, Huang CC, et al. Thiazolidinediones can prevent new onset atrial fibrillation in patients with non-insulin dependent diabetes. Int J Cardiol 2012;156:199–202.
25. Chang SH, Wu LS, Chiou MJ, et al. Association of metformin with lower atrial fibrillation risk among patients with type 2 diabetes mellitus: a population-based dynamic cohort and in vitro studies. Cardiovasc Diabetol 2014;13:123.

26. Fatemi O, Yuriditsky E, Tsioufis C, et al. Impact of intensive glycemic control on the incidence of atrial fibrillation and associated cardiovascular outcomes in patients with type 2 diabetes mellitus (from the Action to Control Cardiovascular Risk in Diabetes Study). Am J Cardiol 2014;114:1217–22.

27. Chen HY, Yang FY, Jong GP, et al. Antihyperglycemic drugs use and new-onset atrial fibrillation in elderly patients. Eur J Clin Invest 2017;47:388–93.

28. Chang CY, Yeh YH, Chan YH, et al. Dipeptidyl peptidase-4 inhibitor decreases the risk of atrial fibrillation in patients with type 2 diabetes: a nationwide cohort study in Taiwan. Cardiovasc Diabetol 2017;16:159.

29. Liou YS, Yang FY, Chen HY, et al. Antihyperglycemic drugs use and new-onset atrial fibrillation: a population-based nested case control study. PLoS One 2018;13:e0197245.

30. Zelniker TA, Bonaca MP, Furtado RHM, et al. Effect of dapagliflozin on atrial fibrillation in patients with type 2 diabetes mellitus: insights from the DECLARE-TIMI 58 Trial. Circulation 2020;141:1227–34.

31. Kume O, Takahashi N, Wakisaka O, et al. Pioglitazone attenuates inflammatory atrial fibrosis and vulnerability to atrial fibrillation induced by pressure overload in rats. Heart Rhythm 2011;8:278–85.

32. Yu O, Azoulay L, Yin H, et al. Sulfonylureas as initial treatment for type 2 diabetes and the risk of severe hypoglycemia. Am J Med 2018;131:317.e11–22.

33. Yun JS, Park YM, Han K, et al. Severe hypoglycemia and the risk of cardiovascular disease and mortality in type 2 diabetes: a nationwide population-based cohort study. Cardiovasc Diabetol 2019;18:103.

34. White WB, Cannon CP, Heller SR, et al. Alogliptin after acute coronary syndrome in patients with type 2 diabetes. N Engl J Med 2013;369:1327–35.

35. Monami M, Nreu B, Scatena A, et al. Glucagon-like peptide-1 receptor agonists and atrial fibrillation: a systematic review and meta-analysis of randomised controlled trials. J Endocrinol Invest 2017;40:1251–8.

36. Usman MS, Siddiqi TJ, Memon MM, et al. Sodium-glucose co-transporter 2 inhibitors and cardiovascular outcomes: a systematic review and meta-analysis. Eur J Prev Cardiol 2018;25:495–502.

37. Grönberg T, Hartikainen JE, Nuotio I, et al. Can we predict the failure of electrical cardioversion of acute atrial fibrillation? The FinCV study. Pacing Clin Electrophysiol 2015;38:368–75.

38. Ebert M, Stegmann C, Kosiuk J, et al. Predictors, management, and outcome of cardioversion failure early after atrial fibrillation ablation. Europace 2018;20:1428–34.

39. Forleo GB, Mantica M, De Luca L, et al. Catheter ablation of atrial fibrillation in patients with diabetes mellitus type 2: results from a randomized study comparing pulmonary vein isolation versus antiarrhythmic drug therapy. J Cardiovasc Electrophysiol 2009;20:22–8.

40. Veglio M, Bruno G, Borra M, et al. Prevalence of increased QT interval duration and dispersion in type 2 diabetic patients and its relationship with coronary heart disease: a population-based cohort. J Intern Med 2002;251:317–24.

41. Anselmino M, Matta M, D'ascenzo F, et al. Catheter ablation of atrial fibrillation in patients with diabetes mellitus: a systematic review and meta-analysis. Europace 2015;17:1518–25.

42. Gu J, Liu X, Wang X, et al. Beneficial effect of pioglitazone on the outcome of catheter ablation in patients with paroxysmal atrial fibrillation and type 2 diabetes mellitus. Europace 2011;13:1256–61.

43. Lu ZH, Liu N, Bai R, et al. HbA1c levels as predictors of ablation outcome in type 2 diabetes mellitus and paroxysmal atrial fibrillation. Herz 2015;40(Suppl 2):130–6.

44. Yang PS, Kim TH, Uhm JS, et al. High plasma level of soluble RAGE is independently associated with a low recurrence of atrial fibrillation after catheter ablation in diabetic patient. Europace 2016;18:1711–8.

45. Providência R, Adragão P, de Asmundis C, et al. Impact of body mass index on the outcomes of catheter ablation of atrial fibrillation: a European observational multicenter study. J Am Heart Assoc 2019;8:e012253.

46. Donnellan E, Aagaard P, Kanj M, et al. Association between pre-ablation glycemic control and outcomes among patients with diabetes undergoing atrial fibrillation ablation. JACC Clin Electrophysiol 2019;5:897–903.

47. Creta A, Providência R, Adragão P, et al. Impact of type-2 diabetes mellitus on the outcomes of catheter ablation of atrial fibrillation (European observational multicentre study). Am J Cardiol 2020;125:901–6.

48. Tang RB, Dong JZ, Liu XP, et al. Safety and efficacy of catheter ablation of atrial fibrillation in patients with diabetes mellitus-single center experience. J Interv Card Electrophysiol 2006;17:41–6.

49. Bogossian H, Frommeyer G, Brachmann J, et al. Catheter ablation of atrial fibrillation and atrial flutter in patients with diabetes mellitus: who benefits and who does not? Data from the German ablation registry. Int J Cardiol 2016;214:25–30.

50. Ross DS, Burch HB, Cooper DS, et al. 2016 American Thyroid Association Guidelines for diagnosis and management of hyperthyroidism and other causes of thyrotoxicosis. Thyroid 2016;26:1343–421.

51. Selmer C, Hansen ML, Olesen JB, et al. New-onset atrial fibrillation is a predictor of subsequent hyperthyroidism: a nationwide cohort study. PLoS One 2013;8:e57893.

52. Agner T, Almdal T, Thorsteinsson B, et al. A reevaluation of atrial fibrillation in thyrotoxicosis. Dan Med Bull 1984;31:157–9.
53. Siddiqui AS, D'Costa DF, Moore-Smith B. Covert hypothyroidism with weight loss and atrial fibrillation. Br J Clin Pract 1993;47:268.
54. Wong PS, Hee FL, Lip GY. Atrial fibrillation and the thyroid. Heart 1997;78:623–4.
55. Zhang Y, Dedkov EI, Teplitsky D, et al. Both hypothyroidism and hyperthyroidism increase atrial fibrillation inducibility in rats. Circ Arrhythm Electrophysiol 2013;6:952–9.
56. Watanabe H, Ma M, Washizuka T, et al. Thyroid hormone regulates mRNA expression and currents of ion channels in rat atrium. Biochem Biophys Res Commun 2003;308:439–44.
57. Hu Y, Jones SV, Dillmann WH. Effects of hyperthyroidism on delayed rectifier K+ currents in left and right murine atria. Am J Physiol Heart Circ Physiol 2005;289:1448–55.
58. Rohrer D, Dillmann WH. Thyroid hormone markedly increases the mRNA coding for sarcoplasmic reticulum Ca2+-ATPase in the rat heart. J Biol Chem 1988;263:6941–4.
59. Arai M, Otsu K, MacLennan DH, et al. Effect of thyroid hormone on the expression of mRNA encoding sarcoplasmic reticulum proteins. Circ Res 1991;69:266–76.
60. Dudley SC Jr, Baumgarten CM. Bursting of cardiac sodium channels after acute exposure to 3,5,3'-triiodo-L-thyronine. Circ Res 1993;73:301–13.
61. Shimoni Y, Fiset C, Clark RB, et al. Thyroid hormone regulates postnatal expression of transient K+ channel isoforms in rat ventricle. J Physiol 1997;500:65–73.
62. Chen YC, Chen SA, Chen YJ, et al. Effects of thyroid hormone on the arrhythmogenic activity of pulmonary vein cardiomyocytes. J Am Coll Cardiol 2002;39:366–72.
63. Wustmann K, Kucera JP, Zanchi A, et al. Activation of electrical triggers of atrial fibrillation in hyperthyroidism. J Clin Endocrinol Metab 2008;93:2104–8.
64. Lozano-Velasco E, Wangensteen R, Quesada A, et al. Hyperthyroidism, but not hypertension, impairs PITX2 expression leading to Wnt-microRNA-ion channel remodeling. PLoS One 2017;12:e0188473.
65. Chen WJ, Lin KH, Lee YS. Molecular characterization of myocardial fibrosis during hypothyroidism: evidence for negative regulation of the pro-alpha1(I) collagen gene expression by thyroid hormone receptor. Mol Cell Endocrinol 2000;162:45–55.
66. Nakazawa HK, Sakurai K, Hamada N, et al. Management of atrial fibrillation in the post-thyrotoxic state. Am J Med 1982;72:903–6.
67. Zhou ZH, Ma LL, Wang LX. Risk factors for persistent atrial fibrillation following successful hyperthyroidism treatment with radioiodine therapy. Intern Med 2011;50:2947–51.
68. Huang JH, Lin YK, Hsieh MH, et al. Thyroxine monotherapy without amiodarone enhances atrial fibrillation recurrences in amiodarone-induced hypothyroidism. Int J Cardiol 2011;152:277–8.
69. Ma CS, Liu X, Hu FL, et al. Catheter ablation of atrial fibrillation in patients with hyperthyroidism. J Interv Card Electrophysiol 2007;18:137–42.
70. Machino T, Tada H, Sekiguchi Y, et al. Prevalence and influence of hyperthyroidism on the long-term outcome of catheter ablation for drug-refractory atrial fibrillation. Circ J 2012;76:2546–51.
71. Mikhaylov EN, Orshanskaya VS, Lebedev AD, et al. Catheter ablation of paroxysmal atrial fibrillation in patients with previous amiodarone-induced hyperthyroidism: a case-control study. J Cardiovasc Electrophysiol 2013;24:888–93.
72. Sousa PA, Providência R, Albenque JP, et al. Impact of free thyroxine on the outcomes of left atrial ablation procedures. Am J Cardiol 2015;116:1863–8.
73. Wongcharoen W, Lin YJ, Chang SL, et al. History of hyperthyroidism and long-term outcome of catheter ablation of drug-refractory atrial fibrillation. Heart Rhythm 2015;12:1956–62.
74. Wang MJ, Cai SL, Sun L, et al. Safety and efficacy of early radiofrequency catheter ablation in patients with paroxysmal atrial fibrillation complicated with amiodarone-induced thyrotoxicosis. Cardiol J 2016;23:416–21.
75. Patti G, Lucerna M, Cavallari I, et al. Insulin-requiring versus noninsulin-requiring diabetes and thromboembolic risk in patients with atrial fibrillation: PREFER in AF. J Am Coll Cardiol 2017;69:409–19.
76. Itzhaki Ben Zadok O, Eisen A. Use of non-vitamin K oral anticoagulants in people with atrial fibrillation and diabetes mellitus. Diabet Med 2018;35:548–56.
77. Siu CW, Pong V, Zhang X, et al. Risk of ischemic stroke after new-onset atrial fibrillation in patients with hyperthyroidism. Heart Rhythm 2009;6:169–73.
78. Bruere H, Fauchier L, Bernard Brunet A, et al. History of thyroid disorders in relation to clinical outcomes in atrial fibrillation. Am J Med 2015;128:30–7.

Obesity and Metabolic Syndrome in Atrial Fibrillation
Cardiac and Noncardiac Adipose Tissue in Atrial Fibrillation

Rajiv Mahajan, MD, PhD[a,b,c,*], Christopher X. Wong, MBBS, MSc, PhD[a,b]

KEYWORDS

• Obesity • Metabolic syndrome • Atrial fibrillation • Adipose tissue

KEY POINTS

- The characterization of adiposity beyond body mass index has allowed for new insights into the separate effects of cardiac and noncardiac adipose tissue.
- Increases in generalized, noncardiac adipose tissue are associated with deleterious metabolic, neurohormonal, hemodynamic, and structural changes.
- Cardiac adipose tissue, such as epicardial fat, is a powerful predictor of atrial fibrillation and leads to myocardial fatty infiltration and adipokine-induced fibrosis.
- Weight loss leads to a regression of adiposity-related fibrosis, improvements in structural abnormalities, and normalization of atrial conduction and heterogeneity.
- Aggressive weight loss and risk factor treatment in patients with atrial fibrillation is now an established pillar of management and guideline recommended.

INTRODUCTION

The prevalence and health effects of excess adiposity represent a growing challenge for clinical care. Data estimate that at least 600 million adults and 100 million children worldwide are obese, as measured by elevated body mass index (BMI).[1] The consequence of these increasing trends is a rising burden of adiposity-related disease and death. The influential role of adiposity and the related metabolic syndrome in the development and maintenance of atrial fibrillation (AF) is therefore of great importance. However, our understanding of this relationship has continued to evolve in recent years with the emergence of new data. In this review, the authors summarize the epidemiology, mechanisms, and clinical implications of adiposity, the metabolic syndrome, and AF, with a focus particularly on information of relevance and interest to health care professionals involved in arrhythmia management.

EPIDEMIOLOGY OF OBESITY, METABOLIC SYNDROME, AND ATRIAL FIBRILLATION

Several population studies have established that generalized obesity, as indicated by elevated BMI, is a strong and independent risk factor for

Sources of Funding: Dr C.X. Wong is supported by a Postdoctoral Fellowship from the National Heart Foundation of Australia and a Mid-Career Fellowship from The Hospital Research Foundation. Dr R. Mahajan is supported by a Mid-Career Fellowship from The Hospital Research Foundation.
a The University of Adelaide, Adelaide, Australia; b South Australian Health and Medical Research Institute, Adelaide, Australia; c Lyell McEwin Hospital, Adelaide, Australia
* Corresponding author. University of Adelaide Precinct, Lyell McEwin Hospital, Haydown Road, Elizabeth Vale, Adelaide, South Australia 5112, Australia.
E-mail address: rajiv.mahajan@adelaide.edu.au
Twitter: Rajiv_EP (R.M.)

Card Electrophysiol Clin 13 (2021) 77–86
https://doi.org/10.1016/j.ccep.2020.11.006
1877-9182/21/© 2020 Elsevier Inc. All rights reserved.

incident AF.[2,3] In the Framingham Heart Study, obesity was associated with a 1.5-fold increase in incident AF, even after adjustment for other risk factors.[2] This association was even more significant in the Danish Diet, Cancer, and Health Study, where obesity was associated with a 2-fold greater hazard in incident AF.[3] Incremental increases in adiposity were also associated with increasing arrhythmogenic risk, with every 5-unit BMI increase conferring a 29% greater risk of AF.[4] Furthermore, analyses suggest that the percentage of AF cases in the population that are attributable to elevated BMI (16.9%) may be second only to hypertension (19.5%).[5] These figures may also underestimate the influence of adiposity as determined by BMI and considering the causal role of adiposity in other AF risk factors. Consequently, little doubt exists on the epidemiologic impact of obesity on AF risk and thus its potential importance in clinical management.

Although definitions vary, metabolic syndrome represents a cluster of interrelated cardiometabolic factors including abdominal adiposity, dyslipidemia, hypertension, and glucose intolerance.[6] Metabolic syndrome has also been shown to be associated with AF in several reports.[7,8] In the Niigata Preventive Medicine Study, the presence of metabolic syndrome was associated with a 1.6-fold greater hazard of incident AF in a Japanese population, with obesity and blood pressure components contributing most to the increased risk.[7] The Atherosclerosis Risk in Communities Study demonstrated similar results, with a 1.7-fold greater hazard of incident AF, with a similar increase in risk among both black and white individuals.[8] Furthermore, the incidence of AF seems to increase as the number of metabolic syndrome components are met.[7,8] This relationship has important clinical implications, given the high prevalence of metabolic syndrome in many populations.

CARDIAC AND NONCARDIAC ADIPOSE TISSUE

Although BMI is a convenient method to define obesity for clinical and epidemiologic purposes, it is an imprecise measurement that only approximates generalized adiposity. As for metabolic syndrome, clinical measures of abdominal adiposity have been purported to more accurately reflect abnormal body fat distribution. Indeed, both waist circumference and waist-to-hip ratio have been demonstrated to be associated with AF.[9] However, whether these measurements of abdominal adiposity are clearly more strongly related to AF compared with BMI remains uncertain. For example, one meta-analysis suggested that the standardized association of waist-to-hip ratio with AF may be modestly greater, whereas the association of waist circumference with AF may be less strong, compared with that of BMI and AF.[10] Such variable findings are commensurate with the fact that these dimensions are clinical measurements that incompletely reflect the underlying biology of adipose tissue.

In recent years, the evolution and increasing availability of noninvasive imaging techniques, such as computed tomography (CT) and MRI, has transformed the field of body fat distribution. In comparison to crude clinical measurements, direct quantification of specific adipose tissue depots is now possible. This distinction is relevant, as different adipose tissue depots seem to have varying biology and subsequent metabolic effects. Although both visceral and subcutaneous adipose tissue compartments correlate with adverse risk profiles, the former seems to be more strongly and consistently associated with cardiometabolic disease.[11] Thus, although BMI, waist circumference, and waist-to-hip ratio are suitable measurements for clinical assessment, they cannot distinguish and are influenced by both of these adipose tissue compartments.

Of potentially greater relevance to cardiovascular disease and AF is adipose tissue that is anatomically adjacent to the heart. It has long been suspected that atrial arrhythmias may be associated with excess adipose tissue within and surrounding the heart.[12] The terminology for different "cardiac adipose tissues" has varied and often been used interchangeably; these include epicardial fat, pericardial fat, cardiac ectopic fat, intrapericardial fat, extrapericardial fat, mediastinal fat, and intrathoracic fat.[12] These are considered part of the total-body visceral adipose tissue compartment. Anatomically, epicardial fat is that adipose tissue located between the myocardium and visceral pericardium without any fascial boundaries. This fat depot is most accurately quantified volumetrically with CT or MRI. However, others have used these or echocardiographic methods to assess less precise single-dimension thicknesses or 2-dimensional areas.[13] In contrast, pericardial fat is the sum of the aforementioned epicardial fat and the paracardial fat layer, which is that adipose tissue external to the visceral pericardium. Several studies have consistently shown that pericardial fat is associated with the presence and severity of AF.[14–17] Pericardial fat also associated with left atrial dimensions, AF symptoms, and recurrent AF.[17] Also, associations of both epicardial and pericardial fat with AF are significantly stronger than those of overall adiposity (as defined by BMI) and abdominal adiposity (either via waist circumference and waist-to-hip ratio or via imaging-defined visceral abdominal fat).[10,16] Furthermore, in a systematic review and meta-analysis of 64 studies, associations of epicardial fat with AF were approximately 2-fold greater than those of pericardial fat, which is consistent with a biologically plausible effect of former being anatomically contiguous to myocardium.[10] Thus, there seems to be a consistently increasing risk gradient, as progressively more relevant fat depots are specifically defined on a continuum from general adiposity (BMI) to abdominal adiposity (waist-to-hip ratio), visceral adipose tissue, pericardial fat, and finally, epicardial adipose tissue (**Fig. 1**).

MECHANISTIC LINKS BETWEEN OBESITY, METABOLIC SYNDROME, AND ATRIAL FIBRILLATION

An abnormal atrial substrate characterized by structural remodeling, atrial fibrosis, and conduction abnormalities is the end product that results from sustained obesity, hypertension, and metabolic syndrome, similar to that observed in multiple other conditions predisposing to AF.[18–21] This substrate that develops after prolonged exposure to obesity, metabolic syndrome, and related entities is characterized clinically by macroscopic abnormalities of left atrial size and function, with

left atrial enlargement, hypertrophy, pressure overload, and dysfunction being consistent findings in studies of obese individuals.[22]

Multiple pathophysiologic mechanisms have been postulated to mediate the association between epicardial fat and an abnormal atrial substrate (**Fig. 2**). Preclinical studies have shown that myocardial infiltration from adjacent epicardial adipocytes (**Fig. 3**) may facilitate arrhythmogenesis by promoting reentry and facilitating paracrine effect of secreted adipocytokines. Such fatty infiltration from overlying epicardial fat seems to be more pronounced in the presence of obesity.[18,23] The expansion of epicardial fat and resultant fatty infiltration is associated with nonhomogenous reduction in voltage, reductions in conduction velocities, increases in conduction heterogeneity, and electrogram fractionation, leading to greater propensity electrical reentry and AF.[18] Similar atrial substrate has been observed in obese patients with AF.[24] Basic evidence also suggests that epicardial adipocytes influence atrial electrophysiology by modulating cellular currents in myocytes.[25] Epicardial fat also promotes fibrosis of neighboring myocardium via the free diffusion of adipokines, cytokines, and reactive oxygen species, such as Activin A and matrix metalloproteinases, and this fibrosis also seems greater in obese states.[18,26] Thus, a combination of fibrofatty infiltration is likely to contribute to conduction slowing and heterogeneity in atrial myocardium

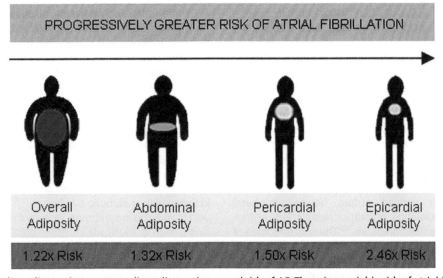

Fig. 1. Cardiac adipose tissue, noncardiac adipose tissue, and risk of AF. There is a variable risk of atrial fibrillation (AF) associated with different adipose tissue compartments. Risk estimates are per 1-standard deviation increases in body mass index (for overall adiposity), waist circumference (for abdominal adiposity), pericardial fat (for pericardial adiposity), and epicardial fat (for epicardial adiposity). The strength of associations increases progressively from overall, abdominal, pericardial, and epicardial adiposity.

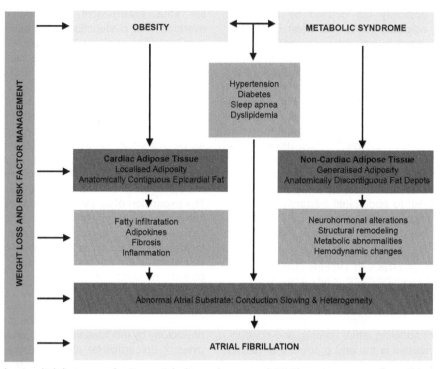

Fig. 2. Mechanism link between obesity, metabolic syndrome, and AF. There is a range of possible mechanisms mediating associations between obesity, metabolic syndrome, and atrial fibrillation (AF). The end-result of these pathways are the formation of an abnormal atrial substrate that is characterized by conduction slowing and heterogeneity, predisposing to AF. Weight loss and risk factor management has salutatory effects on multiple steps in this pathologic cascade.

that can predispose to arrhythmogenesis. This has been confirmed by human studies that have shown that epicardial fat is independently associated with local and global atrial conduction properties.[24,27]

Separate to the local effects of cardiac-specific adipose tissue, it is likely that generalized adiposity also contributes to structural remodeling via systemic neurohormonal, metabolic, and hemodynamic changes.[18,20,28] Experimental studies have suggested that neurohormonal and metabolic abnormalities include activation of the sympathetic nervous system and the renin-angiotensin-aldosterone system among others.[29] Hemodynamic alterations from obesity also include increases in cardiac output, lower peripheral vascular resistance, and an increase in left ventricular end-diastolic pressure.[28] The sum sequelae of these changes include left ventricular enlargement, hypertrophy, and abnormal geometry, which subsequently can lead to both diastolic and systolic dysfunction. Finally, excess adiposity is associated with increase in both lean body mass and myocardial mass.[30] Lean body mass has been shown to be a strong predictor of AF and may contribute to the

causal pathway between obesity and AF by increasing atrial size and volume overload.[31–33]

Of the other components of metabolic syndrome, hypertension and diabetes are also established independent risk factors for AF. Hypertension leads to atrial and ventricular dilatation, macrophage infiltration, and fibrosis, resulting in conduction heterogeneity.[21] In diabetes, there is an increased production of advanced glycation end products, greater expression of transforming growth factor beta, and higher production of reactive oxygen species that leads to interstitial fibrosis and conduction abnormalities.[34] Associations of low high-density lipoprotein or high triglyceride levels with AF are inconsistent and less convincing in those with metabolic syndrome.[7,35] In a similar vein to metabolic syndrome, obesity frequently co-exists with a multitude of other cardiometabolic conditions; these include obstructive sleep apnea and obesity hypoventilation, pulmonary hypertension, and frank heart failure. These also seem to be independently associated with AF, although the specific mechanisms of these individual conditions in contributing to an abnormal atrial substrate is beyond the scope of this review.

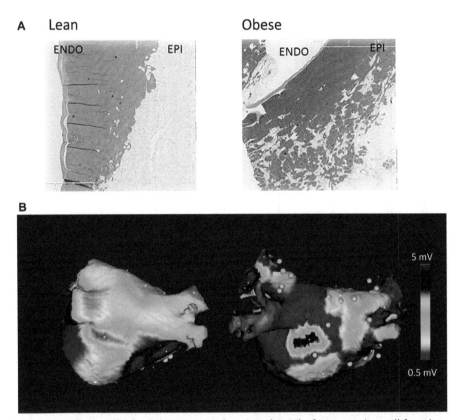

Fig. 3. AF substrate and epicardial fat. (*A*) H&E stained sections (X1.25) of LA posterior wall from lean and obese sheep. There is extensive infiltration of the posterior left atrium with fat cells from the adjoining epicardial fat in the obese sheep. Arrow shows infiltration of atrial musculature with fat cells. (*B*) Representative left atrial voltage maps (PA view) of the lean and obese patients with AF demonstrating distribution of low-voltage areas and increased fractionation in the obese patients. The voltage scale was set to 0.5 to 5 mV with red representing low voltage. The fractionated potentials are marked in pink and double potentials in blue. H&E, hematoxylin and eosin, PA, posteroanterior. ([*A*] *Adapted from* Mahajan R, Lau DH, Brooks AG, et al. Electrophysiological, Electro-anatomical and Structural Remodeling of the Atria as a Consequence of Sustained Obesity. *J Am Coll Cardiol.* 2015;66(1):1-11; and [*B*] Mahajan R, Nelson A, Pathak RK, et al. Electroanatomical Remodeling of the Atria in Obesity: Impact of Adjacent Epicardial Fat. *JACC Clin Electrophysiol.* 2018;4(12):1529-1540; with permission.)

REVERSIBILITY OF OBESITY-RELATED ATRIAL FIBRILLATION SUBSTRATE

Adiposity is now established as an important and independent determinant of AF. However, it also plays a causal role in the development and persistence of other AF risk factors, including hypertension, diabetes, sleep apnea, to name only a few related conditions. As a result, minimizing the effects of adiposity holds great clinical and population potential as a treatment strategy for AF. Indeed, this theoretic possibility has been borne out in both mechanistic and clinical studies, resulting in weight loss assuming a central role in the management of individuals with AF.

From a pathophysiological point of view, weight loss leads to a reduction in epicardial fat and a reversal of obesity-related abnormalities in the abnormal atrial substrate that predisposes to

AF.[36,37] In an ovine model of weight loss, the effects of both incremental weight gain and subsequently weight loss were assessed. Major reductions in adiposity were associated with a significant reduction in atrial fibrosis, improvement in connexin-43 expression, and resultant normalization of atrial conduction and heterogeneity.[37] These changes were also associated with a reduction in AF inducibility.

The above-mentioned weight-loss–related substrate reversal provides the mechanistic basis and explanation for the clinical benefits that have been observed with weight loss in individuals with AF (**Table 1**). In a clinical trial, overweight and obese patients with symptomatic AF were randomized to weight management intervention with low-calorie diet, exercise uptitration, and behavioral modification, or a control group who received general lifestyle advice.[38] In this trial,

Table 1
Clinical studies demonstrating benefit of weight reduction and risk factor management in patients with atrial fibrillation

Study, Year	Population	Intervention	Follow-up	Results
Abed et al,[38] 2013	150 with symptomatic pAF or persAF	Weight and risk factor management intervention or control	12 mo	Reduction in AF symptom scores and AF episode number/duration with intervention
ARREST-AF[41] 2014	149 patients with AF undergoing ablation	Weight and risk factor management intervention or control	42 mo	Reduction in AF frequency, duration, symptoms, and arrhythmia-free survival with intervention
LEGACY[39] 2015	825 with symptomatic pAF or persAF	Weight and risk factor management intervention	48 mo	Greater weight loss and less weight fluctuation associated with arrhythmia-free survival
Mohanty et al,[44] 2018	90 patients with long-standing persAF	Weight loss intervention or control	9 mo	Improved quality-of-life scores but no change in AF symptoms or arrhythmia-free survival with intervention
RACE 3[43] 2018	245 patients with early persAF	Targeted therapy for underlying conditions, including dietary restrictions	12 mo	Reduction in AF episodes and improvement in arrhythmia-free survival associated with intervention
REVERSE-AF[40] 2018	825 with symptomatic pAF or persAF	Weight and risk factor management intervention	48 mo	Greater weight loss associated with less progression from pAF to persAF and more regression from persAF to pAF or no AF

Abbreviations: pAF, paroxysmal AF; persAF, persistent AF.

weight loss and risk factor management improved symptoms and arrhythmia burden.[38] The subsequent LEGACY study showed that persistent weight loss and lesser weight fluctuation were associated with superior AF freedom over long-term follow-up.[39] For those who lost greater than or equal to 10% of weight, there was a 6-fold greater probability of arrhythmia-free survival. However, if weight fluctuation exceeded 5%, there was a 2-fold increased risk of arrhythmia recurrence. In the REVERSE-AF study, patients who achieved substantial weight loss ($\geq$10%) were less likely to progress from paroxysmal to persistent AF (3% of individuals) and more likely to reverse from persistent to paroxysmal or no AF (88% of individuals).[40] This was in contrast to those who had less than 3% of weight loss, 41% of whom progressed from paroxysmal to persistent AF, and only 26% reversing from persistent to paroxysmal or no AF. Finally, even in those

Table 2
Selected guideline recommendations for weight loss and risk factor management

Year	Organization	Guideline	Recommendation	Classification
2019	AHA/ACC/HRS	Focused Update of the 2014 AHA/ACC/HRS Guideline for the Management of Patients with Atrial Fibrillation	7.13 For overweight and obese patients with AF, weight loss, combined with risk factor modification, is recommended.	Class 1 Evidence B-R
2018	CCS	Focused Update of the Canadian Cardiovascular Society Guidelines for the Management of Atrial Fibrillation	18. We suggest that, in addition to implementing appropriate rate or rhythm control measures, an approach targeting modifiable risk markers and conditions associated with AF should be applied to prevent recurrence of the arrhythmia and/or decrease its symptom burden.	Strength: weak Quality: low
2018	NHF/CSANZ	Australian Clinical Guidelines for the Diagnosis and Management of Atrial Fibrillation	4.5.4. Intensive management of weight—to a target of greater than or equal to 10% body weight loss, aiming for a BMI less than 27—and concomitant management of associated cardiovascular risk factors to target levels should be performed in overweight and obese individuals with AF.	Strength: strong Quality: moderate
2016	ESC	Guidelines for the Management of Atrial Fibrillation Developed in Collaboration with EACTS	7.5. In obese patients with AF, weight loss together with management of other risk factors should be considered to reduce AF burden and symptoms.	Class IIa Level B

individuals who require antiarrhythmic or ablation therapy for symptomatic AF, aggressive risk factor management and weight loss was shown in the ARREST study to be highly beneficial for arrhythmia-free survival.[41] This approach has been shown to be not only clinically superior but also cost-effective.[42] In the RACE-3 trial, patients with persistent AF underwent targeted therapy for underlying conditions, including dietary restrictions, which was associated with a 1.3 kg weight difference between groups and a 1.8 greater odds of maintaining sinus rhythm at 1 year.[43] Contrastingly, in 90 patients with long-standing persistent AF undergoing ablation, those who volunteered for a weight loss intervention demonstrated superior quality of life but no improvement in AF-free survival.[44] These findings raise the possibility that the substrate associated with prolonged obesity and arrhythmia may be in part or wholly irreversible, supporting the importance of early intervention. Importantly, it should be noted from a mechanistic perspective that it is challenging to disentangle the effects of weight loss from that of other related risk factors. Although weight loss was a central strategy of the aforementioned studies, concurrent attention was paid to strict control of other risk factors. This also reflects the fact that many cardiometabolic risk factors are interrelated. However, from a practical point of view, risk factors are rarely treated in isolation. As a result, weight loss and risk factor control is now considered the "fourth pillar" of AF management, alongside the other cornerstones of anticoagulation, rhythm therapies, and rate control, and is recommended in international guidelines (**Table 2**).[45,46]

FUTURE DIRECTIONS

Thus far, the relation of adiposity with incident and recurrent AF has been well described and established. There is now a priority to use this understanding to guide management in patients with or at risk of AF. However, ongoing research is required to facilitate a greater understanding of how to implement and maximize the effectiveness of adiposity-related interventions across heterogenous settings and populations. Although dietary and exercise strategies for weight loss can be successful in many motivated individuals, others may potentially benefit from pharmacologic assistance or even bariatric surgery.[47] Furthermore, a better characterization of underlying mechanisms by which adiposity leads to arrhythmogenesis is likely to lead to novel insights. For example, recent interest is now turning to the potential role of adiposity-related inflammation, which can be indirectly quantified in vivo via positron emission or CT. It may be the case that binary distinctions of obesity, as defined by crude clinical measurements, may be eventually replaced by more detailed quantification of adiposity burden and function, allowing for more powerful risk stratification and guidance of management.

SUMMARY

Obesity and the related metabolic syndrome are important and influential predictors of AF. Both local cardiac adiposity and noncardiac adiposity have pathogenic effects on the atrial substrate that leads to arrhythmogenesis. Aggressive weight loss and risk factor management are now guideline recommended in the treatment of patients with AF. Ongoing research is likely to further our understanding of adiposity-related mechanisms and refine our approach to the management of patients with obesity, metabolic syndrome, and AF.

POTENTIAL CONFLICT OF INTEREST

Dr C.X. Wong reports that the University of Adelaide has received on his behalf lecture, travel, and/or research funding from Abbott Medical, Bayer, Boehringer Ingelheim, Medtronic, Novartis, Servier, and St. Jude Medical. Dr R. Mahajan reports having served on the advisory board of Abbott Medical and Medtronic. Dr R. Mahajan reports that the University of Adelaide has received on his behalf lecture fees from Medtronic, Abbott Medical, Pfizer, and Bayer. Dr R. Mahajan also reports that the University of Adelaide has received on his behalf research funding from Medtronic, Abbott Medical, and Bayer.

CLINICS CARE POINTS

- General adiposity and cardiac adipose tissue are associated with increased risk of incident AF.
- Weight loss results in reversal of obesity related AF substrate, reduction in AF burden and may modify the natural progression of AF.

REFERENCES

1. Collaborators GBDO, Afshin A, Forouzanfar MH, et al. Health effects of overweight and obesity in 195 countries over 25 years. N Engl J Med 2017; 377(1):13–27.
2. Wang TJ, Parise H, Levy D, et al. Obesity and the risk of new-onset atrial fibrillation. JAMA 2004; 292(20):2471–7.

3. Frost L, Hune LJ, Vestergaard P. Overweight and obesity as risk factors for atrial fibrillation or flutter: the Danish diet, cancer, and health study. Am J Med 2005;118(5):489–95.

4. Wong CX, Sullivan T, Sun MT, et al. Obesity and the risk of incident, post-operative, and post-ablation atrial fibrillation: a meta-analysis of 626,603 individuals in 51 studies. JACC Clin Electrophysiol 2015; 1(3):139–52.

5. Schnabel RB, Yin X, Gona P, et al. 50 year trends in atrial fibrillation prevalence, incidence, risk factors, and mortality in the Framingham Heart Study: a cohort study. Lancet 2015;386(9989):154–62.

6. Alberti KG, Eckel RH, Grundy SM, et al. Harmonizing the metabolic syndrome: a joint interim statement of the international diabetes federation task force on epidemiology and prevention; national heart, lung, and blood institute; American heart association; world heart federation; international atherosclerosis society; and international association for the study of obesity. Circulation 2009; 120(16):1640–5.

7. Watanabe H, Tanabe N, Watanabe T, et al. Metabolic syndrome and risk of development of atrial fibrillation: the Niigata preventive medicine study. Circulation 2008;117(10):1255–60.

8. Chamberlain AM, Agarwal SK, Ambrose M, et al. Metabolic syndrome and incidence of atrial fibrillation among blacks and whites in the Atherosclerosis Risk in Communities (ARIC) Study. Am Heart J 2010; 159(5):850–6.

9. Long MJ, Jiang CQ, Lam TH, et al. Atrial fibrillation and obesity among older Chinese: the Guangzhou biobank cohort study. Int J Cardiol 2011;148(1):48–52.

10. Wong CX, Sun MT, Odutayo A, et al. Associations of epicardial, abdominal, and overall adiposity with atrial fibrillation. Circ Arrhythm Electrophysiol 2016; 9(12):e004378.

11. Fox CS, Massaro JM, Hoffmann U, et al. Abdominal visceral and subcutaneous adipose tissue compartments: association with metabolic risk factors in the Framingham Heart Study. Circulation 2007;116(1):39–48.

12. Wong CX, Ganesan AN, Selvanayagam JB. Epicardial fat and atrial fibrillation: current evidence, potential mechanisms, clinical implications, and future directions. Eur Heart J 2016;38(17):1294–302.

13. Mahajan R, Kuklik P, Grover S, et al. Cardiovascular magnetic resonance of total and atrial pericardial adipose tissue: a validation study and development of a 3 dimensional pericardial adipose tissue model. J Cardiovasc Magn Reson 2013;15:73.

14. Al Chekakie MO, Welles CC, Metoyer R, et al. Pericardial fat is independently associated with human atrial fibrillation. J Am Coll Cardiol 2010;56(10):784–8.

15. Batal O, Schoenhagen P, Shao M, et al. Left atrial epicardial adiposity and atrial fibrillation. Circ Arrhythm Electrophysiol 2010;3(3):230–6.

16. Thanassoulis G, Massaro JM, O'Donnell CJ, et al. Pericardial fat is associated with prevalent atrial fibrillation: the Framingham heart study. Circ Arrhythm Electrophysiol 2010;3(4):345–50.

17. Wong CX, Abed HS, Molaee P, et al. Pericardial fat is associated with atrial fibrillation severity and ablation outcome. J Am Coll Cardiol 2011;57:1745–51.

18. Mahajan R, Lau DH, Brooks AG, et al. Electrophysiological, electroanatomical and structural remodeling of the atria as a consequence of sustained obesity. J Am Coll Cardiol 2015;66(1):1–11.

19. Iwasaki YK, Shi Y, Benito B, et al. Determinants of atrial fibrillation in an animal model of obesity and acute obstructive sleep apnea. Heart Rhythm 2012;9(9):1409–1416 e1401.

20. Mahajan R, Lau DH, Sanders P. Impact of obesity on cardiac metabolism, fibrosis, and function. Trends Cardiovasc Med 2015;25(2):119–26.

21. Lau DH, Shipp NJ, Kelly DJ, et al. Atrial arrhythmia in ageing spontaneously hypertensive rats: unraveling the substrate in hypertension and ageing. PloS one 2013;8(8):e72416.

22. Lavie CJ, Pandey A, Lau DH, et al. Obesity and atrial fibrillation prevalence, pathogenesis, and prognosis: effects of weight loss and exercise. J Am Coll Cardiol 2017;70(16):2022–35.

23. Hatem SN, Sanders P. Epicardial adipose tissue and atrial fibrillation. Cardiovasc Res 2014;102(2):205–13.

24. Mahajan R, Nelson A, Pathak RK, et al. Electroanatomical remodeling of the atria in obesity: impact of adjacent epicardial fat. JACC Clin Electrophysiol 2018;4(12):1529–40.

25. Lin YK, Chen YC, Chen JH, et al. Adipocytes modulate the electrophysiology of atrial myocytes: implications in obesity-induced atrial fibrillation. Basic Res Cardiol 2012;107(5):293.

26. Venteclef N, Guglielmi V, Balse E, et al. Human epicardial adipose tissue induces fibrosis of the atrial myocardium through the secretion of adipo-fibrokines. Eur Heart J 2013;36(13):795–805.

27. Friedman DJ, Wang N, Meigs JB, et al. Pericardial fat is associated with atrial conduction: the Framingham Heart Study. J Am Heart Assoc 2014;3(2): e000477.

28. Alpert MA, Omran J, Bostick BP. Effects of obesity on cardiovascular hemodynamics, cardiac morphology, and ventricular function. Curr Obes Rep 2016;5(4):424–34.

29. Lavie CJ, Alpert MA, Arena R, et al. Impact of obesity and the obesity paradox on prevalence and prognosis in heart failure. JACC Heart Fail 2013;1(2):93–102.

30. Nattel S. Atrial fibrillation and body composition: is it fat or lean that ultimately determines the risk? J Am Coll Cardiol 2017;69(20):2498–501.

31. Larsson SC, Back M, Rees JMB, et al. Body mass index and body composition in relation to 14

cardiovascular conditions in UK Biobank: a Mendelian randomization study. Eur Heart J 2020;41(2):221–6.

32. Tikkanen E, Gustafsson S, Knowles JW, et al. Body composition and atrial fibrillation: a Mendelian randomization study. Eur Heart J 2019;40(16):1277–82.

33. Fenger-Gron M, Overvad K, Tjonneland A, et al. Lean body mass is the predominant anthropometric risk factor for atrial fibrillation. J Am Coll Cardiol 2017;69(20):2488–97.

34. Zhang Q, Liu T, Ng CY, et al. Diabetes mellitus and atrial remodeling: mechanisms and potential upstream therapies. Cardiovasc Ther 2014;32(5):233–41.

35. Nystrom PK, Carlsson AC, Leander K, et al. Obesity, metabolic syndrome and risk of atrial fibrillation: a Swedish, prospective cohort study. PloS one 2015;10(5):e0127111.

36. Rabkin SW, Campbell H. Comparison of reducing epicardial fat by exercise, diet or bariatric surgery weight loss strategies: a systematic review and meta-analysis. Obes Rev 2015;16(5):406–15.

37. Mahajan R, Brooks AG, Shipp N, et al. AF and obesity: impact of weight reduction on the atrial substrate. Heart Rhythm 2013;(10):S484.

38. Abed HS, Wittert GA, Leong DP, et al. Effect of weight reduction and cardiometabolic risk factor management on symptom burden and severity in patients with atrial fibrillation: a randomized clinical trial. JAMA 2013;310(19):2050–60.

39. Pathak RK, Middeldorp ME, Meredith M, et al. Long-term effect of goal directed weight management in an atrial fibrillation cohort: a long-term follow-up StudY (LEGACY Study). J Am Coll Cardiol 2015;65(20):2159–69.

40. Middeldorp ME, Pathak RK, Meredith M, et al. PREVEntion and regReSsive effect of weight-loss and risk factor modification on atrial fibrillation: the REVERSE-AF study. Europace 2018;20(12):1929–35.

41. Pathak RK, Middeldorp ME, Lau DH, et al. Aggressive risk factor reduction study for atrial fibrillation and implications for the outcome of ablation: the ARREST-AF cohort study. J Am Coll Cardiol 2014;64(21):2222–31.

42. Pathak RK, Evans M, Middeldorp ME, et al. Cost-effectiveness and clinical effectiveness of the risk factor management clinic in atrial fibrillation: the CENT study. JACC Clin Electrophysiol 2017;3(5):436–47.

43. Rienstra M, Hobbelt AH, Alings M, et al. Targeted therapy of underlying conditions improves sinus rhythm maintenance in patients with persistent atrial fibrillation: results of the RACE 3 trial. Eur Heart J 2018;39(32):2987–96.

44. Mohanty S, Mohanty P, Natale V, et al. Impact of weight loss on ablation outcome in obese patients with longstanding persistent atrial fibrillation. J Cardiovasc Electrophysiol 2018;29(2):246–53.

45. Mahajan R, Pathak RK, Thiyagarajah A, et al. Risk factor management and atrial fibrillation clinics: saving the best for last? Heart Lung Circ 2017;26(9):990–7.

46. January CT, Wann LS, Calkins H, et al. 2019 AHA/ACC/HRS focused update of the 2014 AHA/ACC/HRS guideline for the management of patients with atrial fibrillation: a report of the american college of cardiology/American heart association task force on clinical practice guidelines and the heart rhythm society in collaboration with the society of thoracic surgeons. Circulation 2019;140(2):e125–51.

47. Jamaly S, Carlsson L, Peltonen M, et al. Bariatric surgery and the risk of new-onset atrial fibrillation in Swedish obese subjects. J Am Coll Cardiol 2016;68(23):2497–504.

Sleep Apnea and Atrial Fibrillation

Dominik Linz, MD, PhD[a,b,c,d],*, Stanley Nattel, MD[e,f,g], Jonathan M. Kalman, MBBS, PhD[h], Prashanthan Sanders, MBBS, PhD[a]

KEYWORDS

- Atrial fibrillation • Sleep apnea • Continuous positive air pressure (CPAP) • Pulmonary vein isolation
- Screening • Polygraphy

KEY POINTS

- Obstructive sleep apnea (OSA) creates a complex and dynamic substrate for atrial fibrillation (AF).
- OSA is present in up to 74% of patients with AF and nonrandomized studies suggest that treatment of OSA may help to maintain sinus rhythm.
- Because most patients with AF with OSA do not report daytime sleepiness, sleep-study evaluation may be reasonable for all patients being considered for a rhythm control strategy.
- Management of OSA in patients with AF requires a close interdisciplinary collaboration within an integrated care approach.
- Randomized controlled trials are needed to confirm the benefits of routine screening and treatment of OSA in patients with AF.

INTRODUCTION

Obstructive sleep apnea (OSA) is present in 21% to 74% of patients with atrial fibrillation (AF),[1–6] is an independent predictor of stroke,[7] and reduces the efficacy of catheter-based and pharmacologic rhythm-control therapy.[8,9] In observational studies, treatment of OSA by continuous positive airway pressure (CPAP) was associated with reduced recurrence of AF after electrical cardioversion and improved catheter-ablation success rates.[10–15]

This review summarizes the current understanding of the pathophysiology of OSA and highlights diagnostic and therapeutic considerations in patients with AF with OSA.

PATHOPHYSIOLOGY

OSA is characterized by repetitive partial (obstructive hypopnea) or complete (obstructive apnea) collapse of the upper airway during sleep.[16,17] Hypopneas typically represent the larger proportion of sleep apnea events; obstructive as well as central respiratory events may both occur in the same patient and even during the same night. In addition to high-frequency intermittent deoxygenation-reoxygenation, negative intrathoracic pressure fluctuations (up to −60 mm Hg)

[a] Centre for Heart Rhythm Disorders, South Australian Health and Medical Research Institute, University of Adelaide and Royal Adelaide Hospital, Adelaide, Australia; [b] Department of Cardiology, Maastricht University Medical Centre and Cardiovascular Research Institute, Maastricht, the Netherlands; [c] Department of Cardiology, Radboud University Medical Centre, Nijmegen, the Netherlands; [d] Department of Biomedical Sciences, Faculty of Health and Medical Sciences, University of Copenhagen, Copenhagen, Denmark; [e] Department of Medicine, Montreal Heart Institute and Université de Montréal, Montréal, Quebec, Canada; [f] Department of Pharmacology and Therapeutics, McGill University, 3655 Prom. Sir Willian Osler, Montreal, Quebec H3G 1Y6, Canada; [g] Institute of Pharmacology, West German Heart and Vascular Center, Faculty of Medicine, University Duisburg-Essen, Essen, Germany; [h] Department of Cardiology, Royal Melbourne Hospital and Department of Medicine, University of Melbourne, 300 Grattan Street, Melbourne, Victoria, Australia
* Corresponding author. Department of Cardiology, Centre for Heart Rhythm Disorders, Royal Adelaide Hospital, Adelaide 5000, Australia.
E-mail address: Dominik.Linz@adelaide.edu.au

Card Electrophysiol Clin 13 (2021) 87–94
https://doi.org/10.1016/j.ccep.2020.10.003

cardiacEP.theclinics.com

during inspiration against an occluded upper airway result in changes in transmural pressure gradients and myocardial stretch.[16]

Long-term exposure to OSA results in structural remodeling processes. Intermittent airway-obstruction episodes in rats older than 4 weeks produce connexin dysregulation and atrial fibrosis, which were associated with atrial conduction abnormalities and increased AF susceptibility/duration.[18] Correspondingly, patients with long-term OSA show marked atrial structural changes and conduction abnormalities, without any changes in atrial refractoriness, forming a substrate for AF vulnerability.[19,20]

Although atrial structural remodeling is important in maintaining AF, nocturnal AF paroxysms are often temporally related to individual respiratory obstructive events.[21,22] In the VARIOSA study, patients with implanted pacemakers showed a considerable night-to-night variability in sleep apnea severity, and the more severe sleep apnea nights conferred a 1.7-fold increased risk of having at least 5 min of AF during the same day compared with the best sleep nights.[23,24] This observation suggests that acute transient arrhythmogenic changes during apneas may further contribute to AF development. In a pig model of OSA, application of negative tracheal pressure during tracheal occlusion reproducibly and reversibly shortened atrial refractory period and enhanced AF inducibility.[25] In rats, obstructive respiratory events mimicked by intermittently stopping the ventilator and closing the airway for 40 seconds resulted in substantial negative intrathoracic pressure, acute left atrial dilation, and increased AF inducibility.[26] In a sheep model, the transition from hypercapnia back to normal blood gases was characterized by increased atrial vulnerability due to a differential recovery of atrial refractoriness and atrial conduction properties.[27]

OSA may also increase trigger formation. Combined sympathovagal activation during apneas contributes to the acute and transient arrhythmogenic electrophysiologic changes and increased frequency of premature atrial contractions with the potential to initiate AF in a vulnerable substrate.[28] In patients with AF, OSA is associated with increased incidence of extrapulmonary vein triggers,[20] and in atrial myocardium of patients with sleep apnea, increased calcium/calmodulin-dependent protein kinase II–dependent phosphorylation of the cardiac voltage-gated sodium channel (Nav1.5) results in proarrhythmic activity.[29]

The complex and dynamic substrate for AF induced by OSA, which is characterized by structural remodeling as a result of long-term OSA as well as transient and acute apnea-associated transient atrial electrophysiological changes, is summarized in **Fig. 1**.

ASSESSMENT AND DIAGNOSIS OF SLEEP APNEA IN PATIENTS WITH ATRIAL FIBRILLATION

Questionnaires, such as the Epworth sleepiness scale, can help to assess the neurobehavioral impact of sleep apnea, in particular subjective daytime sleepiness, but the absence of subjective sleepiness is not a reliable means of ruling out OSA in patients with AF.[6,30,31] In an ambulatory AF population in the SNOOZE study, OSA was common but most patients reported low daytime sleepiness levels, suggesting that lack of excessive daytime sleepiness should not preclude patients from being investigated for the potential presence of concomitant sleep apnea.[30] Difficult-to-treat AF or a predominance of nocturnal AF episodes should be considered a sign of possible OSA and should trigger a sleep evaluation (high probability), particularly in patients with symptomatic AF for whom a rhythm control strategy is intended. Polysomnography (level I: in-laboratory, technician-attended or level II: outside of the laboratory, technician not present, complete polysomnography) is the gold standard for the diagnosis and assessment of sleep-disordered breathings. However, polygraphy (level III: airflow, respiratory effort, oxygen saturation, no sleep stages recorded) is a suitable method to ensure patient access and to implement screening for OSA in the standard work-up of patients with AF. Overnight oximetry (level IV: oxygen saturation ± airflow) can be used as a prescreening tool to rule out OSA.[32] In patients with AF with a negative result in one overnight sleep recording, a repeated multiple-night sleep test may make sense if OSA probability remains high. A possible decision pathway is shown in **Fig. 2** and **Table 1**, which summarize the predictive value of the available screening modalities for OSA in patients with AF.

PREVALENCE OF SLEEP APNEA IN PATIENTS WITH ATRIAL FIBRILLATION

The prevalence of OSA is assessed by the apnea-hypopnea index (AHI), which represents the number of apnea and hypopnea events per hour of sleep. Cross-sectional studies reporting on the prevalence of OSA in patients with AF used different AHI threshold for the diagnosis of sleep apnea, the diagnosis was not always excluded in

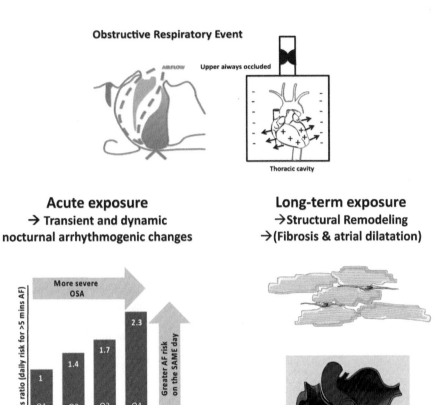

Fig. 1. Obstructive respiratory events transiently expose the heart to intermittent hypoxia and intrathoracic pressure swings. Acute exposure results in transient and dynamic nocturnal arrhythmogenic changes, which determine daily AF risk. The more severe the daily OSA is, the greater the AF risk on the same day is. Long-term exposure results in a structural remodeling characterized by atrial fibrosis and left atrial dilatation.

non-OSA groups, and clinical history or diagnostic questionnaires formed the basis of OSA diagnosis in some studies. Notwithstanding these methodological limitations, the estimated prevalence of sleep apnea in patients with AF has been found to be much higher (21%–74%) than in controls without AF (3%–49%).[1–6]

SLEEP APNEA REDUCES THE EFFECTIVENESS OF ATRIAL FIBRILLATION TREATMENT

The patients with atrial fibrillation with severe OSA show a lower response-rate to antiarrhythmic drug therapy than those with milder OSA.[21] A prospective analysis by Kanagala and colleagues[2] demonstrated that patients with OSA have a higher recurrence rate of AF after initially successful cardioversion than those without OSA. Meta-analyses of observational studies with a total of around 1000 patients show that patients with OSA have a 31% greater AF recurrence rate after pulmonary vein isolation (PVI).[8,9]

TREATMENT OF SLEEP APNEA IN PATIENTS WITH ATRIAL FIBRILLATION
Continuous Positive Airway Pressure Treatment

In nonrandomized, observational studies, CPAP use was associated with maintenance of sinus rhythm in patients with AF with OSA. Among 39 patients with OSA undergoing cardioversion for AF, patients receiving CPAP treatment were less likely to have AF recurrences at 12 months compared with the untreated group.[2] This finding, however, was not confirmed by a small prospective study.[33] In patients with OSA and AF undergoing PVI (n = 62), CPAP treatment was associated with lower AF recurrence rate at 12 months after the procedure (28%, vs 63% without CPAP) and almost similar to patients without OSA.[11] In meta-analyses of several nonrandomized studies, the use of CPAP was associated with a 42% decreased risk of AF recurrence (pooled risk ratio of 8 studies: 0.58; 95% confidence interval, 0.47–0.70; P <.001).[14,15]

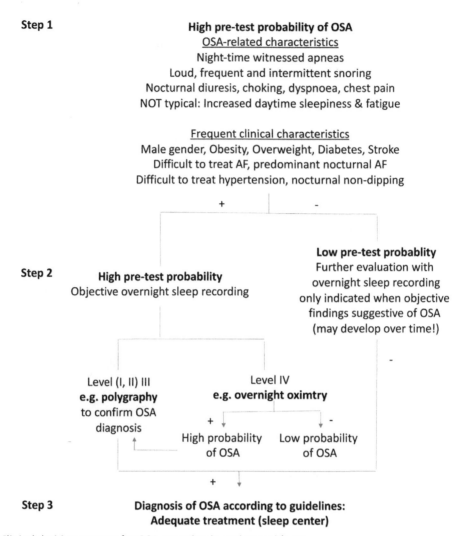

Step 1
High pre-test probability of OSA
OSA-related characteristics
Night-time witnessed apneas
Loud, frequent and intermittent snoring
Nocturnal diuresis, choking, dyspnoea, chest pain
NOT typical: Increased daytime sleepiness & fatigue

Frequent clinical characteristics
Male gender, Obesity, Overweight, Diabetes, Stroke
Difficult to treat AF, predominant nocturnal AF
Difficult to treat hypertension, nocturnal non-dipping

+   -

Step 2
High pre-test probability
Objective overnight sleep recording

Low pre-test probablity
Further evaluation with
overnight sleep recording
only indicated when objective
findings suggestive of OSA
(may develop over time!)

Level (I, II) III
e.g. polygraphy
to confirm OSA
diagnosis

Level IV
e.g. overnight oximtry

+   -
High probability   Low probability
of OSA   of OSA

+

Step 3
Diagnosis of OSA according to guidelines:
Adequate treatment (sleep center)

Fig. 2. Clinical decision support for OSA screening in patients with AF.

Noncontinuous Positive Airway Pressure Interventions

Sleep positional therapy and the use of mandibular advancement devices may be effective in patients with OSA who refuse or are intolerant of CPAP treatment. Weight loss by behavioral changes or bariatric surgery, as well as alcohol abstinence, have beneficial effects on OSA[34,35] and have been shown to promote sinus-rhythm maintenance in patients with AF.[36–39] Nevertheless, most of the abovementioned studies were not specifically performed in patients with AF with OSA. Whether interventions such as weight loss, cessation of alcohol, or other non-CPAP interventions show antiarrhythmic effects in patients with OSA is unknown and needs to be further investigated.

CLINICAL PRACTICE IMPLICATIONS

International professional societies recommend interrogation for clinical symptoms and signs of OSA and the use of CPAP treatment in confirmed cases to help maintain sinus rhythm.[40,41] However, most patients with AF with severe OSA do not report typical OSA-related symptoms such as daytime sleepiness.[6,30,31] Therefore, sleep study evaluation may be reasonable in all patients with symptomatic AF considered for a rhythm control strategy. The implementation of sleep apnea testing and sleep apnea management in AF clinics requires close interdisciplinary collaboration between the electrophysiologist/cardiologist and sleep specialists, ideally within an integrated care model.[42] Although technologies for simple sleep apnea testing are available, hurdles including

Table 1	
Sleep apnea screening and diagnosis in patients with atrial fibrillation	
WHO should be screened	All patients with AF considered for a rhythm control strategy
HOW should we screen	Sleep study evaluation may be reasonable, as patients with AF do not report daytime sleepiness
Diagnostic sleep-study options	
Questionnaire (eg, Epworth Sleepiness Scale [ESS])	Vs polysomnography to detect sleep apnea in patients with AF: sensitivity: 0.32; specificity: 0.54
Portable polygraphy (level III: airflow, respiratory effort, oxygen saturation, no sleep stages recorded)	Vs polysomnography to detect sleep apnea: sensitivity: 0.79 and 0.97; specificity: 0.60 and 0.93
Overnight oximetry (level IV: oxygen saturation)	Vs polysomnography to detect sleep apnea: sensitivity: 0.93; specificity: 0.75

lack of infrastructure, as well as inflexible reimbursement models, prevent the implementation in AF clinics in many centers.[43]

Currently, it remains uncertain how to optimally assess OSA severity in patients with AF and whether incorporation of parameters such as nocturnal hypoxemia or sleep quality in addition to the AHI helps to decide which patients with AF require OSA treatment.[44–46] In addition, instead of the current practice of establishing a categorical diagnosis of OSA from a single overnight sleep study, longitudinal sleep monitoring incorporating the night-to-night variability of OSA may be a better metric to assess the extent of dynamic OSA-related cardiovascular responses such as daily AF risk and cardiovascular outcomes (**Fig. 3**).[47]

Once sleep apnea is diagnosed and a treatment is initiated, limited CPAP tolerance and adherence (ca. 50%)[48] due to adverse effects such as poor mask fit, improper pressure levels, social unacceptability, claustrophobia, agitated pets, skin abrasion or rash, contact dermatitis (facial and/or scalp), keratitis from air leaks, and nasal folliculitis (nasal pillows) represents another challenge. Future risk-factor modification models should implement longitudinal assessment and optimization of CPAP adherence to ensure optimal benefit from CPAP treatment and non-CPAP interventions.

Finally, randomized prospective controlled trials are required and are on their way (eg, SLEEP-AF: ACTRN12616000088448) to confirm the relationship between OSA and AF, and the benefits of

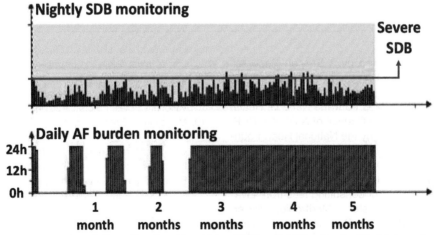

Fig. 3. Longitudinal combined sleep-disordered breathing (SDB) and AF burden monitoring in patients with implanted pacemakers reveals a high nightly SDB variability, which relates to daily AF burden.

treatment of OSA, to make further recommendations.

SUMMARY

Sleep-related breathing disturbances, particularly OSA, are a major treatable risk factor for AF. Further work is needed to better clarify mechanisms, optimal diagnostic approaches, and the effectiveness of both preventive and remedial treatment modalities. Research and clinical implementation in this area presents important opportunities for improving AF outcomes.

CLINICS CARE POINTS: EVIDENCE-BASED PEARLS AND PITFALLS

- OSA is present in up to 74% of patients with AF.[1–6]
- Nonrandomized studies suggest that treatment of OSA may help to maintain sinus rhythm.[8–15]
- Most patients with AF with OSA do not report daytime sleepiness; therefore, OSA questionnaires cannot identify OSA in patients with AF.[6,30,31]
- Sleep-study evaluation may be reasonable for all patients being considered for a rhythm control strategy.[42]
- Management of OSA in patients with AF requires a close interdisciplinary collaboration within an integrated care approach.[42]
- Randomized controlled trials are needed to confirm the benefits of routine screening and treatment of OSA in patients with AF.

DISCLOSURE

Dr D. Linz is supported by a Beacon Research Fellowship by the University of Adelaide. Drs J.M. Kalman and P. Sanders are supported by Practitioner Fellowships from the National Health and Medical Research Council of Australia. Dr P. Sanders is supported by the National Heart Foundation of Australia. Dr D. Linz reports having served on the advisory board of LivaNova, Respicardia, and Medtronic. Dr D. Linz reports having received lecture and/or consulting fees from LivaNova, Biosense-Webster, Medtronic, Pfizer, Bayer, and ResMed. Dr D. Linz reports having received research funding from Sanofi, ResMed, and Medtronic. Dr P. Sanders reports having served on the advisory board of Biosense-Webster, Medtronic, St Jude Medical, Boston Scientific, and CathRx. Dr P. Sanders reports having received lecture and/or consulting fees from Biosense-Webster, Medtronic, St Jude Medical, and Boston Scientific. Dr P. Sanders reports having received research funding from Medtronic, St Jude Medical, Boston Scientific, Biotronik, and Sorin. The other authors have nothing to disclose.

REFERENCES

1. Heinzer R, Vat S, Marques-Vidal P, et al. Prevalence of sleep-disordered breathing in the general population: the HypnoLaus study. Lancet Respir Med 2015; 3:310–8.
2. Kanagala R, Murali NS, Friedman PA, et al. Obstructive sleep apnea and the recurrence of atrial fibrillation. Circulation 2003;107:2589–94.
3. Gami AS, Pressman G, Caples SM, et al. Association of atrial fibrillation and obstructive sleep apnea. Circulation 2004;110:364–7.
4. Stevenson IH, Teichtahl H, Cunnington D, et al. Prevalence of sleep-disordered breathing in paroxysmal and persistent atrial fibrillation patients with normal left ventricular function. Eur Heart J 2008;29:1662–9.
5. Bitter T, Langer C, Vogt J, et al. Sleep-disordered breathing in patients with atrial fibrillation and normal systolic left ventricular function. Dtsch Arztebl Int 2009;106:164–70.
6. Traaen GM, Øverland B, Aakerøy L, et al. Prevalence, risk factors, and type of sleep apnea in patients with paroxysmal atrial fibrillation. Int J Cardiol Heart Vasc 2019;26:100447.
7. Yaranov DM, Smyrlis A, Usatii N, et al. Effect of obstructive sleep apnea on frequency of stroke in patients with atrial fibrillation. Am J Cardiol 2015; 115:461–5.
8. Ng CY, Liu T, Shehata M, et al. Meta-analysis of obstructive sleep apnea as predictor of atrial fibrillation recurrence after catheter ablation. Am J Cardiol 2011;108:47–51.
9. Li L, Wang ZW, Li J, et al. Efficacy of catheter ablation of atrial fibrillation in patients with obstructive sleep apnoea with and without continuous positive airway pressure treatment: a meta-analysis of observational studies. Europace 2014;16:1309–14.
10. Monahan K, Brewster J, Wang L, et al. Relation of the severity of obstructive sleep apnea in response to anti-arrhythmic drugs in patients with atrial fibrillation or atrial flutter. Am J Cardiol 2012;110:369–72.
11. Fein AS, Shvilkin A, Shah D, et al. Treatment of obstructive sleep apnea reduces the risk of atrial fibrillation recurrence after catheter ablation. J Am Coll Cardiol 2013;62:300–5.
12. Jongnarangsin K, Chugh A, Good E, et al. Body mass index, obstructive sleep apnea, and outcomes

of catheter ablation of atrial fibrillation. J Cardiovasc Electrophysiol 2008;19:668–72.

13. Naruse Y, Tada H, Satoh M, et al. Concomitant obstructive sleep apnea increases the recurrence of atrial fibrillation following radiofrequency catheter ablation of atrial fibrillation: clinical impact of continuous positive airway pressure therapy. Heart Rhythm 2013;10:331–7.

14. Shukla A, Aizer A, Holmes D, et al. Effect of obstructive sleep apnea treatment on atrial fibrillation recurrence: a meta-analysis. JACC Clin Electrophysiol 2015;1:41–51.

15. Qureshi WT, Nasir UB, Alqalyoobi S, et al. Meta-analysis of continuous positive airway pressure as a therapy of atrial fibrillation in obstructive sleep apnea. Am J Cardiol 2015;116:1767–73.

16. Linz D, Linz B, Hohl M, et al. Atrial arrhythmogenesis in obstructive sleep apnea: therapeutic implications. Sleep Med Rev 2016;26:87–94.

17. Linz D, McEvoy RD, Cowie MR, et al. Associations of obstructive sleep apnea with atrial fibrillation and continuous positive airway pressure treatment: a review. JAMA Cardiol 2018;3:532–40.

18. Iwasaki YK, Kato T, Xiong F, et al. Atrial fibrillation promotion with long-term repetitive obstructive sleep apnea in a rat model. J Am Coll Cardiol 2014;64:2013–23.

19. Dimitri H, Ng M, Brooks AG, et al. Atrial remodeling in obstructive sleep apnea: implications for atrial fibrillation. Heart Rhythm 2011;9:321–7.

20. Anter E, Di Biase L, Contreras-Valdes FM, et al. Atrial substrate and triggers of paroxysmal atrial fibrillation in patients with obstructive sleep apnea. Circ Arrhythm Electrophysiol 2017;10:e005407.

21. Monahan K, Storfer-Isser A, Mehra R, et al. Triggering of nocturnal arrhythmias by sleep-disordered breathing events. J Am Coll Cardiol 2009;54:1797–804.

22. Mehra R, Benjamin EJ, Shahar E, et al. Association of nocturnal arrhythmias with sleep-disordered breathing: the sleep heart Health study. Am J Respir Crit Care Med 2006;173:910–6.

23. Linz D, Brooks AG, Elliott AD, et al. Variability of sleep apnea severity and risk of atrial fibrillation: the VARIOSA-AF study. JACC Clin Electrophysiol 2019;5:692–701.

24. Linz D, Brooks AG, Elliott AD, et al. Nightly variation in sleep apnea severity as atrial fibrillation risk. J Am Coll Cardiol 2018;72:2406–7.

25. Linz D, Schotten U, Neuberger HR, et al. Negative tracheal pressure during obstructive respiratory events promotes atrial fibrillation by vagal activation. Heart Rhythm 2011;8:1436–43.

26. Iwasaki YK, Shi Y, Benito B, et al. Determinants of atrial fibrillation in an animal model of obesity and acute obstructive sleep apnea. Heart Rhythm 2012;9:1409–16.

27. Stevenson IH, Roberts-Thomson KC, Kistler PM, et al. Atrial electrophysiology is altered by acute hypercapnia but not hypoxemia: implications for promotion of atrial fibrillation in pulmonary disease and sleep apnea. Heart Rhythm 2010;7:1263–70.

28. Linz D, Hohl M, Ukena C, et al. Obstructive respiratory events increase premature atrial contractions after cardioversion. Eur Respir J 2015;45:1332–40.

29. Lebek S, Pichler K, Reuthner K, et al. Enhanced CaMKII-dependent late INa induces atrial proarrhythmic activity in patients with sleep-disordered breathing. Circ Res 2020;126:603–15.

30. Albuquerque FN, Calvin AD, Sert Kuniyoshi FH, et al. Sleep-disordered breathing and excessive daytime sleepiness in patients with atrial fibrillation. Chest 2012;141:967–73.

31. Kadhim K, Middeldorp ME, Elliott AD, et al. Self-reported daytime sleepiness and sleep-disordered breathing in patients with atrial fibrillation: SNOozE-AF. Can J Cardiol 2019;35:1457–64.

32. Linz D, Kadhim K, Brooks AG, et al. Diagnostic accuracy of overnight oximetry for the diagnosis of sleep-disordered breathing in atrial fibrillation patients. Int J Cardiol 2018;272:155–61.

33. Caples SM, Mansukhani MP, Friedman PA, et al. The impact of continuous positive airway pressure treatment on the recurrence of atrial fibrillation post cardioversion: a randomized controlled trial. Int J Cardiol 2019;278:133–6.

34. Scanlan MF, Roebuck T, Little PJ, et al. Effect of moderate alcohol upon obstructive sleep apnoea. Eur Respir J 2000;16:909–13.

35. Araghi MH, Chen YF, Jagielski A, et al. Effectiveness of lifestyle interventions on obstructive sleep apnea (OSA): systematic review and meta-analysis. Sleep 2013;36:1553–62.

36. Pathak RK, Middeldorp ME, Lau DH, et al. Aggressive risk factor reduction study for atrial fibrillation and implications for the outcome of ablation: the ARREST-AF cohort study. J Am Coll Cardiol 2014;64:2222–31.

37. Pathak RK, Middeldorp ME, Meredith M, et al. Long-term effect of goal-directed weight management in an atrial fibrillation cohort: a long-term follow-up study (LEGACY). J Am Coll Cardiol 2015;65:2159–69.

38. Abed HS, Wittert GA, Leong DP, et al. Effect of weight reduction and cardiometabolic risk factor management on symptom burden and severity in patients with atrial fibrillation: a randomized clinical trial. JAMA 2013;310:2050–60.

39. Jamaly S, Carlsson L, Peltonen M, et al. Bariatric surgery and the risk of new-onset atrial fibrillation in Swedish obese subjects. J Am Coll Cardiol 2016;68:2497–504.

40. Calkins H, Hindricks G, Cappato R, et al. 2017 HRS/EHRA/ECAS/APHRS/SOLAECE expert consensus

statement on catheter and surgical ablation of atrial fibrillation. Heart Rhythm 2017;14:e275–444.

41. Andrade JG, Verma A, Mitchell LB, et al. 2018 focused update of the Canadian cardiovascular society guidelines for the management of atrial fibrillation. Can J Cardiol 2018;34:1371–92.

42. Desteghe L, Hendriks JML, McEvoy RD, et al. The why, when and how to test for obstructive sleep apnea in patients with atrial fibrillation. Clin Res Cardiol 2018;107:617–31.

43. Desteghe L, Linz D, Hendriks JM. Sleep apnea testing and management in patients with atrial fibrillation: why is it so difficult? J Cardiovasc Nurs 2020; 35:324–6.

44. Linz D, Baumert M, Catcheside P, et al. Assessment and interpretation of sleep disordered breathing severity in cardiology: clinical implications and perspectives. Int J Cardiol 2018;271:281–8.

45. Baumert M, Immanuel SA, Stone KL, et al. Composition of nocturnal hypoxaemic burden and its prognostic value for cardiovascular mortality in older community-dwelling men. Eur Heart J 2020;41: 533–41.

46. Linz D, Kadhim K, Kalman JM, et al. Sleep and cardiovascular risk: how much is too much of a good thing? Eur Heart J 2019;40:1630–2.

47. Linz D, Baumert M, Desteghe L, et al. Nightly sleep apnea severity in patients with atrial fibrillation: potential applications of long-term sleep apnea monitoring. Int J Cardiol Heart Vasc 2019;24:100424.

48. Weaver TE, Grunstein RR. Adherence to continuous positive airway pressure therapy: the challenge to effective treatment. Proc Am Thorac Soc 2008;5: 173–8.

Renal Disease and Atrial Fibrillation

Maria Stefil, BSc, MBBS, MRes[a,b], Katarzyna Nabrdalik, MD, PhD[b,c],
Gregory Y.H. Lip, MD, FRCP[b,c,d,*]

KEYWORDS

- Atrial fibrillation • Chronic kidney disease • Risk stratification • Management

KEY POINTS

- Atrial fibrillation (AF) is associated with higher prevalence of chronic kidney disease (CKD) and vice versa.
- Renal impairment further increases the risk of ischemic stroke and systemic thromboembolism in patients with AF but also paradoxically predisposes to bleeding.
- Although patients with AF with CKD are at high risk of stroke, inclusion of renal function markers did not significantly improve the predictive value of currently approved stroke risk stratification tools.
- Patients with AF and CKD scoring high on bleeding risk stratification scores may still benefit from dose-adjusted oral anticoagulation therapy but require frequent follow-up and close monitoring of renal function.

INTRODUCTION

Atrial fibrillation (AF) and chronic kidney disease (CKD) often coexist and have a poorly understood epidemiologic and pathophysiologic interaction. CKD is defined as reduction in renal function as shown by a decline in estimated glomerular filtration rate (eGFR) less than 60 mL/min/1.73 m^2 or abnormalities in kidney structure present for more than 3 months.[1] AF is known to predispose to the development and progression of CKD and vice versa, with a bidirectional relationship between the 2 pathologic entities.

The presence of CKD poses multiple challenges for the pharmacologic as well as procedural management of AF. There is uncertainty regarding the best treatment strategy and safety profile of the conventional AF therapies in the context of end-stage kidney disease (ESKD), because these patients have historically been underrepresented in large-scale randomized trials[2] and many gaps in knowledge still exist.

This article identifies and discusses key issues surrounding the risk stratification and management of AF in patients with CKD.

METHODS

Electronic databases (PubMed, MEDLINE, EMBASE, Cochrane Database of Systematic Reviews) were searched for completed, peer-reviewed meta-analysis manuscripts published in, or translated into, English. The following text words and Medical Subject Headings (MeSH) were used as search terms: atrial fibrillation; renal impairment; chronic kidney disease. Reference lists of included publications were screened to identify further relevant literature.

EPIDEMIOLOGY OF ATRIAL FIBRILLATION AND CHRONIC KIDNEY DISEASE

The worldwide incidence and prevalence of AF are rapidly growing. It is estimated that the global incidence of AF in 2017 was at 403 new cases and

[a] Department of Cardiology, Royal Liverpool Hospital, Prescot Street, Liverpool, L7 8XP, UK; [b] Liverpool Centre for Cardiovascular Science, University of Liverpool and Liverpool Heart & Chest Hospital, Liverpool L14 3PE, UK; [c] Department of Internal Medicine, Diabetology and Nephrology, Faculty of Medical Sciences in Zabrze, Medical University of Silesia, Katowice, Poland; [d] Aalborg Thrombosis Research Unit, Department of Clinical Medicine, Aalborg University, Aalborg, Denmark
* Corresponding author. Liverpool Centre for Cardiovascular Science, University of Liverpool and Liverpool Heart & Chest Hospital, Liverpool L14 3PE, UK.
E-mail address: Gregory.Lip@liverpool.ac.uk

Card Electrophysiol Clin 13 (2021) 95–112
https://doi.org/10.1016/j.ccep.2020.11.001

prevalence at 4977 cases per million inhabitants, both figures increasing by about 17% and 30% compared with 2007 and 1997 respectively.[3] Similarly, CKD is becoming more prevalent, affecting about 10% of the adult population worldwide.[4] The burden of AF among patients with CKD is higher compared with those with preserved kidney function, with an estimated prevalence of AF in patients with non–end-stage kidney disease (NESKD) being in the range of 16% to 21%[5-8] and, in patients receiving renal replacement therapy (RRT), reaching 15% to 40%.[8-12]

There is an abundance of evidence suggesting that AF is associated with a higher risk of incident CKD and more rapid progression to ESKD,[13-16] and, in contrast, large-scale meta-analyses of cross-sectional and cohort studies showed that the risk of incident AF increases with more advanced renal dysfunction (**Table 1**). This finding can partially be explained by the shared multifactorial pathophysiologic pathways and presence of common risk factors such as increasing age, male gender, obesity, smoking, sedentary lifestyle, hypertension, diabetes mellitus, heart failure, and cardiovascular disease, which all in turn contribute to systemic inflammation, oxidative stress, and fibrotic changes (**Fig. 1**).[17]

ISCHEMIC STROKE AND BLEEDING IN PATIENTS WITH ATRIAL FIBRILLATION AND CHRONIC KIDNEY DISEASE

Both AF and CKD are independent risk factors for ischemic stroke [18-22]; however, it remains unclear as to how best to stratify risk of stroke when both conditions coexist. Both NESKD and ESKD

Table 1
Epidemiologic interaction between atrial fibrillation and chronic kidney disease

Authors (Year)	Included Studies	Studies/Participants (N)	Findings
Prevalence of CKD in Patients with AF			
Zimmerman et al,[8] 2012	Cross-sectional and cohort studies	25 studies, 253,589 participants	Prevalence of AF in patients with ESKD: 11.6% Incidence of AF in patients with ESKD: 2.7/100 patient-years
Shang et al,[122] 2016	Prospective cohort studies	7 studies, 400, 189 participants	CKD vs no CKD adjusted HR (95% CI) for new-onset AF: 1.47 (1.21–1.78)
Bansal et al,[123] 2017	Cohort studies	3 studies, 16,769 participants	Participants with eGFR 60–89 vs eGFR >90 adjusted HR (95% CI) for incident AF: 1.09 (0.97–1.24) Participants with eGFR 45–59 vs eGFR >90 adjusted HR (95% CI) for incident AF: 1.17 (1.00–1.38) Participants with eGFR 30–44 vs eGFR >90 adjusted HR (95% CI) for incident AF: 1.59 (1.28–1.98) Participants with eGFR <30 vs eGFR >90 adjusted HR (95% CI) for incident AF: 2.03 (1.40–2.96)
Prevalence/Incidence of AF in Patients with CKD			
Odutayo et al,[124] 2016	Cohort studies	104 studies, 9,686,513 participants (3 studies involving 467,000 patients examined CKD as an outcome, 20,312 adults with AF)	AF vs no AF RR (95% CI) for CKD: 1.64 (1.41–1.91)

Abbreviations: CI, confidence interval; HR, hazard ratio; RR, risk ratio.

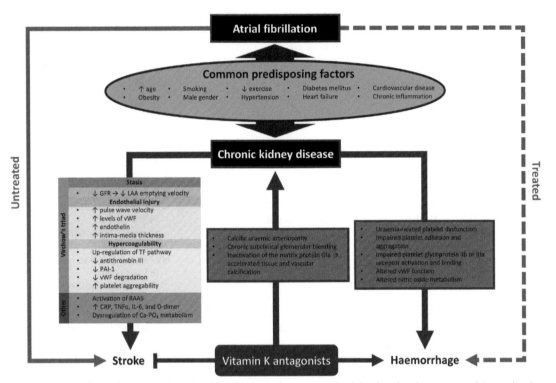

Fig. 1. Epidemiologic factors and pathophysiologic pathways involved in the development and interplay between AF, CKD, ischemic stroke, and hemorrhage. AF and CKD share a list of predisposing factors and are epidemiologically tightly interlinked. CKD independently increases the risk of thromboembolic events such as ischemic stroke by inducing changes consistent with the Virchow triad principles of hemostasis, endothelial injury, and hypercoagulability; CKD also contributes to the thrombogenesis via pathophysiologic changes that are not in the Virchow triad. Renal impairment paradoxically increases the hemorrhagic tendency by interfering with coagulation cascade components and thrombogenesis. Patients with AF commonly receive vitamin K antagonist agents such as warfarin that decrease the risk of stroke but at the same time add to the increased risk of bleeding in the context of CKD; vitamin K antagonist use can lead to changes in microvasculature that in turn can cause glomerular dysfunction and promote accelerated decline in renal function. CRP, C-reactive protein; GFR, glomerular filtration rate; IL-6, interleukin-6; LAA, left atrial appendage; PAI-1, plasminogen-activator inhibitor 1; RAAS, renin-angiotensin-aldosterone system; TF, tissue factor; TNFα, tumor necrosis factor alpha; vWF, von Willebrand factor.

aggravate the risk of ischemic stroke and systemic embolism when present on the background of AF but they also lead to more adverse outcomes following stroke.[23,24] The increase in relative risk of death can reach as high as 60% to 70% in patients with both conditions, which is largely a result of a higher propensity for thromboembolic events.[8,25,26] Proteinuria and worsening glomerular filtration rate (GFR) are associated with hypercoagulability and, in the The AnTicoagulation and Risk factors In Atrial fibrillation (ATRIA) study, patients with AF and documented proteinuria had a 57% higher risk of experiencing thromboembolic events, whereas those with AF and eGFR less than 45 mL/min/1.73 m^2 had a 39% higher risk of stroke compared with their counterparts with preserved renal function.[18]

Two large-scale meta-analyses have shown that patients with concurrent AF and CKD have at least double the risk of sustaining a thromboembolic event compared with patients with AF without CKD, and those with AF and ESKD have twice the risk of mortality compared with patients with ESKD with no AF (**Table 2**). This relationship is universally observed in different populations worldwide. Data derived from Danish and Swedish national cohort studies as well as multiple studies performed in Asia have attested to a higher risk of stroke and thromboembolism but also hemorrhage and death, associated with concomitant AF and CKD.[19,27–30]

Compared with patients with preserved renal function, the risk of stroke is doubled in those with ESKD requiring RRT[29] and those with rapidly declining renal function (ie, absolute eGFR reduction of ≥25–30 mL/min/1.73 m^2 or relative reduction of ≥25% over a period of 6 months or less)[31] regardless of anticoagulation status.[32]

Table 2
Risk of stroke and mortality in patients with AF and CKD

Authors (Year)	Included Studies	Studies/Participants (N)	Findings
Zimmerman et al,[8] 2012	Cross-sectional and cohort studies	25 studies, 253,589 participants	Risk of mortality in patients with ESKD with vs without AF: 26.9/100 patient-years vs 13.4/100 patient-years Risk of stroke in patients with ESKD with vs without AF: 5.2/100 patient-years vs 1.9/100 patient-years
Providência et al,[22] 2014	RCTs and cohort studies	19 studies, 379,506 patients with AF and CKD	NVAF and CKD vs no CKD HR (95% CI) for thromboembolism: 1.46 (1.20–1.76) NVAF and ESKD vs no ESKD HR (95% CI) for thromboembolism: 1.83 (1.56–2.14)
Zeng et al,[125] 2015	RCTs and cohort studies	18 studies, 538,479 patients with NVAF	AF and eGFR <60 mL/min vs eGFR ≥60 mL/min RR (95% CI) for thromboembolic event: 1.62 (1.40–1.87)

Abbreviation: NVAF, nonvalvular AF.

There is potential additive value from considering renal function markers for the purposes of determining the risk of central and systemic thromboembolic events in patients with AF and CKD. However, the reports of stroke risk in this patient population are varied; this could be a reflection of the complexity of the interaction between AF and worsening renal function but also the presence of competing risk of death in advanced CKD and potentially high prevalence of undetected AF.

Paradoxically, CKD is also known to be associated with hemorrhagic tendency because reduced renal function has been linked to increased risk of intracranial and gastrointestinal (GI) bleeding in patients with AF.[19] Worsening renal function leads to progressive vascular dysfunction, which in turn leads to microvascular changes intracerebrally. Patients receiving RRT are at a higher risk of GI bleeding as well as intracranial hemorrhagic events,[33] which is thought to be attributed to the uremia-related impairment of platelet adhesion and aggregation, glycoprotein IIb or IIIa receptor activation, von Willebrand factor function, and nitric oxide metabolism.[34–36] These secondary changes in the coagulation system are commonly exacerbated by the concomitant use of antiplatelet and nonsteroidal antiinflammatory drugs as well as exposure to heparin as part of hemodialysis. In patients with CKD, oral anticoagulation

(OAC) treatment of concomitant AF can therefore be associated with an increased risk of major bleeding and clinically significant minor bleeding.

According to the Japanese CIRC (Circulatory Risk in Communities) study and the Rotterdam study, renal impairment of GFR less than 60 mL/min/1.73 m^2 increases the risk of total stroke, and especially hemorrhagic stroke, in men and ischemic stroke in female patients,[37,38] whereas those on maintenance dialysis show a 10-fold increase in risk of intracerebral hemorrhage.[39] Worsening renal function is correlated with higher frequency and recurrence rates of AF but also with greater severity of hemorrhagic events.[34–36]

RISK STRATIFICATION TOOLS

There is evidence that suggests the utility and prognostic value of conventional stroke prediction scores such as CHADS$_2$ (congestive heart failure, hypertension, age, diabetes, prior stroke) or CHA$_2$-DS$_2$-VASc (congestive heart failure; hypertension; age ≥75 years; diabetes mellitus; prior stroke, TIA, or thromboembolism; vascular disease; age 65–74 years; sex category) in patients receiving dialysis treatment is comparable with patients with no CKD[10,20,40,41]; however, the reliability of these tools in patients with mild and moderate renal impairment remains undetermined owing to inconclusive data from most studies that incorporated CKD into risk scores.[30,42]

Although patients with AF with CKD are at high risk of stroke, inclusion of renal function markers did not significantly improve the predictive value of currently approved stroke risk stratification tools. In a post hoc analysis of a selected clinical trial cohort involving anticoagulated patients with NESKD with AF, GFR less than 60 mL/min was integrated into the CHADS$_2$ score (R$_2$CHADS$_2$) but did not produce a clinically meaningful improvement in the C-statistic, a measure of discrimination between low-risk and high-risk patients[21]; however, there was improvement in the net reclassification index (NRI), a measure for evaluating the improvement in prediction performance.[43] Further studies involving nonanticoagulated AF cohorts and ESKD cohorts failed to significantly improve predictive value by the addition of renal impairment to clinical risk scores.[42,44–47]

The ATRIA score, which accounts for renal function, has been shown to be associated with marginal improvement in NRI and C-statistic compared with CHADS$_2$ and CHA$_2$DS$_2$-VASc,[48] although uncertainty remains with regard to the clinical significance of these findings.[49] A potential explanation for the lack of added predictive value from inclusion of renal dysfunction into the existing scoring systems is the close links between CKD and the individual components of the risk scoring schemes currently in use.[50] For now, the CHA$_2$DS$_2$-VASc and CHADS$_2$ scores remain the best of the widely recommended stroke risk stratification tools in patients with AF with and without CKD.[51]

Aside from stroke risk, there are also bleeding risk stratification scores such as HAS-BLED (hypertension, abnormal renal/liver function, stroke, bleeding history or predisposition, labile International Normalized Ratio [INR], elderly, drugs/alcohol concomitantly), ATRIA, ORBIT, and HEMORR$_2$HAGES.[52] All aforementioned bleeding risk stratification tools incorporate CKD measures, but, although these tools are designed to aid clinical decision making, high bleeding risk scores are not interpreted as an absolute contraindication to anticoagulation. However, high scores warrant closer monitoring and frequent follow-up and should prompt more careful consideration of the modifiable bleeding risk factors such as poorly controlled hypertension, unstable INR (for warfarin), alcohol consumption, and the use of medications that predispose to bleeding. Proactive assessment of bleeding risk using the HAS-BLED score was associated with the mitigation of modifiable bleeding risk factors, reduced bleeding rates on anticoagulation, and an overall increase in OAC use over follow-up, compared with usual care.[53]

Recommencement of suspended OAC agents following GI bleeding is associated with improved survival benefit as well as reduced rate of thromboembolic events in patients with CKD, including patients with ESKD.[54–56]

THROMBOPROPHYLAXIS IN PATIENTS WITH ATRIAL FIBRILLATION AND NON–END-STAGE KIDNEY DISEASE

Increased risk of ischemic stroke and systemic embolism in patients with AF and CKD is thought to arise as a result of shared contribution from cardioembolic as well as noncardioembolic factors.[57] The presence of 1 or more stroke risk factors in men, or 2 or more stroke risk factors in women, as quantified by the CHA$_2$DS$_2$-VASc scoring system, warrants anticoagulation therapy[58,59]; the latter is in the form of a tightly monitored vitamin K antagonist (VKA) such as warfarin, or direct oral anticoagulants (DOACs) such as apixaban, dabigatran, edoxaban, or rivaroxaban. Several meta-analyses involving patients with AF with NESKD have established survival benefit and reduction in the risk of ischemic stroke, systemic embolism, and overall mortality associated with the use of VKAs compared with nonuse (**Table 3**).

The efficacy and safety of VKA use in patients with CKD largely depend on the time in therapeutic range (TTR) measure. Multiple studies have suggested that lower risks of thromboembolism as well as hemorrhage can be achieved through boosting of TTR to greater than 70% in patients with CKD on warfarin.[30,60,61] Benefits derived from VKA therapy are difficult to balance with the adverse effects of VKA-related accelerated tissue and vascular calcification,[62] secondary calcific uremic arteriopathy,[63] and chronic subclinical glomerular bleeding,[64] processes implicated in the acceleration of CKD progression and predisposition to noncardiogenic thromboembolism (see **Fig. 1**).

In contrast with VKA use, there may be potential renoprotective effect related to DOAC use, which was observed in a post hoc analysis of the Randomized Evaluation of Long-term anticoagulation therapY (RE-LY) trial with dabigatran as well as in Rivaroxaban Once-daily, oral, direct factor Xa inhibition Compared with Vitamin K antagonism for prevention of stroke and Embolism Trial in Atrial Fibrillation (ROCKET-AF) trial with rivaroxaban.[65,66] Nonetheless, a post hoc analysis of the Apixaban for Reduction In STroke and Other ThromboemboLic Events in atrial fibrillation (ARISTOTLE) trial with apixaban indicated a small decline in renal function.[67] More comparative data are needed.

Table 3
Oral vitamin K antagonist compared with no anticoagulation in patients with atrial fibrillation and chronic kidney disease

Authors (Year)	Included Studies	Studies/Participants (N)	Findings
Non–end-stage CKD			
Providência et al,[22] 2014	RCTs and cohort studies	19 studies, 379,506 patients with AF and CKD	Warfarin vs no warfarin HR (95% CI) for stroke or systemic embolism: 0.39 (0.18–0.86)
Bai et al,[126] 2016	RCTs and cohort studies	12 studies, 212,393 patients with AF and CKD	Warfarin vs placebo/antiplatelet drugs HR (95% CI) for major bleeding: 1.05 (0.74–1.36)
Dahal et al,[127] 2016	Cohort studies	13 studies, 51,901 patients with AF and CKD	Warfarin vs no warfarin HR (95% CI) for ischemic stroke/thromboembolism: 0.70 (0.54–0.89) Warfarin vs no warfarin HR (95% CI) for mortality: 0.65 (0.59–0.72) Warfarin vs no warfarin HR (95% CI) for major bleeding: 1.15 (0.88–1.49)
He et al,[76] 2019	Retrospective cohort studies	7 studies, 24,794 older patients with AF and CKD	Anticoagulants vs no anticoagulation RR (95% CI) for all-cause death: 0.66 (0.54–0.79) Anticoagulants vs no anticoagulation RR (95% CI) for ischemic stroke/TIA: 0.91 (0.46–1.79) Anticoagulants vs no anticoagulation RR (95% CI) for bleeding: 1.17 (0.86–1.60)
Malhotra et al,[128] 2019	RCTs and cohort studies	15 studies, 78,053 patients with AF and CKD	Warfarin vs no anticoagulation adjusted HR (95% CI) for ischemic stroke: 0.42 (0.24–0.72) Warfarin vs no anticoagulation adjusted HR (95% CI) for mortality: 0.68 (0.61–0.76) Warfarin vs no anticoagulation adjusted HR (95% CI) for major bleeding: 1.14 (0.88–1.47)

(continued on next page)

Table 3 *(continued)*			
Authors (Year)	**Included Studies**	**Studies/Participants (N)**	**Findings**
ESKD			
Dahal et al,[127] 2016	Cohort studies	13 studies, 51,901 patients with AF and CKD	Warfarin vs no warfarin HR (95% CI) for major bleeding: 1.30 (1.08–1.56) Warfarin vs no warfarin HR (95% CI) for stroke: 1.12 (0.69–1.82) Warfarin vs no warfarin HR (95% CI) for mortality: 0.96 (0.81–1.13)
Tan et al,[129] 2016	Cohort studies	20 studies, 56,146 patients with ESKD and AF	Warfarin vs no warfarin HR (95% CI) for all-cause stroke: 0.92 (0.74–1.16) Warfarin vs no warfarin HR (95% CI) for any stroke: 1.01 (0.81–1.26) Warfarin vs no warfarin HR (95% CI) for ischemic stroke: 0.80 (0.58–1.11) Warfarin vs no warfarin HR (95% CI) for all-cause bleeding: 1.21 (1.01–1.44) Warfarin vs no warfarin HR (95% CI) for major bleeding: 1.18 (0.82–1.69) Warfarin vs no warfarin HR (95% CI) for GI bleeding: 1.19 (0.81–1.76) Warfarin vs no warfarin HR (95% CI) for any bleeding: 1.21 (0.99–1.48)
He et al,[76] 2019	Retrospective cohort studies	7 studies, 24,794 older patients with AF and CKD	Anticoagulants vs no anticoagulation RR (95% CI) for bleeding: 1.37 (1.09–1.74) Anticoagulants vs no anticoagulation RR (95% CI) for ischemic stroke/TIA: 1.18 (0.88–1.58) Anticoagulants vs no anticoagulation RR (95% CI) for death: 0.87 (0.60–1.27)

(continued on next page)

Authors (Year)	Included Studies	Studies/Participants (N)	Findings
Malhotra et al,[128] 2019	RCTs and cohort studies	15 studies, 78,053 patients with AF and CKD	Warfarin vs no anticoagulation unadjusted RR (95% CI) for ischemic stroke: 0.55 (0.37–0.81)
Randhawa et al,[130] 2020	Cohort studies	15 studies, 47,480 patients with AF and ESRD (10,445 receiving warfarin)	Warfarin vs no warfarin HR (95% CI) for ischemic stroke: 0.96 (0.82–1.13) Warfarin vs no warfarin HR (95% CI) for major bleeding: 1.20 (0.99–1.47) Warfarin vs no warfarin HR (95% CI) for overall mortality: 0.95 (0.83–1.09) Warfarin vs no warfarin HR (95% CI) for hemorrhagic stroke: 1.49 (1.03–1.94)

Table 3 *(continued)*

Abbreviation: TIA, transient ischemic attack.

Several meta-analyses included in this review indicate that VKAs might be associated with a nonsignificant increase in the risk of bleeding in patients with NESKD (see **Table 3**). Increased bleeding tendency and the protective effect against ischemic stroke associated with VKA use in patients with NESKD can be balanced effectively by implementing a dose-adjusted approach.[19,22,29,68] However, it is not an easy task to obtain good TTR in such a population given that severe renal dysfunction is a strong predictor for overanticoagulation or poor anticoagulation control.[69]

Multiple large-scale randomized controlled trials, such as RE-LY, ROCKET-AF, ARISTOTLE, and ENGAGE AF-TIMI 48, have shown noninferiority of DOACs at reducing the rate of ischemic stroke, and some produced evidence to suggest DOACs are superior to VKAs in the risk reduction of major bleeding.[70–76] However, these large trials did not focus on patients with CKD and excluded patients with Cockcroft-Gault estimated creatinine clearance (CrCL) less than 30 mL/min, except for the ARISTOTLE trial, which excluded patients with CrCL less than 25 mL/min.[67] In a subgroup analysis of the ARISTOTLE trial focusing on patients with CrCL 25 to 30 mL/min compared with those with CrCl greater than 30 mL/min, the findings were consistent with the overall trial where apixaban treatment was associated with less bleeding compared with warfarin.[77]

Numerous meta-analyses and observational studies have reiterated the comparative efficacy and safety profile of DOACs in the CKD population (**Table 4**). At present, there is a lack of head-to-head comparison data, and therefore no robust understanding of the risk/benefit profile of each individual DOAC in this population exists.[75,78–82] The approved prescribing recommendations that are available at the moment are based on pharmacologic modeling studies rather than clinical trial data. Nonetheless, the official guidance states that all 4 types of DOACs are safe to use in patients with AF with mild to moderate renal impairment,[83] with advised caution when using edoxaban in patients with very good kidney function; namely, CrCL greater than 95 mL/min in the United States.[84] It is also advised that decisions regarding the dose of DOACs ought to be based on markers of renal function as per manufacturer's recommendations, where renal function is estimated using the Cockcroft-Gault calculation.

THROMBOPROPHYLAXIS IN PATIENTS WITH ATRIAL FIBRILLATION AND END-STAGE KIDNEY DISEASE

Patients with ESKD are known to have suboptimal TTR regardless of the INR monitoring intensity[85] and therefore are at higher risk of experiencing complications as a result of VKA therapy.[86] There is a wide variation in prescription trends between

Table 4
Direct oral anticoagulants compared with vitamin K antagonists in patients with atrial fibrillation and chronic kidney disease

Authors (Year)	Included Studies	Studies/Participants (N)	Findings
Non–end-stage CKD			
Harel et al,[131] 2014	RCTs	8 studies, 10,616 patients with CKD with AF or VTE	DOACs vs VKAs RR (95% CI) for stroke and systemic thromboembolism: 0.64 (0.39–1.04). DOACs vs VKAs RR (95% CI) for recurrent thromboembolism or thromboembolism-related death: 0.97 (0.43–2.15). DOACs vs VKAs RR (95% CI) for major bleeding or clinically relevant nonmajor bleeding: 0.89 (0.68–1.16)
Providência et al,[22] 2014	RCTs and cohort studies	19 studies, 379,506 patients with AF and CKD	DOACs vs warfarin HR (95% CI) for stroke or systemic embolism: 0.80 90.66–0.96)
Bai et al,[126] 2016	RCTs and cohort studies	12 studies, 212,393 patients with AF and CKD	DOACs vs dose-adjusted warfarin RR (95% CI) for composite of GI bleeding, intracranial hemorrhage, and other fatal or nonfatal bleeding: 0.81 (0.75–0.88)
Andò et al,[132] 2017	RCTs	5 studies, 13,878 patients with AF with moderate CKD	DOACs vs warfarin OR (95% CrI) for stroke/systemic embolism: 0.79 (0.67–0.94). DOACs vs warfarin OR (95% CrI) for major bleeding: 0.74 (0.65–0.86)
Kimachi et al,[133] 2017	RCTs	5 studies, 12,545 patients with AF and CKD stage III and IV	DOACs vs warfarin RR (95% CI) for stroke and systemic embolism events: 0.81 (0.65–1.00). DOACs vs warfarin RR (95% CI) for major bleeding events: 0.79 (0.59–1.04)

(continued on next page)

Table 4
(continued)

Authors (Year)	Included Studies	Studies/Participants (N)	Findings
Malhotra et al,[128] 2019	RCTs and cohort studies	15 studies, 78,053 patients with AF and CKD	DOACs vs warfarin adjusted HR (95% CI) for ICH: 0.39 (0.30–0.50) DOACs vs warfarin adjusted HR (95% CI) for stroke or systemic embolism: 0.75 (0.65–0.88) DOACs vs warfarin adjusted HR (95% CI) for major bleeding: 0.85 (0.71–1.01) DOACs vs warfarin adjusted HR (95% CI) for mortality: 0.92 (0.82–1.04)
ESKD			
Chan K.E et al,[101] 2015	Observational	1 study, 29.977 patients with AF	Dabigatran vs warfarin RR (95% CI) for major bleeding: 1.76 (1.44–2.15) Dabigatran vs warfarin RR (95% CI) for total embolic events: 1.71 (0.97–2.99) Rivaroxaban vs warfarin RR (95% CI) for major bleeding: 1.4 (1.09–1.93) Rivaroxaban vs warfarin RR (95% CI) for total embolic events: 1.8 (0.89–3.64)
Kuno et al.[102] 2020	observational	16 studies, 71.877 patients with AF and long-term dialysis	Apixaban 5 mg vs warfarin HR (95% CI) for mortality: 0.65 (0.45–0.93)

Abbreviations: CrI, credible interval; OR, odds ratio; VTE, venous thromboembolism.

different countries, which is an indication of lack of consensus on the OAC use strategy in patients with terminal renal disease.[30] The balance between risks and benefits of VKA use in patients with ESKD is more ambiguous, with various meta-analyses providing opposing evidence (see **Table 3**).

Some observational data suggest there is a reduction in the risk of ischemic stroke, with well-managed VKA use producing good-quality anticoagulation control in patients with ESKD[29,87,88]; however, very few studies have been able to produce evidence of survival benefit,[89,90] and some reported no difference or potential negative net clinical effect with the use of VKAs, especially in patients older than 75 years.[10,68,91–99] RRT use is associated with inadequate control of OAC quality, as shown by suboptimal TTR.[30] The type of RRT may also have a bearing on the outcomes following VKA use, because warfarin therapy in the context of peritoneal dialysis has not been associated with poor clinical outcomes, unlike in hemodialysis patients, leading to a lower risk of ischemic stroke and lower rate of hemorrhagic stroke.[41]

There is no sufficient evidence base that would warrant recommendations of routine use of VKA therapy in patients with ESKD with AF and, as a result, the debate around the efficacy, safety, and optimal dosing of DOACs as an alternative option is ongoing. There are no data from randomized controlled trials related to the use of DOACs in patients with severe or end-stage CKD. Some reports suggest that there is no need for dose reduction in patients with ESKD, whereas others have raised safety concerns over the use of DOACs in patients with ESKD altogether.

The recent 2019 update of the 2014 American Heart Association (AHA)/American College of Cardiology (ACC)/Heart Rhythm Society (HRS) guideline for the management of patients with AF states that apixaban might be reasonable in dialysis patients, but the need for further studies is stressed.[100] The first study that evaluated DOACs (dabigatran and rivaroxaban) compared with warfarin in patients on maintenance dialysis had an observational design where the drugs were prescribed to the patients with ESKD off label, despite US Food and Drug Administration (FDA) warning of caution in renal failure: there was excess morbidity and mortality from bleeding associated with DOAC use, with no significant difference in the incidence of total embolic events (embolic stroke and arterial embolism) in patients on dabigatran or on rivaroxaban compared with warfarin.[101]

In a meta-analysis of observational studies of the efficacy and safety of OAC in patients with AF on long-term dialysis (only 2 studies included DOACs), OACs were not associated with reduced risk of thromboembolism but a higher risk of bleeding in patients treated with warfarin, dabigatran, and rivaroxaban, compared with apixaban or no anticoagulant. Apixaban 5 mg twice daily was linked to significantly lower risk of death compared with apixaban 2.5 mg twice daily, warfarin, and nonanticoagulation[102] (see **Table 4**).

Ha and colleagues[103] performed a systematic review and meta-analysis evaluating VKA and DOAC in patients with CKD stages 3 to 5, including dialysis patients, who were prescribed those drugs for various indications (11 trials included OAC prescribed for AF) and found that, among patients with advanced CKD or ESKD, there was insufficient evidence to determine harms and benefits of VKAs or DOAC.

Challenges surrounding the choice of DOAC dose can be partially explained by all DOACs being more or less renally excreted and therefore being thought to be unsafe in severe renal dysfunction. Dialysis-dependent, as well as non–dialysis-dependent, patients with AF and with Cockcroft-Gault estimated CrCL (eCrCl) of less than 30 mL/min have been historically underrepresented in randomized trials and there is a shortage of data in these categories of patients.[50,83,104]

Renal function can be labile in these patients and sudden decline, if unnoticed, can result in DOAC overdosing and lead to fatal bleeding.[105] Particular care should be taken during intercurrent acute illnesses, which can cause drastic fluctuations in renal function.[106] Therefore, regular monitoring of kidney function and dose adjustment on an individual basis have been advocated, and a multidisciplinary approach to decision making regarding the choice of OAC is advised.[107]

Ongoing trials that aim to address this gap in the literature related to the safety of DOAC in patients with severe renal impairment include AVKDIAL (https://clinicaltrials.gov/ct2/show/NCT028869 62 Oral Anticoagulation in Haemodialysis Patients), evaluating VKA versus no OAC; SAFE-D (NCT03987711; Strategies for the Management of Atrial Fibrillation in Patients Receiving Dialysis), comparing warfarin, apixaban, and no anticoagulation; and AXADIA (https://clinicaltrials.gov/ct2/show/NCT02933697; Compare Apixaban and Vitamin-K Antagonists in Patients With AF and ESKD), comparing phenprocoumon and apixaban.

There is only 1 randomized controlled trial that has been presented and unpublished: RENAL-AF (Renal Hemodialysis Patients Allocated Apixaban vs Warfarin in Atrial Fibrillation; https://clinicaltrials.gov/ct2/show/NCT02942407), evaluating apixaban versus VKA in patients with ESKD, which has prematurely stopped because of problems related to enrollment.[108]

OTHER CONSIDERATIONS: DEVICES, RATE AND RHYTHM CONTROL

Rate and rhythm control constitute symptomatic treatment of AF. In patients with CKD, the most important consideration is reduced clearance and increased half-life of water-soluble antiarrhythmic and rate-controlling agents that may require dose modification.[109] In contrast, dialysis may lead to rapid removal of medication from circulation and result in drastic troughs in concentration, which in turn can increase the risk of rebound arrhythmic episodes, particularly on a background of electrolyte imbalance.[110] The choice of a rate versus rhythm control strategy should be guided by the clinical picture and individual patient circumstances and preferences. In general, patients with NESKD tend to receive rhythm control, whereas those at the more severe end of the spectrum are more likely to receive rate control management.[111]

It is also apparent that patients with severe CKD and AF are less likely to undergo ablation therapy[111] owing to the lack of evidence of long-term benefit and high rate of AF recurrence postprocedure, particularly in those with declining renal function.[112–114] Electrical cardioversion also seems to be less effective at producing sinus rhythm in patients with CKD, who have a high recurrence rate.[115]

Left atrial appendage (LAA) occluders, such as Watchman or Amplatzer Cardiac Plug, are considered an effective alternative to OAC in patients in whom OAC is contraindicated. Patients with CKD can safely undergo the procedure of device insertion; however, trials assessing the safety and efficacy of LAA occluders did not report on the proportion of patients with CKD among the enrolled subjects.[116,117] In addition, the need for antiplatelet therapy following the insertion of the device may render this strategy unacceptable because of the associated risk of bleeding in patients with advanced kidney disease.

SUMMARY

Prevalence of AF among patients with CKD is higher than among individuals with normal kidney function. Although patients with AF with CKD are at high risk of stroke, inclusion of renal function markers did not significantly improve the predictive value of currently approved stroke risk stratification tools. Also, CKD is independently associated with a greater bleeding propensity, which complicates the decision-making process regarding anticoagulation strategy. Nonetheless, bleeding risk estimation forms an important part of follow-up and should inform renal function monitoring intensity, particularly in patients with rapidly declining renal markers or advanced kidney disease.

Both VKAs and DOACs are effective to use in patients with mild to moderate renal impairment and have been shown to reduce stroke-related morbidity and mortality; however, DOACs are superior to VKAs in their lower rate of hemorrhagic events. VKA use in patients with ESKD may lead to a reduced risk of cardioembolic stroke, but the associated risk of major bleeding outweighs the benefit. The safety profile of VKAs is inferior to that of DOACs owing to suboptimal TTR in dialysis-dependent patients and an increased risk of noncardioembolic thrombotic events caused by VKA-induced vascular changes. Thromboembolic and hemorrhagic risks are greater in patients with ESKD receiving RRT compared with patients with more preserved renal function. Thus far, no head-to-head analysis involving patients with ESKD has been performed to provide comparative efficacy and safety data on each individual DOAC. Patients with AF and renal dysfunction across the whole spectrum should receive a dose-adjusted regimen if a DOAC is chosen to provide thromboprophylaxis. With both AF and CKD growing in incidence and in prevalence among older patients, the proportion of patients living with both diagnoses will increase progressively over the coming years.

CLINICS CARE POINTS

- The risk of stroke in patients with AF and CKD must be assessed by an approved risk stratification tool such as CHA_2DS_2-VASc. A score of 2 or more in women and 1 or more in men should prompt consideration of OAC.[118]

- A risk of bleeding assessment is advised in patients with AF and CKD. However, high scores do not necessarily preclude the use of OAC, but they indicate the need for minimizing the modifiable bleeding risk factors as well as more frequent monitoring of coagulation and renal function markers.[119,120]

- The grade of chronic kidney dysfunction should be assessed before initiation of OAC during a period of renal function stability and not at the time of acute kidney injury.[83]

- For the purpose of estimation of kidney function and therefore assessment of renal clearance capacity, CrCL should be estimated using the Cockcroft-Gault method.[83]

- Renal function markers should be reassessed at least annually in patients with an existing diagnosis of AF in order to screen for CKD; worsening renal impairment, multimorbidity, old age, and intercurrent acute illness should trigger more frequent monitoring.[83,118]

- Patients with CKD are at an increased risk of AF and should be systematically screened for AF with an electrocardiogram, regardless of history or symptoms of AF.[118]

- VKAs and DOACs are both safe and effective at preventing stroke and systemic thromboembolic events in patients with mild and moderate CKD. Compared with dose-adjusted DOACs, VKAs are associated with less benefit and higher risk of adverse events in patients with ESKD.[118]

- All available DOACs are excreted renally to a varying extent, and acute kidney injury warrants discontinuation of all types of DOACs and substitution with parenteral anticoagulation as per local guidance.[83]

- A structured multidisciplinary approach, involving primary care, cardiology, and nephrology, is advised in the management of patients with AF and CKD.[121]

DISCLOSURE

Professor G.Y.H. Lip discloses serving as a consultant for Bayer/Janssen, BMS/Pfizer, Medtronic, Boehringer Ingelheim, Novartis, Verseon, and Daiichi Sankyo, and serving as a speaker for Bayer, BMS/Pfizer, Medtronic, Boehringer Ingelheim, and Daiichi Sankyo. K. Nabrdalik has received remunerations/fees for activities on behalf of Abbott, Astra-Zeneca, Boehringer Ingelheim, Mundipharma, Eli Lilly, Novo Nordisk, and Polfa. This research did not receive any specific grant from funding agencies in the public, commercial, or not-for-profit sectors.

REFERENCES

1. KIDGO. Kidney disease: improving global outcomes (KDIGO) CKD Work Group. Kidney Int Suppl 2013;3(1):4.
2. Charytan D, Kuntz RE. The exclusion of patients with chronic kidney disease from clinical trials in coronary artery disease. Kidney Int 2006;70(11):2021–30.
3. Lippi G, Sanchis-Gomar F, Cervellin G. Global epidemiology of atrial fibrillation: an increasing epidemic and public health challenge. Int J Stroke 2020. https://doi.org/10.1177/1747493019897870. 174749301989787.
4. Bikbov B, Purcell CA, Levey AS, et al. Global, regional, and national burden of chronic kidney disease, 1990–2017: a systematic analysis for the Global Burden of Disease Study 2017. Lancet 2020;395(10225):709–33.
5. McManus DD, Corteville DC, Shlipak MG, et al. Relation of kidney function and albuminuria with atrial fibrillation (from the heart and soul study). Am J Cardiol 2009;104(11):1551–5.
6. Ananthapanyasut W, Napan S, Rudolph EH, et al. Prevalence of atrial fibrillation and its predictors in nondialysis patients with chronic kidney disease. Clin J Am Soc Nephrol 2010;5(2):173.
7. Soliman EZ, Prineas RJ, Go AS, et al. Chronic kidney disease and prevalent atrial fibrillation: the Chronic Renal Insufficiency Cohort (CRIC). Am Heart J 2010;159(6):1102.
8. Zimmerman D, Sood MM, Rigatto C, et al. Systematic review and meta-analysis of incidence, prevalence and outcomes of atrial fibrillation in patients on dialysis. Nephrol Dial Transpl 2012;27(10):3816.
9. Genovesi S, Pogliani D, Faini A, et al. Prevalence of atrial fibrillation and associated factors in a population of long-term hemodialysis patients. Am J Kidney Dis 2005;46(5):897.
10. Wizemann V, Tong L, Satayathum S, et al. Atrial fibrillation in hemodialysis patients: clinical features and associations with anticoagulant therapy. Kidney Int 2010;77(12):1098–106.
11. Wetmore JB, Mahnken JD, Rigler SK, et al. The prevalence of and factors associated with chronic atrial fibrillation in Medicare/Medicaid-eligible dialysis patients. Kidney Int 2012;81(5):469.
12. Königsbrügge O, Posch F, Antlanger M, et al. Prevalence of atrial fibrillation and antithrombotic therapy in hemodialysis patients: cross-sectional results of the vienna InVestigation of AtriaL fibrillation and thromboembolism in patients on HemoDIalysis (VIVALDI). PLoS One 2017;12(1):e0169400.
13. Watanabe H, Watanabe T, Sasaki S, et al. Close bidirectional relationship between chronic kidney disease and atrial fibrillation: the Niigata preventive medicine study. Am Heart J 2009;158(4):629.
14. Bansal N, Xie D, Tao K, et al. Atrial fibrillation and risk of ESRD in adults with CKD. Clin J Am Soc Nephrol 2016;11(7):1189.
15. Bansal N, Fan D, Hsu CY, et al. Incident atrial fibrillation and risk of end-stage renal disease in adults with chronic kidney disease. Circulation 2013;127(5):569.
16. O'Neal WT, Tanner RM, Efird JT, et al. Atrial fibrillation and incident end-stage renal disease: the REasons for Geographic and Racial Differences in Stroke (REGARDS) study. Int J Cardiol 2015;185:219.
17. Turakhia MP, Blankestijn PJ, Carrero JJ, et al. Chronic kidney disease and arrhythmias: Conclusions from a kidney disease: improving global outcomes (KDIGO) Controversies conference. Eur Heart J 2018;39(24):2314–25.
18. Go AS, Fang MC, Udaltsova N, et al. Impact of proteinuria and glomerular filtration rate on risk of thromboembolism in atrial fibrillation: the anticoagulation and risk factors in atrial fibrillation (ATRIA) study. Circulation 2009;119(10):1363–9.
19. Olesen JB, Lip GY, Kamper AL, et al. Stroke and bleeding in atrial fibrillation with chronic kidney disease. N Engl J Med 2012;367(7):625.
20. Wetmore JB, Ellerbeck EF, Mahnken JD, et al. Atrial fibrillation and risk of stroke in dialysis patients. Ann Epidemiol 2013;23(3):112.
21. Piccini JP, Stevens SR, Chang Y, et al. Renal dysfunction as a predictor of stroke and systemic embolism in patients with nonvalvular atrial fibrillation: Validation of the R2CHADS2 index in the ROCKET AF. Circulation 2013.
22. Providência R, Marijon E, Boveda S, et al. Meta-analysis of the influence of chronic kidney disease on the risk of thromboembolism among patients with nonvalvular atrial fibrillation. Am J Cardiol 2014;114(4):646.
23. Yahalom G, Schwartz R, Schwammenthal Y, et al. Chronic kidney disease and clinical outcome in patients with acute stroke. Stroke 2009;40(4):1296.
24. Kumai Y, Kamouchi M, Hata J, et al. Proteinuria and clinical outcomes after ischemic stroke. Neurology 2012;78(24):1909.

25. Nelson SE, Shroff GR, Li S, et al. Impact of chronic kidney disease on risk of incident atrial fibrillation and subsequent survival in medicare patients. J Am Heart Assoc 2012;1(4):e002097.

26. Hwang HS, Park MW, Yoon HE, et al. Clinical significance of chronic kidney disease and atrial fibrillation on morbidity and mortality in patients with acute myocardial infarction. Am J Nephrol 2014; 40(4):345.

27. Akazawa T, Nishihara H, Iwata H, et al. Preoperative plasma brain natriuretic peptide level is an independent predictor of postoperative atrial fibrillation following off-pump coronary artery bypass surgery. J Anesth 2008;22(4):347.

28. Chinda J, Nakagawa N, Kabara M, et al. Impact of decreased estimated glomerular filtration rate on Japanese acute stroke and its subtype. Intern Med 2012;51(13):1661.

29. Bonde AN, Lip GY, Kamper AL, et al. Net clinical benefit of antithrombotic therapy in patients with atrial fibrillation and chronic kidney disease: a nationwide observational cohort study. J Am Coll Cardiol 2014;64(23):2471.

30. Friberg L, Benson L, Lip GY. Balancing stroke and bleeding risks in patients with atrial fibrillation and renal failure: the Swedish Atrial Fibrillation Cohort study. Eur Heart J 2015;36(5):297.

31. Guo Y, Wang H, Zhao X, et al. Sequential changes in renal function and the risk of stroke and death in patients with atrial fibrillation. Int J Cardiol 2013; 168(5):4678.

32. Roldán V, Marín F, Fernández H, et al. Renal impairment in a "real-life" cohort of anticoagulated patients with atrial fibrillation (implications for thromboembolism and bleeding). Am J Cardiol 2013;111(8):1159.

33. Huang KW, Leu HB, Luo JC, et al. Different peptic ulcer bleeding risk in chronic kidney disease and end-stage renal disease patients receiving different dialysis. Dig Dis Sci 2014;59(4):807.

34. Sood P, Kumar G, Nanchal R, et al. Chronic kidney disease and end-stage renal disease predict higher risk of mortality in patients with primary upper gastrointestinal bleeding. Am J Nephrol 2012;35(3):216.

35. Luo JC, Leu HB, Hou MC, et al. Nonpeptic ulcer, nonvariceal gastrointestinal bleeding in hemodialysis patients. Am J Med 2013;126(3):264.

36. Kuo CC, Kuo HW, Lee IM, et al. The risk of upper gastrointestinal bleeding in patients treated with hemodialysis: a population-based cohort study. BMC Nephrol 2013;14:15.

37. Bos MJ, Koudstaal PJ, Hofman A, et al. Decreased glomerular filtration rate is a risk factor for hemorrhagic but not for ischemic stroke: the Rotterdam Study. Stroke 2007;38(12):3127–32.

38. Shimizu Y, Maeda K, Imano H, et al. Chronic kidney disease and drinking status in relation to risks of stroke and its subtypes: the circulatory risk in communities study (CIRCS). Stroke 2011;42(9):2531.

39. Iseki K, Kinjo K, Kimura Y, et al. Evidence for high risk of cerebral hemorrhage in chronic dialysis patients. Kidney Int 1993;44(5):1086.

40. Chao TF, Liu CJ, Wang KL, et al. Incidence and prediction of ischemic stroke among atrial fibrillation patients with end-stage renal disease requiring dialysis. Heart Rhythm 2014;11(10):1752.

41. Chan PH, Huang D, Yip PS, et al. Ischaemic stroke in patients with atrial fibrillation with chronic kidney disease undergoing peritoneal dialysis. Europace 2016;18(5):665.

42. Roldán V, Marín F, Manzano-Fernández S, et al. Does chronic kidney disease improve the predictive value of the CHADS2 and CHA2DS2-VASc stroke stratification risk scores for atrial fibrillation? Thromb Haemost 2013;109(5):956.

43. Pepe MS, Fan J, Feng Z, et al. The net reclassification index (NRI): a Misleading measure of prediction improvement even with independent test data Sets. Stat Biosci 2015;7(2):282.

44. Banerjee A, Fauchier L, Vourc'H P, et al. Renal impairment and ischemic stroke risk assessment in patients with atrial fibrillation: the Loire valley atrial fibrillation project. J Am Coll Cardiol 2013; 61(20):2079.

45. Kornej J, Hindricks G, Kosiuk J, et al. Renal dysfunction, stroke risk scores (CHADS2, CHA2DS2-VASc, and R2CHADS2), and the risk of thromboembolic events after catheter ablation of atrial fibrillation: the Leipzig Heart Center AF Ablation Registry. Circ Arrhythm Electrophysiol 2013;6(5):868.

46. Bautista J, Bella A, Chaudhari A, et al. Advanced chronic kidney disease in non-valvular atrial fibrillation: Extending the utility of R2CHADS2 to patients with advanced renal failure. Clin Kidney J 2015; 8(2):226.

47. Abumuaileq RR, Abu-Assi E, López-López A, et al. Comparison between CHA2DS2-VASc and the new R2CHADS2 and ATRIA scores at predicting thromboembolic event in non-anticoagulated and anticoagulated patients with non-valvular atrial fibrillation. BMC Cardiovasc Disord 2015;15:156.

48. Singer DE, Chang Y, Borowsky LH, et al. A new risk scheme to predict ischemic stroke and other thromboembolism in atrial fibrillation: the ATRIA study stroke risk score. J Am Heart Assoc 2013; 2(3):e000250.

49. Kerr KF, Wang Z, Janes H, et al. Net reclassification indices for evaluating risk-prediction instruments: a critical Review NIH public access. Epidemiology 2014;25(1):114–21.

50. Lau YC, Proietti M, Guiducci E, et al. Atrial fibrillation and thromboembolism in patients with chronic kidney disease. J Am Coll Cardiol 2016;68(13): 1452–64.

51. Borre ED, Goode A, Raitz G, et al. Predicting thromboembolic and bleeding event risk in patients with non-valvular atrial fibrillation: a systematic review. Thromb Haemost 2018;118(12):2171–87.

52. Zulkifly H, Lip GYH, Lane DA. Bleeding risk scores in atrial fibrillation and venous thromboembolism. Am J Cardiol 2017;120(7):1139.

53. Guo Y, Lane DA, Chen Y, et al. Regular bleeding risk assessment associated with reduction in bleeding outcomes: the mAFA-II randomized trial. Am J Med 2020;133(10):1195–202.e2.

54. Khalid F, Qureshi W, Qureshi S, et al. Impact of restarting warfarin therapy in renal disease anticoagulated patients with gastrointestinal hemorrhage. Ren Fail 2013;35(9):1228.

55. Sengupta N, Feuerstein JD, Patwardhan VR, et al. The risks of thromboembolism vs. recurrent gastrointestinal bleeding after interruption of systemic anticoagulation in hospitalized inpatients with gastrointestinal bleeding: a prospective study. Am J Gastroenterol 2015;110(2):328.

56. Staerk L, Lip GY, Olesen JB, et al. Stroke and recurrent haemorrhage associated with antithrombotic treatment after gastrointestinal bleeding in patients with atrial fibrillation: nationwide cohort STUDY. BMJ 2015;351:h5876.

57. Kamel H, Okin PM, Elkind MS, et al. Atrial fibrillation and mechanisms of stroke: time for a new model. Stroke 2016;47(3):895.

58. Lip G, Freedman B, De Caterina R, et al. Stroke prevention in atrial fibrillation: Past, present and future. Comparing the guidelines and practical decision-making. Thromb Haemost 2017;117(7):1230–9.

59. Nielsen PB, Skjøth F, Overvad TF, et al. Female sex is a risk modifier rather than a risk factor for stroke in atrial fibrillation. Circulation 2018;137(8):832–40.

60. Proietti M, Lane DA, Lip GYH. Chronic kidney disease, time in therapeutic range and adverse clinical outcomes in anticoagulated patients with non-valvular atrial fibrillation: observations from the SPORTIF trials. EBioMedicine 2016;8:309.

61. Szummer K, Gasparini A, Eliasson S, et al. Time in therapeutic range and outcomes after warfarin initiation in newly diagnosed atrial fibrillation patients with renal dysfunction. J Am Heart Assoc 2017;6:3.

62. Holden RM, Booth SL. Vascular calcification in chronic kidney disease: the role of vitamin K. Nat Clin Pract Nephrol 2007;3(10):522.

63. Hayashi M, Takamatsu I, Kanno Y, et al. A case-control study of calciphylaxis in Japanese end-stage renal disease patients. Nephrol Dial Transpl 2012;27(4):1580.

64. Brodsky SV, Nadasdy T, Rovin BH, et al. Warfarin-related nephropathy occurs in patients with and without chronic kidney disease and is associated with an increased mortality rate. Kidney Int 2011; 80(2):181.

65. Böhm M, Ezekowitz MD, Connolly SJ, et al. Changes in renal function in patients with atrial fibrillation: an analysis from the RE-LY Trial. J Am Coll Cardiol 2015;65(23):2481–93.

66. FC B, HA S, Yuliya L, et al. On-treatment outcomes in patients with worsening renal function with rivaroxaban compared with warfarin. Circulation 2016; 134(1):37–47.

67. Hijazi Z, Hohnloser SH, Andersson U, et al. Efficacy and safety of apixaban compared with warfarin in patients with atrial fibrillation in relation to renal function over time: insights from the ARISTOTLE randomized clinical trial. JAMA Cardiol 2016 Jul; 1(4):451–60.

68. Shah M, Avgil Tsadok M, Jackevicius CA, et al. Warfarin use and the risk for stroke and bleeding in patients with atrial fibrillation undergoing dialysis. Circulation 2014;129(11):1196.

69. Martín-Pérez M, Gaist D, De Abajo F, et al. Predictors of over-anticoagulation in warfarin users in the UK general population: a nested case-control study in a primary health care database. Thromb Haemost 2019;119(01):066–76.

70. Connolly SJ, Ezekowitz MD, Yusuf S, et al. Dabigatran versus warfarin in patients with atrial fibrillation. N Engl J Med 2009;361(12):1139.

71. Connolly SJ, Eikelboom J, Joyner C, et al. Apixaban in patients with atrial fibrillation. N Engl J Med 2011;364(9):806.

72. Patel MR, Mahaffey KW, Garg J, et al. Rivaroxaban versus warfarin in nonvalvular atrial fibrillation. N Engl J Med 2011;365(10):883.

73. Granger CB, Alexander JH, McMurray JJ, et al. Apixaban versus warfarin in patients with atrial fibrillation. N Engl J Med 2011;365(11):981.

74. Giugliano RP, Ruff CT, Braunwald E, et al. Edoxaban versus warfarin in patients with atrial fibrillation. N Engl J Med 2013;369(22):2093.

75. Hijazi Z, Hohnloser SH, Oldgren J, et al. Efficacy and safety of dabigatran compared with warfarin in relation to baseline renal function in patients with atrial fibrillation: a RE-LY (Randomized evaluation of long-term anticoagulation therapy) trial analysis. Circulation 2014;129(9):961.

76. He W, Zhang H, Zhu W, et al. Effect of anticoagulation therapy in older patients with chronic kidney disease and atrial fibrillation: a meta-analysis. Medicine (Baltimore) 2019;98(42):e17628.

77. Stanifer JW, Pokorney SD, Chertow GM, et al. Apixaban versus warfarin in patients with atrial fibrillation and advanced chronic kidney disease. Circulation 2020;141(17):1384–92.

78. Hart RG, Pearce LA, Asinger RW, et al. Warfarin in atrial fibrillation patients with moderate chronic kidney disease. Clin J Am Soc Nephrol 2011;6(11): 2599.

79. Fox KA, Piccini JP, Wojdyla D, et al. Prevention of stroke and systemic embolism with rivaroxaban compared with warfarin in patients with non-valvular atrial fibrillation and moderate renal impairment. Eur Heart J 2011;32(19):2387.

80. Hohnloser SH, Hijazi Z, Thomas L, et al. Efficacy of apixaban when compared with warfarin in relation to renal function in patients with atrial fibrillation: insights from the ARISTOTLE trial. Eur Heart J 2012; 33(22):2821.

81. Eikelboom JW, Connolly SJ, Gao P, et al. Stroke risk and efficacy of apixaban in atrial fibrillation patients with moderate chronic kidney disease. J Stroke Cerebrovasc Dis 2012;21(6):429.

82. Bohula EA, Giugliano RP, Ruff CT, et al. Impact of renal function on outcomes with edoxaban in the ENGAGE AF-TIMI 48 trial. Circulation 2016; 134(1):24.

83. Steffel J, Verhamme P, Potpara TS, et al. The 2018 European Heart Rhythm Association Practical Guide on the use of non-Vitamin K antagonist oral anticoagulants in patients with atrial fibrillation. Eur Heart J 2018;39(16):1330–93.

84. Yu HT, Yang PS, Kim TH, et al. Impact of renal function on outcomes with edoxaban in real-world patients with atrial fibrillation a nationwide cohort study. Stroke 2018;49(10):2421–9.

85. Yang F, Hellyer JA, Than C, et al. Warfarin utilisation and anticoagulation control in patients with atrial fibrillation and chronic kidney disease. Heart 2017;103(11):818–26.

86. Winkelmayer WC, Turakhia MP. Warfarin treatment in patients with atrial fibrillation and advanced chronic kidney disease: Sins of omission or commission? JAMA 2014;311(9):913.

87. Olesen JB, Lip GY, Lindhardsen J, et al. Risks of thromboembolism and bleeding with thromboprophylaxis in patients with atrial fibrillation: a net clinical benefit analysis using a "real world" nationwide cohort study. Thromb Haemost 2011;106(4):739.

88. Genovesi S, Rossi E, Gallieni M, et al. Warfarin use, mortality, bleeding and stroke in haemodialysis patients with atrial fibrillation. Nephrol Dial Transpl 2015;30(3):491.

89. Abbott KC, Trespalacios FC, Taylor AJ, et al. Atrial fibrillation in chronic dialysis patients in the United States: risk factors for hospitalization and mortality. BMC Nephrol 2003;4:1.

90. Carrero JJ, Evans M, Szummer K, et al. Warfarin, kidney dysfunction, and outcomes following acute myocardial infarction in patients with atrial fibrillation. JAMA 2014;311(9):919.

91. Shen JI, Montez-Rath ME, Lenihan CR, et al. Outcomes after warfarin initiation in a cohort of hemodialysis patients with newly diagnosed atrial fibrillation. Am J Kidney Dis 2015;66(4):677–88.

92. Wiesholzer M, Harm F, Tomasec G, et al. Incidence of stroke among chronic hemodialysis patients with nonrheumatic atrial fibrillation. Am J Nephrol 2001; 21(1):35–9.

93. Chan KE, Lazarus JM, Thadhani R, et al. Warfarin use associates with increased risk for stroke in hemodialysis patients with atrial fibrillation. J Am Soc Nephrol 2009;20(10):2223.

94. Phelan PJ, O'Kelly P, Holian J, et al. Warfarin use in hemodialysis patients: what is the risk? Clin Nephrol 2011;75(3):204.

95. Winkelmayer WC, Liu J, Setoguchi S, et al. Effectiveness and safety of warfarin initiation in older hemodialysis patients with incident atrial fibrillation. Clin J Am Soc Nephrol 2011;6(11):2662.

96. Knoll F, Sturm G, Lamina C, et al. Coumarins and survival in incident dialysis patients. Nephrol Dial Transpl 2012;27(1):332.

97. Sood MM, Larkina M, Thumma JR, et al. Major bleeding events and risk stratification of antithrombotic agents in hemodialysis: results from the DOPPS. Kidney Int 2013;84(3):600.

98. Chen JJ, Lin LY, Yang YH, et al. Anti-platelet or anticoagulant agent for the prevention of ischemic stroke in patients with end-stage renal disease and atrial fibrillation–a nation-wide database analyses. Int J Cardiol 2014;177(3):1008.

99. Wakasugi M, Kazama JJ, Tokumoto A, et al. Association between warfarin use and incidence of ischemic stroke in Japanese hemodialysis patients with chronic sustained atrial fibrillation: a prospective cohort study. Clin Exp Nephrol 2014;18(4):662.

100. JC T, Samuel WL, Hugh C, et al. 2019 AHA/ACC/HRS focused update of the 2014 AHA/ACC/HRS guideline for the management of patients with atrial fibrillation: a report of the American College of cardiology/American heart association task Force on clinical Practice guidelines and the heart R. Circulation 2019;140(2):e125–51.

101. Chan KE, Edelman ER, Wenger JB, et al. Dabigatran and rivaroxaban use in atrial fibrillation patients on hemodialysis. Circulation 2015;131(11): 972–9.

102. Kuno T, Takagi H, Ando T, et al. Oral anticoagulation for patients with atrial fibrillation on long-term hemodialysis. J Am Coll Cardiol 2020;75(3): 273–85.

103. Ha JT, Neuen BL, Cheng LP, et al. Benefits and harms of oral anticoagulant therapy in chronic kidney disease: a systematic review and meta-analysis. Ann Intern Med 2019;171(3):181–9.

104. Qamar A, Bhatt DL. Anticoagulation therapy: balancing the risks of stroke and bleeding in CKD. Nat Rev Nephrol 2015;11(4):200.

105. Yao X, Shah ND, Sangaralingham LR, et al. Non–Vitamin K antagonist oral anticoagulant dosing in

patients with atrial fibrillation and renal dysfunction. J Am Coll Cardiol 2017;69(23):2779.

106. Andreu-Cayuelas JM, Pastor-Pérez FJ, Puche CM, et al. Impact of variations in kidney function on non-vitamin K oral anticoagulant dosing in patients with atrial fibrillation and recent acute heart failure. Rev Esp Cardiol (Engl Ed) 2016;69(2):134.

107. Kirchhof P, Breithardt G, Bax J, et al. A roadmap to improve the quality of atrial fibrillation management: Proceedings from the fifth Atrial Fibrillation Network/European Heart Rhythm Association consensus conference. Europace 2015;18(1): 37–50.

108. SD. P. Renal hemodialysis patients allocated apixaban versus warfarin in atrial fibrillation—RENAL-AF.Presented at the American Heart Association Annual Scientific Sessions; November 16, 2019; Philadelphia, PA.

109. Boriani G, Savelieva I, Dan GA, et al. Chronic kidney disease in patients with cardiac rhythm disturbances or implantable electrical devices: clinical significance and implications for decision making-a position paper of the European Heart Rhythm Association endorsed by the Heart Rhythm Society and the Asia Pacific Heart Rhythm Society. Europace 2015;17(8):1169.

110. Khouri Y, Stephens T, Ayuba G, et al. Understanding and managing atrial fibrillation in patients with kidney disease. J Atr Fibrillation 2015;7(6):1069.

111. Potpara TS, Lenarczyk R, Larsen TB, et al. Management of atrial fibrillation in patients with chronic kidney disease in Europe results of the European heart rhythm association survey. Europace 2015; 17(12):1862–7.

112. Li M, Liu T, Luo D, et al. Systematic review and meta-analysis of chronic kidney disease as predictor of atrial fibrillation recurrence following catheter ablation. Cardiol J 2014;21(1):89.

113. Hayashi M, Kaneko S, Shimano M, et al. Efficacy and safety of radiofrequency catheter ablation for atrial fibrillation in chronic hemodialysis patients. Nephrol Dial Transpl 2014;29(1):160.

114. Kornej J, Hindricks G, Banerjee A, et al. Changes in renal function after catheter ablation of atrial fibrillation are associated with CHADS2and CHA2DS2-VASc scores and arrhythmia recurrences. Heart 2015;101(2):126–31.

115. Diemberger I, Genovesi S, Massaro G, et al. Meta-analysis of clinical outcomes of electrical cardioversion and catheter ablation in patients with atrial fibrillation and chronic kidney disease. Curr Pharm Des 2018;24(24):2794–801.

116. Kefer J, Tzikas A, Freixa X, et al. Impact of chronic kidney disease on left atrial appendage occlusion for stroke prevention in patients with atrial fibrillation. Int J Cardiol 2016;207:335.

117. Reddy VY, Doshi SK, Kar S, et al. 5-Year outcomes after left atrial appendage closure: from the PRE-VAIL and PROTECT AF trials. J Am Coll Cardiol 2017;70(24):2964–75.

118. Kirchhof P, Benussi S, Kotecha D, et al. 2016 2016 ESC Guidelines for the management of atrial fibrillation developed in collaboration with EACTS. Eur Heart J 2016;37(38):2893.

119. Boriani G, Proietti M, Laroche C, et al. Contemporary stroke prevention strategies in 11 096 European patients with atrial fibrillation: a report from the EURObservational Research Programme on atrial fibrillation (EORP-AF) long-term general Registry. Europace 2018;20(5):747–57.

120. Potpara TS, Dan GA, Trendafilova E, et al. Stroke prevention in atrial fibrillation and "real world" adherence to guidelines in the Balkan region: the BALKAN-AF survey. Sci Rep 2016;6: 20432.

121. Gallagher C, Elliott AD, Wong CX, et al. Integrated care in atrial fibrillation: a systematic review and meta-analysis. Heart 2017;103(24):1947–53.

122. Shang W, Li L, Huang S, et al. Chronic kidney disease and the risk of new- onset atrial fibrillation: a meta-analysis of prospective cohort studies. PLoS One 2016;11(5):1–10.

123. Bansal N, Zelnick LR, Alonso A, et al. eGFR and albuminuria in relation to risk of incident atrial fibrillation: a meta-analysis of the jackson heart study, the multi-ethnic study of atherosclerosis, and the cardiovascular health study. Clin J Am Soc Nephrol 2017;12(9):1386–98.

124. Odutayo A, Wong CX, Hsiao AJ, et al. Atrial fibrillation and risks of cardiovascular disease, renal disease, and death: systematic review and meta-analysis. BMJ 2016;354:i4482.

125. Zeng WT, Sun XT, Tang K, et al. Risk of thromboembolic events in atrial fibrillation with chronic kidney disease. Stroke 2015;46(1):157–63.

126. Bai Y, Chen H, Yang Y, et al. Safety of antithrombotic drugs in patients with atrial fibrillation and non-end-stage chronic kidney disease: meta-analysis and systematic review. Thromb Res 2016;137:46–52.

127. Dahal K, Kunwar S, Rijal J, et al. Stroke, major bleeding, and mortality outcomes in warfarin users with atrial fibrillation and chronic kidney disease: a meta-analysis of observational studies. Chest 2016;149(4):951–9.

128. Malhotra K, Ishfaq MF, Goyal N, et al. Oral anticoagulation in patients with chronic kidney disease: a systematic review and meta-analysis. Neurology 2019;92(21):e2421–31.

129. Tan J, Liu S, Segal JB, et al. Warfarin use and stroke, bleeding and mortality risk in patients with end stage renal disease and atrial fibrillation: a

systematic review and meta-analysis. BMC Nephrol 2016;17(1):157.

130. Randhawa MS, Vishwanath R, Rai MP, et al. Association between use of warfarin for atrial fibrillation and outcomes among patients with end-stage renal disease: a systematic review and meta-analysis. JAMA Netw Open 2020;3(4):e202175.

131. Harel Z, Sholzberg M, Shah PS, et al. Comparisons between novel oral anticoagulants and vitamin K antagonists in patients with CKD. J Am Soc Nephrol 2014;25(3):431–42.

132. Andò G, Capranzano P. Non-vitamin K antagonist oral anticoagulants in atrial fibrillation patients with chronic kidney disease: a systematic review and network meta-analysis. Int J Cardiol 2017; 231:162–9.

133. Kimachi M, Furukawa TA, Kimachi K, et al. Direct oral anticoagulants versus warfarin for preventing stroke and systemic embolic events among atrial fibrillation patients with chronic kidney disease. Cochrane Database Syst Rev 2017;11(11): CD011373.

Atrial Fibrillation in Valvular Heart Disease

Bobby John, MBBS, MD, DM, PhD, FHRS[a,b,c,*], Chu-Pak Lau, MD[d]

KEYWORDS

- Atrial fibrillation • Rheumatic heart disease • Remodeling • Embolism

KEY POINTS

- Atrial fibrillation in rheumatic heart disease increases the embolic risk several folds compared with the nonvalvular group.
- Prompt identification of atrial fibrillation and institution of oral anticoagulation is imperative to reduce morbidity and mortality.
- Identification of a high-risk subset that is prone to develop atrial fibrillation may prevent its devastating complications.
- Substrate maintaining atrial fibrillation may be reversible in the early stages.

PREVALENCE OF RHEUMATIC HEART DISEASE

The prevalence of rheumatic heart disease (RHD) declined in the developed world after the industrial revolution.[1,2] However, it continues to be a major health problem in the developing world. Even in developed countries, pockets of indigenous population may remain affected, as for example, in the aboriginal population of Australia and the New Zealand Maori.[3] It is estimated that 15.6 million suffer from RHD and 3%.0 to 7.5% of all strokes in developing countries are directly related to RHD.[4–6]

The 3 main factors that have been reported to determine the prevalence of RHD in a community are (1) the environmental factors; (2) virulence of the organism, that is, Group A *Streptococcus*; and (3) the host. Lower socioeconomic status and overcrowding are associated with higher prevalence of RHD, especially in children living in households of more than 8. The virulence of the organism contributed to the resurgence of rheumatic fever in the United States.[7,8] Racial difference in prevalence of RHD within the same geographic location has been observed, but has been attributed to the difference in exposure and treatment rather than genetic susceptibility.[9] In a recent survey, the prevalence of RHD in the aboriginal population was 11.8 per 1000 and 6.5 per 1000 in the Maori population of New Zealand.[3,10] Comparable findings were noted in the Indian population, where the prevalence was 6 per 1000.[11]

The estimated prevalence of RHD in a community depends on the size of the population that has been studied, in addition to the definition, method used to confirm the diagnosis, and the period in which it was undertaken. This was evident in a study conducted by Jose and Gomathi[12] that included 229,829 school-going children. Of the 374 children who were diagnosed by auscultation to have heart disease, only 41.8% (157) were diagnosed to have RHD on color Doppler study, emphasizing that both the population studied and diagnostic tool used would change the prevalence.[12]

An extensive study that uses echocardiogram as the diagnostic tool would involve tremendous financial resource and skilled personal, thus limiting the number of subjects who could be screened. A systematic review by Noubiap and

[a] James Cook University, Townsville, Australia; [b] Cardiology Unit, Townsville University Hospital, 100 Angus Smith Drive, Douglas, Queensland 4814, Australia; [c] Christian Medical College, Vellore, India; [d] Department of Medicine, Queen Mary Hospital, The University of Hong Kong, Suite 1301-3, Central Building, 1 Pedder Street, Central, Hong Kong
* Corresponding author. Cardiology Unit, Townsville University Hospital, 100 Angus Smith Drive, Douglas, QLD 4814, Australia.
E-mail address: bobby.john@health.qld.gov.au

colleagues[13] found that when the auscultatory method was used to screen the population and further confirmation was carried out using echocardiogram, the cumulative prevalence per 1000 was 6.3 (95% confidence interval [CI] 4.02–9.21) in a total population of 774,073, as opposed to 21.23 per 1000 (95% CI 15.26–28.94) using echocardiogram but with screening of a far smaller population of 296,909. This suggests the limitations of auscultation as a tool and also at the same time, the sensitivity of echocardiogram to diagnose borderline cases that may not necessarily progress to chronic RHD with the attendant structural changes. The review highlighted that only 11.3% (95% CI 6.9–16.5) progressed to definite RHD.[13]

PREVALENCE OF ATRIAL FIBRILLATION IN RHEUMATIC HEART DISEASE

Prevalence of the arrhythmia in the rheumatic population is widely variable. This is primarily because of differing periods of study, diagnostic methods used, and the country in which it was reviewed.

Diker and colleagues[14] in 1995, in a retrospective study using echocardiographic criteria, evaluated 1100 patients in Turkey and reported it in 29% of patients with pure mitral stenosis and in 58% of those with mitral stenosis in conjunction with other valvular disease. The prevalence among those with pure aortic valve disease was rare; none seen in those with aortic regurgitation and 5% in those with aortic stenosis.[14] Okello and colleagues,[15] in a cross-sectional study of 309 patients with newly diagnosed RHD attending a tertiary hospital in Africa, found the overall prevalence of atrial fibrillation (AF) was 13.9%. Among these, AF was most prevalent in those with mitral regurgitation (81.4%) and mitral stenosis (58.1%), whereas it was not common in aortic regurgitation (32.6%) and none found in patients with aortic stenosis.[15] Negi and colleagues,[16] while studying 1918 consecutive patients attending a tertiary hospital in India, found that those with tricuspid regurgitation had the highest prevalence of AF (34.9%) as compared with mitral stenosis (31.7%) and mitral regurgitation (25.3%). There was no association of AF with aortic valve disease in this study.

INCIDENCE OF ATRIAL FIBRILLATION IN RHEUMATIC HEART DISEASE

Longitudinal studies of patients with mitral stenosis determining the incidence of AF are very few and far between. One of the earliest studies was done in a Swedish cohort by Olesen.[17] He followed a cohort of patients with isolated mitral stenosis with a mean age of 41.5 (range 14–73) years from 1932 to 1951 and found a prevalence of 57%.[17] In this study, the diagnosis of mitral stenosis was based solely on clinical examination and later confirmed at autopsy in some. The largest series was published by Paul Wood[18] in 1954 involving 300 patients. He reported an incidence of 40%, of which 5% were paroxysmal episodes. It is likely that the incidence of paroxysmal AF was underestimated in this study for lack of very close follow-up.

SEQUEL OF ATRIAL FIBRILLATION

AF in the rheumatic population heralds in greater morbidity and mortality as compared with the nonrheumatic population. It is not uncommon for patients to become symptomatic for the first time with the onset of AF; acute pulmonary edema, as a result of fast ventricular rate and abbreviated diastolic filling time, being one such example.[19] It precipitates cardiac failure and increases mortality.[20,21] The most devastating complication is systemic embolization with 18.0% ± 6.8% of patients having left atrial thrombus.[22] Coulshed and colleagues,[23] in an extensive study involving 737 patients with predominant mitral stenosis, found that 32% of patients with AF developed systemic embolism in contrast to 8% in the sinus rhythm group. The most common site of embolization was the cerebral circulation, being found in 60% to 75%.[18,24] Unlike the nonrheumatic population, AF conferred 17.5-fold increased risk for stroke as opposed to the fivefold risk in the former.[25] Notably, stroke occurs in a much younger population with consequent loss of man power and resultant burden on the economy. In addition, AF is associated with poorer outcome after surgical valvular intervention.

ASYMPTOMATIC ATRIAL FIBRILLATION IN RHEUMATIC HEART DISEASE

Silent AF poses a great risk for thromboembolic events as revealed in a study by Coulshed and colleagues.[23] More than 20% of patients with RHD presenting with ischemic stroke for the first time, were in sinus rhythm.[23] Therefore, it has become apparent that they were not truly in sinus rhythm but would have periods of AF that predisposed them to embolic events. In a cohort of 179 patients who were in sinus rhythm at presentation, 27% had AF lasting 30 seconds recorded on 24-hour ambulatory electrocardiogram monitor.[26] When a broader class of supraventricular arrhythmias were included, such as paroxysmal atrial tachycardia, multifocal atrial tachycardia, and flutter in addition to AF, the number who suffered from the rhythm disturbance was higher; approaching more than 50%.[27] It was even more remarkable to note that 95% of these patients were asymptomatic.[27] These patients, although asymptomatic, remained at risk for embolic complications.

PREDICTORS FOR ATRIAL FIBRILLATION IN RHEUMATIC HEART DISEASE

Publications related to predictors for AF in native rheumatic valvular disease are scant (Table 1). Age at presentation has been an important determinant for prevalence of AF. In a number of studies, it has been consistently found that patients older than 50 years have a high prevalence, between 33% and 57%.[16,28–34]

It would be intuitive to consider functional symptom class to correlate with AF, as it would reflect deleterious hemodynamic effects of the arrhythmia and also duration of the disease in the subject. However, there have been differing observations. Almost one-third of patients who have New York Heart Association (NYHA) class II or more symptoms have been found to have AF in a registry of almost 2000 patients.[16] Kabukcu and colleagues[35] made similar observations in 92 patients. Those with AF were most often in NYHA Class III (74% vs 22%) compared with subjects who maintained sinus rhythm.[35] However, a study of 650 patients undergoing mitral valve intervention in France did not find functional class as a significant predictor for AF.[36]

Left atrial diameter on echocardiogram has shown to be an important parameter to predict AF. Henry and colleagues[37] reported a prevalence of 54% when the left atrial diameter was greater than 4.0 cm. This was further corroborated by Diker and colleagues,[14] in which mean left atrial dimension of 5.7 ± 1.2 cm (P<.0001) was found in those with AF. Recent studies, from India have reported left atrial dimension greater than 22 mm/m^2 and presence of spontaneous echo contrast as significant risk factors for AF and consequently ischemic stroke.[38]

Valve calcification is found in 35% of patients with mitral valve disease and its prevalence increases with age.[39] It is an important marker for embolic events and may well be a manifestation of the length of time the disease process has been established.[23,36] A multivariate analysis including 650 patients found mitral valve calcification as a significant predictor for AF.[36]

There are conflicting reports on the presence of pulmonary hypertension and mitral valve gradient as predictors for AF. Diker and colleagues[14] found that mean mitral valve gradient of 9.5 ± 6.1 mm Hg was strongly associated with AF (P<.05). Gupta

and colleagues,[38] in a case-control design, noted that presence of pulmonary hypertension (75% vs 42.5%, P = .003) conferred higher risk for ischemic stroke. However, Kabukcu and colleagues[35] did not find a correlation with hemodynamic derangements and AF. Similarly, Negi and colleagues[16] in a multivariate analysis did not observe pulmonary hypertension to be a contributor for AF, but tricuspid regurgitation was an important determinant.

The severity of mitral valve stenosis has correlated with AF. Mitral valve area less than 1.0 cm^2 has been found in most patients with AF in a cross-sectional study done in India.[38,40]

STRUCTURALLY REMODELING IN MITRAL STENOSIS

Interstitial fibrosis, degenerative remodeling, and inflammation are hallmarks of pathologic changes in the rheumatic atria.[41–46] The differences in pathology relate to the age of the patient, the site of sampling, and the severity of mitral stenosis. The upstream changes related to elevated atrial pressure in mitral stenosis are not uniform. It affects each of the atria differently and some parts more than others. Shenthar and colleagues[41] studied patients with isolated mitral stenosis undergoing open heart surgery. Intraoperative biopsies of 5 different sites from both atria were sampled. Although interstitial fibrosis was found in all sites, endocardial inflammation was most common in the left atrial appendage. Advanced matrix and subendocardial remodeling was found more extensively in the left atrium than the right atrium by Park and colleagues.[46] On electron microscopy, cells affected by AF revealed widespread loss of contractile elements with marked areas of sarcoplasmic vacuolation.[45] Myocytolysis was seen as opposed to myocyte hypertrophy and glycogen deposition in sinus rhythm.[41]

Fibrogenesis is a complex process. It occurs consequent to deposition of extracellular matrix and activity of connective tissue growth factor. Studies have confirmed that transforming growth factor-β1 (TGF-β1) plays a pivotal role in differentiation of cardiac myofibroblast. TGF-β1 results in phosphorylation of focal adhesion molecule (FAK) and its downstream effects are mediated by AKT/S6K signaling pathway. This was evidenced by suppression of α-smooth muscle actin expression in TGF-β1–induced fibroblasts with FAK and AKT inhibitors in an animal model.[44] In addition, calreticulin and integrin-alpha5 expression has been found to correlate with AF among patients with RHD.[47]

Remodeling of connexins have been explored as another mechanism of AF in patients with

Table 1
Published predictors of atrial fibrillation occurrence in rheumatic mitral stenosis

Risk Factors	Remarks	
Age, y[16,28–34]	<40	21%
	40–54	59%
	55–69	73%
	≥70	85%[34]
NYHA Class[16,35]	≥NYHA Class II increase risk	
Left atrium diameter[14,37,38]	>4 cm 54%[37]	
Valve calcification[36,39]		
Valve area[38,40]	<1 cm²[38,40]	
Mitral valve gradient[14]	>10 mm Hg	
Pulmonary artery hypertension[38]		

Abbreviation: NYHA, New York Heart Association.

RHD. Samples of right atrial appendage were examined. The collagen volume fraction of type 1 (CVF-1) was significantly increased whereas the volume fraction of connexin-43 was reduced in AF, suggesting its role in arrhythmogenesis.[42]

Immunohistochemistry, quantitative real-time polymerase chain reaction, and Western blotting have been used to evaluate the signaling pathway in fibrosis related to RHD.[43] Alpha-actin-2 was upregulated via the TGF-β1/Smad pathway in patients with AF secondary to RHD compared with those in sinus rhythm with congenital heart disease. Angiotensin II/Rac1/STAT3 signaling is the other putative pathway to induce atrial fibrosis in this subset of patients.[48]

ELECTROANATOMICAL REMODELING OF THE ATRIA IN RHEUMATIC MITRAL STENOSIS

Chronic mitral stenosis results in left atrial "stretch" due to elevated pressure. Although left atrial enlargement due to stretch per se may be sufficient to explain the increase in AF in this population, rheumatic process affecting the atrium also results in significant electrical remodeling, thereby creating the substrate for atrial arrhythmias. Dilatation and pressure on the PVs and elsewhere may also increase their firing and serve as triggers. This electrical remodeling has been validated in patients who were undergoing percutaneous mitral commissurotomy (PTMC). The control population consisted of patients who underwent transseptal puncture for ablation of left side accessory pathways.[49]

Patients with mitral stenosis demonstrated the following abnormalities compared with controls (**Fig. 1**):

i. Marked conduction abnormalities within the atria characterized by regions of double potentials, fractionated electrograms, prolonged conduction times, and P-wave duration, and site-specific conduction delay.
ii. No change or an increase in effective refractory period (ERP) with no change in heterogeneity of ERP and preservation of rate adaptation of ERP. This finding is consistent with prior studies evaluating clinical substrates for AF but in contrast to the remodeling attributed to AF itself.
iii. Sinus node remodeling characterized by prolongation of the corrected sinus node recovery times.

Potentially as a consequence of these abnormalities, patients with mitral stenosis developed AF more frequently.

Importantly, although these abnormalities were observed within both atria, their extent was greater in the left atrium than the right atrium. Thus, the electrical substrate for AF in patients with MS is related to the structural abnormalities and the associated widespread and site-specific conduction abnormalities rather than the changes observed in atrial refractoriness.

ACUTE EFFECTS REVERSAL OF CHRONIC ATRIAL STRETCH REVERSAL ON LEFT AND RIGHT ATRIAL ELECTRICAL REMODELING

As demonstrated, severe mitral stenosis results in significant electrical and electroanatomic remodeling of the atria. PTMC has been established to reverse the hemodynamic effects of the stenosed valve with marked reduction in left atrium size and pressure. The effect of acute pressure reduction following PTMC is associated with the following electrophysiological changes (**Fig. 2**):

i. An almost instantaneous reduction in P-wave duration (PWD) suggesting a global improvement in atrial conduction.
ii. Although there was no change in conduction time as evaluated along linearly placed catheters, there was improvement observed in site-specific conduction along the crista terminalis. In particular, there was significant improvement in conduction across this structure while pacing from the left atrium.
iii. There was no significant change in atrial refractoriness.
iv. Improvement in bipolar voltage in both the left atrium and right atrium with no regional specificity.
v. Increased conduction velocity in both the left atrium and right atrium with no regional specificity.

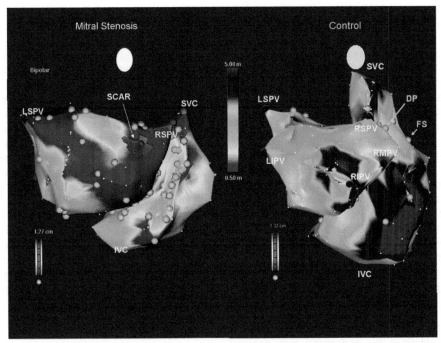

Fig. 1. Electroanatomic bipolar voltage map of a patient with mitral stenosis (*left*) and a representative age-matched control (*right*). Both atria are oriented in the posterior-anterior projection and are of similar scale. The color scale is identical in both images with red representing low voltage areas (≤0.5 mV) and purple being voltages ≥5 mV. The patient with MS (*left image*; left atrium 120 mL, right atrium 58 mL) has a much larger atria than the control patient (left atrium 80 mL, right atrium 100 mL). In addition to having greater regions of low voltage (*red*), the patient with mitral stenosis has regions of spontaneous scar (*gray*), and evidence of conduction abnormalities in the form of fractionated signals (FS; *pink tags*) and double potentials (DS; *blue tags*).

In another study involving 12 patients with mitral stenosis in sinus rhythm following PTMC, there was reduction of conduction delay (CD) and the index of heterogeneity (CoV) of ERP with homogeneous increase in regional ERPs.[50] On the other hand, in those patients with more severe mitral stenosis and AF cardioverted at the time of PTMC, both ERP and CD were unaffected after

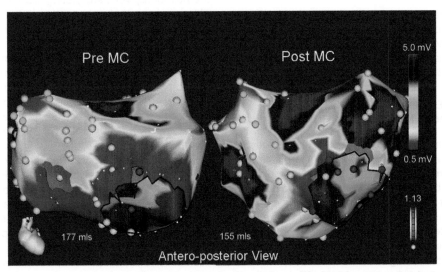

Fig. 2. Electroanatomic voltage map of the left atrium before and immediately after MC. Left is before and the right is after MC. Note the increase in voltage at all sites in left atrium with decrease in volume.

acute left atrium pressure reduction, suggesting chronic changes had already been established. However, both the vulnerability for AF induction and CoV of CD were reduced, suggesting stretch played an important role in AF induction. It is likely that rheumatic process or AF itself has made the atrial substrate more valuable in addition to pressure effect.

These findings suggest that the electroanatomic substrate predisposing to atrial arrhythmias due to chronic atrial stretch may be at least partially reversible with treatments directed at the stretch stimulus before it is established. Importantly, it demonstrates marked improvement in the structural and conduction abnormalities that are considered important elements of the AF substrate. Despite these limited changes, there was a trend for reduced vulnerability for AF.

LONG-TERM EFFECTS OF CHRONIC ATRIAL STRETCH REVERSAL

The long-term effects of chronic stretch reversal were characterized by performing high-density electrophysiological and electroanatomic mapping of the atria 6 months after MC. It revealed the following:

i. Progressive structural changes, which were characterized by a reduction in atrial size and an improvement in the bipolar voltage.
ii. There was widespread and site-specific improvement in conduction velocity associated with a significant reduction in the PWD.
iii. Reduction in atrial refractoriness.
iv. As a result of these changes, there was a reduction in the vulnerability for AF.

These findings stress the importance of treatment directed at reversal of stretch stimulus with progressive reversal of the abnormal electrophysiological and electroanatomic changes consequent to chronic stretch.[51]

SPATIOTEMPORAL ORGANIZATION AND ELECTROGRAM FRACTIONATION

With the increasing recognition that the sources maintaining persistent AF may not be limited to the posterior left atrium, this study sought to determine the bi-atrial characteristics of longstanding, persistent AF in valvular heart disease, a common substrate in which the mechanisms of AF remain incompletely characterized.[52] Using high-density endocardial mapping, the spatiotemporal organization and electrogram fractionation characteristics of longstanding, persistent AF in patients with and without valvular heart disease were

compared. Twenty patients with (n = 10) and without (n = 10) valvular heart disease due to mitral stenosis underwent bi-atrial, high-density contact-mapping during AF. Complex fractionated atrial electrograms were quantified using previously validated software, and activation frequencies and electrical organization characterized by spectral analysis. Slower activation frequencies ($P = .01$) and less fractionation ($P<.001$) was present in valvular AF (**Fig. 3**). Areas of greatest frequency and fractionation were located in the right atrium of valvular AF ($P = .005$ both), whereas these were in the left atrium in nonvalvular AF ($P<.01$ both). Similarly, most high-frequency "clusters" were in the right atrium in valvular AF (82%) as opposed to the left in nonvalvular AF (76%). A right-to-left gradient in organization index was additionally present in valvular AF ($P = .001$). The study suggests that a distinct substrate underlying longstanding, persistent AF is seen in patients with valvular heart disease. In a unique subgroup of patients, dominant right atrial sources were maintaining AF. These observations propose a potential role for ablation within the right atrium beyond current individual, but as yet suboptimally identified, patients who require ablation beyond the left atrium.[52]

REMODELING OF PULMONARY VEINS DUE TO CHRONIC STRETCH

The pulmonary vein has been established as a common source of trigger for AF.[53,54] It possesses distinct properties that promote arrhythmogenesis.[55,56] Pacemakerlike potential and spontaneous after depolarizations have been observed within the pulmonary vein, suggesting focal activity may play an important role in the arrhythmogenesis[57,58]; however, the anatomic structure of the pulmonary vein has been shown to promote heterogeneous conduction implicating reentry, as an alternative mechanism.[56,59] This is further supported by the finding that the pulmonary veins in patients with AF have been noted to possess distinctive electrophysiological properties characterized chiefly by abbreviation of ERP and delay in conduction.[60]

Elimination or isolation of pulmonary vein triggers are the main targets of catheter AF ablation; however, there are very few publications of the PV in AF. Although atrial stretch can lead to atrial electrophysiology change and PV firing, much less is known for RHD.[61,62] The electrophysiological properties of the pulmonary veins in RHD with mitral stenosis (n = 12; 29 ± 7 years) was compared with control group formed by those undergoing left-sided accessory pathway ablation

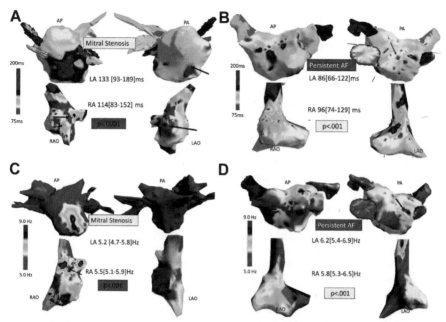

Fig. 3. (*A, B*) Bi-atrial complex fractionated electrograms during AF in valvular and nonvalvular heart disease. High-density color maps demonstrating complex fractionated electrogram during longstanding, persistent AF in a patient with valvular heart disease as compared with the nonvalvular heart disease. Note that areas of fractionation (*red color*) are clustered more often in the right atrium compared with the left atrium in mitral stenosis. (*C, D*) Bi-atrial activation frequencies during AF in valvular and nonvalvular heart disease. High-density color maps demonstrating activation frequencies during longstanding, persistent AF in a patient with valvular heart disease as compared with the nonvalvular heart disease. Note that areas of high frequency (*blue/purple color*) are clustered more often in the right atrium compared with the left atrium in mitral stenosis.

(n = 12; 31 ± 7 years) using multi-electrode basket to perform high-density mapping using the NavX system.[63] The ERP proximal/distal; conduction time (CT); intrapulmonary vein conduction block (CB; ≥30 ms between adjacent poles) resulting in circuitous conduction during the drive (S_1) and preexcited stimulus (S_2); and intrapulmonary vein voltage were determined. Acute stretch was induced in the control group by simultaneous right ventricle and pulmonary vein pacing. This resulted in ERP shortening (240 ± 33–225 ± 39 ms; P = .03), prolonged CT with S_2, which increased further with stretch (77 ± 30–88 ± 37 ms; P = .02). Intrapulmonary vein CB became prominent with S_2 and accentuated with stretch (40 ± 23–59 ± 32 ms; P<.0001). The changes were not site specific. On the other hand, chronic pressure-overload stretch, as seen in mitral stenosis, resulted in following:

i. Marked structural remodeling characterized by a greater region demonstrating low voltage.
ii. Prolongation of the pulmonary vein refractory period.
iii. Conduction slowing and block that was evident in some cases even during sinus rhythm.

These findings implicate stretch as cause for heterogeneous conduction abnormalities within the pulmonary vein that support reentry. Importantly, it provides evidence that the underlying condition can produce remodeling of the pulmonary veins, which in turn have a direct effect on the triggers of AF while creating the milieu for these structures to act as perpetuators or substrate for AF.

SUMMARY

RHD results in significant remodeling of the atria and pulmonary veins that provides the milieu for maintaining AF. Some of the electrical remodeling is reversible and hence early intervention may prove useful. AF in patients with RHD poses a greater risk for embolic event compared with those with nonvalvular AF. Consequently, screening for them early and institution of anticoagulation may reduce the devastating complications that follow. The clinical indicators that would predict the risk of AF in this population would be those older than 50 years, having NYHA functional class II symptoms, with left atrial dimension greater than 4.0 cm on echocardiogram in parasternal long-axis view and gradients across the mitral valve greater than 10 mm Hg.

Studies suggest that the strategy for ablation in this population would differ compared with the nonvalvular group. The extent of atrial fibrosis has been linked to the success of maintaining sinus rhythm after catheter ablation of AF. Although paroxysmal AF might be recorded in patients with MS on Holter, most of them are often persistent, suggesting substrate changes play a dominant role.[26] It is likely that factors contributing to persistent AF will lead to increased fibrosis. Thus, a more extensive ablation on the substrate appears necessary for AF ablation in MS. In addition to isolation of pulmonary veins, targeting complex fractionated electrograms in the right atrium may prove to be efficacious in maintaining sinus rhythm in this population. The 2017 American Heart Association/American College of Cardiology guidelines suggest a full bi-atrial maze procedure at the time of valvular surgery, compared with a lesser ablation procedure, in patients with chronic permanent AF. In addition, molecules that inhibit downstream signaling pathways for fibrogenesis may retard the development of substrate that promotes AF in this vulnerable group.

DISCLOSURE

This study was supported in part by Grant-in-Aid (G.08A.3646) from National Heart foundation of Australia and Indo-Australian strategic research grant (DBT/Indo-Aus/03/16/08); Ministry of Science and Technology, India.

REFERENCES

1. Gordis L. The virtual disappearance of rheumatic fever in the United States: lessons in the rise and fall of disease. T. Duckett Jones memorial lecture. Circulation 1985;72(6):1155–62.
2. WHO programme for the prevention of rheumatic fever/rheumatic heart disease in 16 developing countries: report from Phase I (1986-90). WHO Cardiovascular Diseases Unit and principal investigators. Bull World Health Organ 1992;70(2):213–8.
3. Carapetis JR, Wolff DR, Currie BJ. Acute rheumatic fever and rheumatic heart disease in the top end of Australia's Northern Territory. Med J Aust 1996; 164(3):146–9.
4. Awada A. Stroke in Saudi Arabian young adults: a study of 120 cases. Acta Neurol Scand 1994;89(5): 323–8.
5. Banerjee AK, Varma M, Vasista RK, et al. Cerebrovascular disease in north-west India: a study of necropsy material. J Neurol Neurosurg Psychiatry 1989; 52(4):512–5.
6. Luijckx GJ, Ukachoke C, Limapichat K, et al. Brain infarct causes under the age of fifty: a comparison between an east-Asian (Thai) and a western (Dutch) hospital series. Clin Neurol Neurosurg 1993;95(3): 199–203.
7. Veasy LG, Wiedmeier SE, Orsmond GS, et al. Resurgence of acute rheumatic fever in the intermountain area of the United States. N Engl J Med 1987;316(8): 421–7.
8. Veasy LG, Tani LY, Daly JA, et al. Temporal association of the appearance of mucoid strains of Streptococcus pyogenes with a continuing high incidence of rheumatic fever in Utah. Pediatrics 2004;113(3 Pt 1):e168–72.
9. Carapetis JR, Currie BJ, Mathews JD. Cumulative incidence of rheumatic fever in an endemic region: a guide to the susceptibility of the population? Epidemiol Infect 2000;124(2):239–44.
10. Talbot RG. Rheumatic fever and rheumatic heart disease in the Hamilton health district: I. An epidemiological survey. N Z Med J 1984;97(764):630–4.
11. Padmavati S. Rheumatic heart disease: prevalence and preventive measures in the Indian subcontinent. Heart 2001;86(2):127.
12. Jose VJ, Gomathi M. Declining prevalence of rheumatic heart disease in rural schoolchildren in India: 2001-2002. Indian Heart J 2003;55(2):158–60.
13. Noubiap JJ, Agbor VN, Bigna JJ, et al. Prevalence and progression of rheumatic heart disease: a global systematic review and meta-analysis of population-based echocardiographic studies. Sci Rep 2019;9(1):17022.
14. Diker E, Aydogdu S, Ozdemir M, et al. Prevalence and predictors of atrial fibrillation in rheumatic valvular heart disease. Am J Cardiol 1996;77(1): 96–8.
15. Okello E, Wanzhu Z, Musoke C, et al. Cardiovascular complications in newly diagnosed rheumatic heart disease patients at Mulago Hospital, Uganda. Cardiovasc J Afr 2013;24(3):80–5.
16. Negi PC, Sondhi S, Rana V, et al. Prevalence, risk determinants and consequences of atrial fibrillation in rheumatic heart disease: 6 years hospital based-Himachal Pradesh- Rheumatic Fever/Rheumatic Heart Disease (HP-RF/RHD) Registry. Indian Heart J 2018;70(Suppl 3):S68–73.
17. Olesen KH. The natural history of 271 patients with mitral stenosis under medical treatment. Br Heart J 1962;24:349–57.
18. Wood P. An appreciation of mitral stenosis. Part I. Clinical features. Br Med J 1954;1(4870):1051–63. contd.
19. Selzer A, Cohn KE. Natural history of mitral stenosis: a review. Circulation 1972;45(4):878–90.
20. Selzer A. Effects of atrial fibrillation upon the circulation in patients with mitral stenosis. Am Heart J 1960; 59:518–26.

21. Gajewski J, Singer RB. Mortality in an insured population with atrial fibrillation. JAMA 1981;245(15):1540–4.

22. Davison G, Greenland P. Predictors of left atrial thrombus in mitral valve disease. J Gen Intern Med 1991;6(2):108–12.

23. Coulshed N, Epstein EJ, McKendrick CS, et al. Systemic embolism in mitral valve disease. Br Heart J 1970;32(1):26–34.

24. Casella L, Abelmann WH, Ellis LB. Patients with mitral stenosis and systemic emboli; hemodynamic and clinical observations. Arch Intern Med 1964;114:773–81.

25. Wolf PA, Dawber TR, Thomas HE Jr, et al. Epidemiologic assessment of chronic atrial fibrillation and risk of stroke: the Framingham study. Neurology 1978;28(10):973–7.

26. Karthikeyan G, Ananthakrishnan R, Devasenapathy N, et al. Transient, subclinical atrial fibrillation and risk of systemic embolism in patients with rheumatic mitral stenosis in sinus rhythm. Am J Cardiol 2014;114(6):869–74.

27. Ramsdale DR, Arumugam N, Singh SS, et al. Holter monitoring in patients with mitral stenosis and sinus rhythm. Eur Heart J 1987;8(2):164–70.

28. Hernandez R, Banuelos C, Alfonso F, et al. Long-term clinical and echocardiographic follow-up after percutaneous mitral valvuloplasty with the Inoue balloon. Circulation 1999;99(12):1580–6.

29. Wang A, Krasuski RA, Warner JJ, et al. Serial echocardiographic evaluation of restenosis after successful percutaneous mitral commissurotomy. J Am Coll Cardiol 2002;39(2):328–34.

30. Multicenter experience with balloon mitral commissurotomy. NHLBI balloon valvuloplasty registry report on immediate and 30-day follow-up results. The National Heart, Lung, and Blood Institute Balloon Valvuloplasty Registry Participants. Circulation 1992;85(2):448–61.

31. Palacios IF, Sanchez PL, Harrell LC, et al. Which patients benefit from percutaneous mitral balloon valvuloplasty? Prevalvuloplasty and postvalvuloplasty variables that predict long-term outcome. Circulation 2002;105(12):1465–71.

32. Tomai F, Gaspardone A, Versaci F, et al. Twenty year follow-up after successful percutaneous balloon mitral valvuloplasty in a large contemporary series of patients with mitral stenosis. Int J Cardiol 2014;177(3):881–5.

33. Neumayer U, Schmidt HK, Fassbender D, et al. Early (three-month) results of percutaneous mitral valvotomy with the Inoue balloon in 1,123 consecutive patients comparing various age groups. Am J Cardiol 2002;90(2):190–3.

34. Nunes MC, Nascimento BR, Lodi-Junqueira L, et al. Update on percutaneous mitral commissurotomy. Heart 2016;102(7):500–7.

35. Kabukcu M, Arslantas E, Ates I, et al. Clinical, echocardiographic, and hemodynamic characteristics of rheumatic mitral valve stenosis and atrial fibrillation. Angiology 2005;56(2):159–63.

36. Acar J, Michel PL, Cormier B, et al. Features of patients with severe mitral stenosis with respect to atrial rhythm. Atrial fibrillation in predominant and tight mitral stenosis. Acta Cardiol 1992;47(2):115–24.

37. Henry WL, Morganroth J, Pearlman AS, et al. Relation between echocardiographically determined left atrial size and atrial fibrillation. Circulation 1976;53(2):273–9.

38. Gupta A, Bhatia R, Sharma G, et al. Predictors of ischemic stroke in rheumatic heart disease. J Stroke Cerebrovasc Dis 2015;24(12):2810–5.

39. Kitchin A, Turner R. Calcification of the mitral valve. Results of valvotomy in 100 cases. Br Heart J 1967;29(2):137–61.

40. Sharma SK, Verma SH. A clinical evaluation of atrial fibrillation in rheumatic heart disease. J Assoc Physicians India 2015;63(6):22–5.

41. Shenthar J, Kalpana SR, Prabhu MA, et al. Histopathological study of left and right atria in isolated rheumatic mitral stenosis with and without atrial fibrillation. J Cardiovasc Electrophysiol 2016;27(9):1047–54.

42. Luo MH, Li YS, Yang KP. Fibrosis of collagen I and remodeling of connexin 43 in atrial myocardium of patients with atrial fibrillation. Cardiology 2007;107(4):248–53.

43. Zhang L, Zhang N, Tang X, et al. Increased alpha-actinin-2 expression in the atrial myocardium of patients with atrial fibrillation related to rheumatic heart disease. Cardiology 2016;135(3):151–9.

44. Zhang P, Wang W, Wang X, et al. Focal adhesion kinase mediates atrial fibrosis via the AKT/S6K signaling pathway in chronic atrial fibrillation patients with rheumatic mitral valve disease. Int J Cardiol 2013;168(4):3200–7.

45. Sharma S, Sharma G, Hote M, et al. Light and electron microscopic features of surgically excised left atrial appendage in rheumatic heart disease patients with atrial fibrillation and sinus rhythm. Cardiovasc Pathol 2014;23(6):319–26.

46. Park JH, Lee JS, Ko YG, et al. Histological and biochemical comparisons between right atrium and left atrium in patients with mitral valvular atrial fibrillation. Korean Circ J 2014;44(4):233–42.

47. Zhao F, Zhang S, Shao Y, et al. Calreticulin overexpression correlates with integrin-alpha5 and transforming growth factor-beta1 expression in the atria of patients with rheumatic valvular disease and atrial fibrillation. Int J Cardiol 2013;168(3):2177–85.

48. Xue XD, Huang JH, Wang HS. Angiotensin II activates signal transducers and activators of transcription 3 via Rac1 in the atrial tissue in permanent atrial

fibrillation patients with rheumatic heart disease. Cell Biochem Biophys 2015;71(1):205–13.

49. John B, Stiles MK, Kuklik P, et al. Electrical remodeling of the left and right atria due to rheumatic mitral stenosis. Eur Heart J 2008;29(18):2234–43.

50. Fan K, Lee KL, Chow WH, et al. Internal cardioversion of chronic atrial fibrillation during percutaneous mitral commissurotomy: insight into reversal of chronic stretch-induced atrial remodeling. Circulation 2002;105(23):2746–52.

51. John B, Stiles MK, Kuklik P, et al. Reverse remodeling of the atria after treatment of chronic stretch in humans: implications for the atrial fibrillation substrate. J Am Coll Cardiol 2010;55(12):1217–26.

52. John B, Wong CX, Stiles MK, et al. Differences in left to right atrial gradient of spatiotemporal organization and fractionation in patients with valvular and non valvular atrial fibrillation. Heart Rhythm 2009;6(5):S9.

53. Haissaguerre M, Jais P, Shah DC, et al. Spontaneous initiation of atrial fibrillation by ectopic beats originating in the pulmonary veins. N Engl J Med 1998;339(10):659–66.

54. Chen SA, Hsieh MH, Tai CT, et al. Initiation of atrial fibrillation by ectopic beats originating from the pulmonary veins: electrophysiological characteristics, pharmacological responses, and effects of radiofrequency ablation. Circulation 1999;100(18):1879–86.

55. Verheule S, Wilson EE, Arora R, et al. Tissue structure and connexin expression of canine pulmonary veins. Cardiovasc Res 2002;55(4):727–38.

56. Hocini M, Ho SY, Kawara T, et al. Electrical conduction in canine pulmonary veins: electrophysiological and anatomic correlation. Circulation 2002;105(20):2442–8.

57. Cheung DW. Pulmonary vein as an ectopic focus in digitalis-induced arrhythmia. Nature 1981;294(5841):582–4.

58. Chen YJ, Chen SA, Chen YC, et al. Electrophysiology of single cardiomyocytes isolated from rabbit pulmonary veins: implication in initiation of focal atrial fibrillation. Basic Res Cardiol 2002;97(1):26–34.

59. Ho SY. Pulmonary vein ablation in atrial fibrillation: does anatomy matter? J Cardiovasc Electrophysiol 2003;14(2):156–7.

60. Jais P, Hocini M, Macle L, et al. Distinctive electrophysiological properties of pulmonary veins in patients with atrial fibrillation. Circulation 2002;106(19):2479–85.

61. Tse HF, Pelosi F, Oral H, et al. Effects of simultaneous atrioventricular pacing on atrial refractoriness and atrial fibrillation inducibility: role of atrial mechanoelectrical feedback. J Cardiovasc Electrophysiol 2001;12(1):43–50.

62. Walters TE, Lee G, Spence S, et al. Acute atrial stretch results in conduction slowing and complex signals at the pulmonary vein to left atrial junction: insights into the mechanism of pulmonary vein arrhythmogenesis. Circ Arrhythm Electrophysiol 2014;7(6):1189–97.

63. John B, Brooks AG, Kuklik P, et al. Effect of acute and chronic stretch on the pulmonary veins in humans: implications for arrhythmogenic triggers. Circulation 2008;118(8):S591.

Postoperative Atrial Fibrillation
Features, Mechanisms, and Clinical Management

Martin Aguilar, MD, PhD[a],*, Dobromir Dobrev, MD, PhD[b],
Stanley Nattel, MD[a,b,c]

KEYWORDS

• Postoperative atrial fibrillation • Cardiac surgery • Noncardiac surgery • Perioperative medicine

KEY POINTS

- Postoperative atrial fibrillation (POAF) is an important diagnosis associated with significant short-term and long-term consequences.
- POAF results from the interaction among a subclinical atrial substrate, surgery-induced substrate, and transient postoperative factors.
- Pharmacologic prophylaxis is well established in cardiac surgery, whereas the role of POAF prophylaxis for noncardiac surgery needs further investigation.
- A rate-control strategy is adequate for most asymptomatic patients with POAF and anticoagulation should be initiated for POAF more than 48 to 72 hours after surgery.
- Patients with POAF are at high risk for long-term AF and should be appropriately followed.

INTRODUCTION

Postoperative atrial fibrillation (POAF) is defined as atrial fibrillation (AF) in the postoperative period in a patient without a prior diagnosis of AF. POAF has long been considered as a transient postoperative phenomenon with limited clinical significance. Contemporary developments in our understanding and management of AF, a growing emphasis on perioperative medicine, and evolving surgical standards have reignited an interest in POAF. A number of practice-changing clinical trials have been published in recent years, especially in patients with POAF after cardiac surgery. Moreover, there has been a growing recognition of POAF after noncardiac surgery as a nontrivial entity with a potentially distinct pathophysiology and clinical course. The field of POAF after noncardiac surgery is, however, in its infancy and a large number of clinically relevant questions remain to be explored. In this article, we present a succinct and clinically oriented review of the epidemiology, pathophysiology, prophylaxis, and management of POAF. We conclude with a discussion of the many important areas of uncertainty and potential research directions.

EPIDEMIOLOGY AND RISK FACTORS

POAF generally presents between postoperative days 2 and 4, most often with asymptomatic self-terminating episodes (**Fig. 1**A).[1] Some patients may experience hemodynamic instability, symptoms, or difficult rate control requiring sinus rhythm–maintaining therapies.

a Department of Medicine and Research Center, Montreal Heart Institute and Université de Montréal, 5000 Belanger Street, Montréal, Québec H1T 1C8, Canada; b Institute of Pharmacology, West German Heart and Vascular Center, University Duisburg-Essen, Hufelandstr. 55, Essen 45122, Germany; c IHU LIRYC and Fondation Bordeaux Université, Bordeaux, France
* Corresponding author.
E-mail address: martin.aguilar@mail.mcgill.ca

Card Electrophysiol Clin 13 (2021) 123–132
https://doi.org/10.1016/j.ccep.2020.11.010
1877-9182/21/© 2020 Elsevier Inc. All rights reserved.

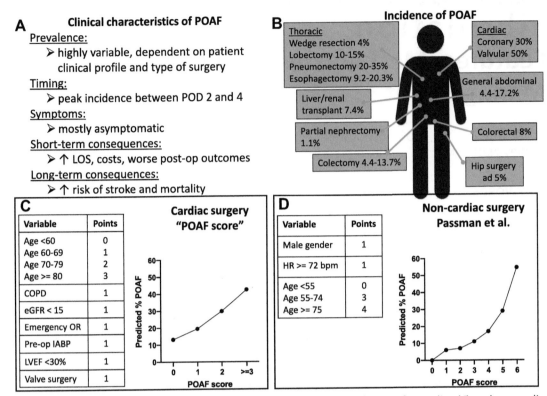

Fig. 1. Clinical characteristics of POAF (*A, B*) and preoperative risk stratification for cardiac (*C*) and noncardiac surgery (*D*). COPD, chronic obstructive pulmonary disease; eGFR, estimated glomerular filtration rate; HR, heart rate; IABP, intra-aortic balloon pump; LOS, length of stay; LVEF, left ventricular ejection fraction; OR, operating room; POD, postoperative day; Pre-op, preoperative.

The incidence of POAF ranges from less than 1% to 60%, depending on the type of surgery (**Fig. 1**B).[2,3] The incidence of POAF increases with increasing proximity of the surgical site to the heart and invasiveness of the procedure. Abdominal surgery is associated with a POAF risk ranging from 1.1% to 18%.[4] After thoracic surgery, the POAF risk increases from 4% for wedge resections to 10% to 15% for lobectomy and 20% to 35% for pneumonectomy,[5,6] whereas esophageal surgery has an intermediate risk (4%–20%).[7,8] Cardiac surgery has the greatest POAF risk, with approximately 30% of patients developing POAF after coronary artery bypass graft (CABG) surgery and up to 50% after combined CABG-valve surgery.[9] Percutaneous coronary revascularization has a much lower AF risk (0.1%) than surgical revascularization.[10] The reported incidences likely underestimate the true POAF burden, as continuous rhythm monitoring is not routine for noncardiac surgery.

A number of risk scores can preoperatively stratify POAF risk. The CHADS-VASc, CHARGE-AF, and STS risk scores predict POAF after cardiac surgery, albeit with limited accuracy (area under the receiver-operator characteristic curve 0.58–0.69).[11–13] The "POAF score" stratifies patients into low (0 points; 13.2%), intermediate (1–2 points; 19.5%–29.9%), and high (≥3 points; 42.5%) risk of POAF and other complications after cardiac surgery (**Fig. 1**C).[14] Similarly, the CHADS-VASc score predicts POAF after lung surgery, although most of the statistical significance is carried by age.[15] Passman and colleagues[16] derived a risk score composed of gender (male), age (<55; 55–74 years and ≥75 years) and heart rate (≥72 beats per minute) with the ability to stratify patients into very low risk (0 points; 0%) to very high risk (6 points; 54.6%) of POAF after noncardiac surgery (**Fig. 1**D). Biomarkers are being studied to improve preoperative POAF risk stratification, including markers of myocardial stretch (brain natriuretic peptide) and inflammation (C-reactive protein, interleukin-6).[17]

MECHANISMS

POAF most likely results from the interaction between a subclinical atrial substrate, surgery-induced substrate, and transient postoperative

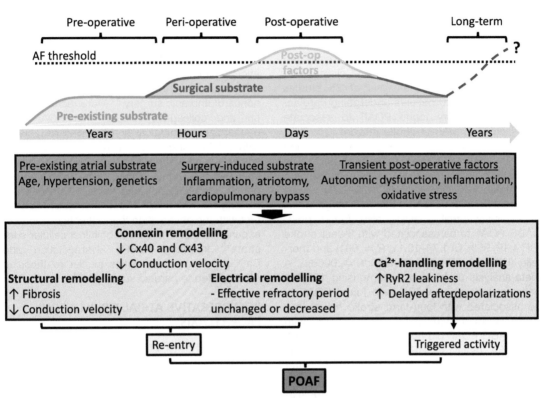

Fig. 2. Mechanisms of POAF. Pre-existing atrial substrate, surgery-induced substrate and transient post-operative factors interact to promote re-entry and triggered activity leading to POAF. Cx, connexin; Cx, connexin; POAF, post-operative atrial fibrillation; RyR2, ryanodine-receptor type-2.

factors (**Fig. 2**), as recently reviewed in detail.[1] Pre-operative activation of the NLRP3-inflammasome and calcium/calmodulin-dependent kinase II pre-dispose the cardiomyocyte calcium-handling apparatus to generate delayed afterdepolariza-tions and AF-triggering ectopic firing under the in-fluence of postoperative inflammation.[18]

The molecular/cellular factors predisposing to POAF are incompletely understood (see **Fig. 2**). There are no differences in action potential (AP) up-stroke velocity, AP-duration (APD), effective refrac-tory period (ERP), and resting membrane potential between patients with POAF and patients without POAF.[19,20] Studies have investigated the cellular determinants of POAF in specimens resected at the time of cardiac surgery. Increases in sarcoplasmic-reticulum Ca^{2+}-leak due to enhanced sarcoplasmic-reticulum Ca^{2+}-release channel (ryanodine-receptor, RyR2) opening are seen in patients who develop POAF, along with NLRP3-inflammasome activation.[1] The combina-tion sensitizes their heart to the proarrhythmic ef-fects of inflammatory mediators.[18] Atrial fibrosis and other structural abnormalities also seem to be increased in patients with POAF, suggesting that a substrate for reentry may also contribute.[21–23]

Animal (sterile pericarditis) and human (biomarker) studies show a robust cardiac surgery–induced inflammatory response. In an an-imal model of pericardiotomy/atriotomy, inflam-mation correlated with conduction heterogeneity, AF inducibility, and AF duration.[24] Other animal studies have found shorter ERPs and impaired conduction with sterile pericarditis.[25–29] Inflammation-induced fibrosis and connexin (Cx)-40/Cx-43 remodeling also appear involved in post-operative conduction disturbances.[26,27,29]

Several noninflammatory postoperative factors also contribute to POAF. Sympathetic-nerve activa-tion (pain, endogenous/exogenous catechol-amines) and autonomic dysfunction may promote triggered activity by shortening APD (parasympa-thetic effect) while prolonging intracellular Ca^{2+}-transients, and promoting Ca^{2+}-loading and RyR2-opening (sympathetic effects) (see **Fig. 2**).[1] Subclinical ischemia may also contribute.[30]

CLINICAL OUTCOMES

POAF is clearly associated with longer intensive care/length of stay, more days on mechanical ventilation, greater risk of intensive care unit readmission, increased hospitalization resource utilization/expenditure, and worse postoperative outcomes.[31,32]

A large number of small trials have investigated the association between POAF and clinical outcomes. A recent meta-analysis of 35 studies including 2,458,010 patients undergoing cardiac/noncardiac surgery found POAF to associate with increased risks of stroke (hazard ratio [HR] 1.37; 95% confidence interval [CI] 1.07–1.77) and mortality (HR 1.37; 95% CI 1.27–1.49).[33] The stroke risk was greater in patients undergoing noncardiac (HR 2.00; 95% CI 1.70–2.35) versus cardiac (HR 1.20; 95% CI 1.07–1.34) surgery.[33] A recent clinical-trial analysis also found post-CABG POAF to be associated with 3-year stroke (HR 4.19; 95% CI 1.74–10.11; $P = .001$) and mortality (HR 3.02; 95% CI 1.60–5.70; $P = .0006$).[10] A meta-analysis of 16 studies comprising 108,711 patients undergoing CABG also found POAF to be associated with long-term stroke risk.[34] In a large Danish registry study, 2108 patients with post-CABG POAF did not have an increased risk of stroke (adjusted HR 1.11; 95% CI 0.94–1.32),[35] but the same group found POAF after left-sided valve surgery to have a thromboembolic risk similar to patients with nonvalvular AF (HR 1.22; 95% CI 0.88–1.68).[36] Moreover, anticoagulation reduced the stroke risk in patients with POAF (HR 0.45; 95% CI 0.22–0.90).[36]

A meta-analysis of 14 studies/3,536,291 patients undergoing noncardiac surgery found POAF to be associated with stroke (risk ratio [RR] 2.51; 95% CI 1.76–3.59); this association was strongest for patients undergoing nonthoracic versus thoracic surgery (RR 3.09; $P = .1$).[2] A post hoc analysis of the combined POISE-1 and -2 trial datasets of patients undergoing noncardiac surgery found POAF to be associated with stroke (adjusted HR 3.34; 95% CI 2.00–5.90), myocardial infarction (adjusted HR 5.10, 95% CI 3.91–6.64), and mortality (adjusted HR 2.51; 95% CI 2.01–3.14).[37] POAF after noncardiac surgery was associated with a thromboembolic risk similar to nonvalvular AF outside the postoperative period (HR 0.95; 95% CI 0.85–1.07) and anticoagulation reduced the stroke risk in patients with POAF (HR 0.52; 95% CI 0.40–0.67).[38] POAF after peripheral orthopedic surgery also appears to be associated with similar adverse prognosis.[39,40]

Attention has recently been directed to the association between POAF and long-term AF. POAF after cardiac surgery increases the risk of long-term AF by up to 8-fold with CABG surgery and 12-fold with combined coronary-valve surgery.[41–43] A Framingham Heart Study found 47% AF recurrence in patients with POAF after cardiothoracic surgery.[44] Two small studies reported 61% and 100% AF recurrence at 2 years post cardiac surgery with implantable continuous monitoring, most of which (93%) were asymptomatic.[45,46] A Framingham Heart Study found a 64% AF-recurrence rate in patients with POAF after noncardiothoracic surgery.[44] More recently, Higuchi and colleagues[47] found that POAF after noncardiac oncological surgery was associated with a 31% AF-recurrence rate, most of which were asymptomatic (92%), versus less than 1% in patients without POAF. The perioperative period, therefore, appears to be a "stress test," for long-term AF risk.[48] These findings are consistent with the observation that patients destined to experience POAF have a subclinical cellular substrate[18] involving NLRP3 dysregulation and Ca^{2+}-handling abnormalities similar to those in AF unrelated to cardiac surgery[49–51]

POSTOPERATIVE ATRIAL FIBRILLATION PROPHYLAXIS

Preoperative POAF prophylaxis includes (1) identifying patients at risk, (2) optimizing hemodynamic and metabolic status, and (3) pharmacologic prophylaxis when appropriate (**Fig. 3**). Several drugs have been studied for POAF prophylaxis including beta-blockers, antiarrhythmic drugs (AADs), intravenous magnesium, statins, polyunsaturated fatty acids, steroids, and colchicine, among others. Intraoperative interventions like posterior pericardiotomy and bi-atrial pacing also have been investigated.

Cardiac Surgery

Beta-blockers clearly reduce the POAF incidence after cardiac surgery (odds ratio [OR] 0.33; 95% CI 0.26–0.43), without affecting length of hospital stay, stroke, or mortality.[52] Society guidelines recommend beta-blockers for POAF prophylaxis in the absence of contraindication.[53–55] Two large retrospective studies of patients undergoing aortic (4592 patients) and CABG surgery (1,231,850 patients) found beta-blockers associated with an *increased* risk of POAF and worse postoperative outcomes[56,57]; however, the role of selection bias cannot be excluded.

Amiodarone also decreases the incidence of POAF after cardiac surgery (OR 0.43; 95% CI 0.34–0.54),[52] an effect maintained in patients on background beta-blockers.[58] Amiodarone is recommended for patients with contraindications to beta-blockers or at very high risk for POAF.[53–55] Other AADs, including class Ia (propafenone), Ic (flecainide and propafenone), and III agents (sotalol and dofetilide), along with more recent

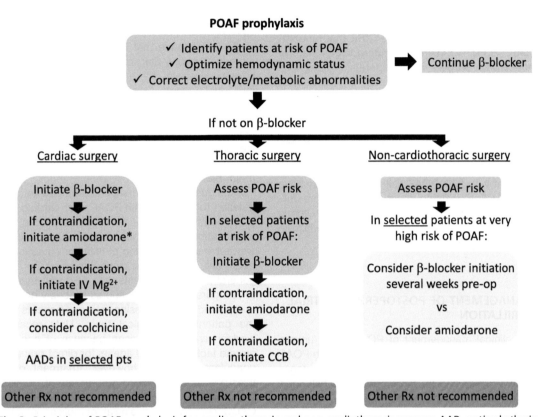

POAF prophylaxis

- ✓ Identify patients at risk of POAF
- ✓ Optimize hemodynamic status
- ✓ Correct electrolyte/metabolic abnormalities

➡ Continue β-blocker

⬇

If not on β-blocker

Cardiac surgery

Initiate β-blocker
⬇
If contraindication, initiate amiodarone*
⬇
If contraindication, initiate IV Mg²⁺
⬇
If contraindication, consider colchicine

AADs in selected pts

Other Rx not recommended

Thoracic surgery

Assess POAF risk
⬇
In selected patients at risk of POAF:
⬇
Initiate β-blocker
⬇
If contraindication, initiate amiodarone
⬇
If contraindication, initiate CCB

Other Rx not recommended

Non-cardiothoracic surgery

Assess POAF risk
⬇
In selected patients at very high risk of POAF:

Consider β-blocker initiation several weeks pre-op

vs

Consider amiodarone

Other Rx not recommended

Fig. 3. Principles of POAF prophylaxis for cardiac, thoracic and non-cardiothoracic surgery. AAD, antiarrhythmic drug; CCB, calcium-channel blocker; POAF, post-operative atrial fibrillation.

molecules like ranolazine and vernakalant, have limited low-quality evidence in favor of use for post cardiac surgery POAF prophylaxis.

A Cochrane meta-analysis supports the use of intravenous magnesium for POAF prophylaxis after cardiac surgery (OR 0.55; 95% CI 0.41–73)[52] but a meta-analysis of only high-quality studies did not find intravenous magnesium to be protective (OR 0.94; 95% CI 0.61–1.44).[59] Intravenous magnesium may be beneficial only in patients without background beta-blocker/amiodarone therapy.[60]

Steroids and statins were initially thought to be beneficial for POAF prophylaxis. However, good-quality trials have not corroborated this. The DECS[61] and SIRS[62] studies, 2 large randomized controlled trials of more than 11,000 patients, found no benefit of glucocorticoids for POAF prophylaxis after cardiac surgery. The STICS trial randomized 1922 patients undergoing elective cardiac surgery to rosuvastatin versus placebo and found no benefit of statin use.[63] In a meta-analysis of 5 trials comprising 1412 patients undergoing cardiac surgery, colchicine reduced the incidence of POAF (RR 0.69; 95% CI 0.57–0.84), although the results were not stratified by background beta-blocker/amiodarone use.[64] Polyunsaturated fatty acids may have modest beneficial effect in patients undergoing CABG surgery.[65] Importantly, currently available agents for POAF prophylaxis have no demonstrable effect on length of stay, stroke, or mortality.

Noncardiac Surgery

The literature on pharmacologic POAF prophylaxis for noncardiac surgery is much less developed. A meta-analysis of 16 trials comprising 2673 patients undergoing a wide range of thoracic surgical procedures found beta-blockade to be the most effective intervention (OR 0.12; 95% CI 0.05–0.27).[66] Angiotensin-converting enzyme inhibitors (OR 0.22; 95% CI 0.08–0.56), amiodarone (OR 0.25; 95% CI 0.14–0.43), intravenous magnesium (OR 0.35%; 95% 0.16–0.74), and calcium-channel blockers (OR 0.52; 95% CI 0.29–0.85) were also found to have statistically significant effects on POAF after thoracic surgery,[66] but the quality of all the data is limited. No data support the use of other antiarrhythmic or anti-inflammatory drugs. Additional studies are needed in this patient population.

Data on POAF prophylaxis for noncardiothoracic surgery are scarce. The POISE trial randomized 8351 patients undergoing elective noncardiac surgery to preoperative metoprolol versus placebo and found a borderline-significant reduction in POAF with metoprolol (HR 0.76; 95% CI 0.58–0.99) but at the cost of excess stroke (HR 2.17; 95% CI 1.26–3.74) and mortality (HR 1.33; 95% CI 1.03–1.74).[67] Hence, beta-blockers should not be routinely used to prevent POAF in noncardiothoracic surgeries. Patients at very high POAF risk for POAF may have beta-blockers initiated several weeks before surgery. There are no studies on other antiarrhythmic or anti-inflammatory drugs for POAF prophylaxis in noncardiothoracic surgeries.

MANAGEMENT OF POSTOPERATIVE ATRIAL FIBRILLATION

The clinical management of POAF offers unique challenges and opportunities. Patients with POAF should be assessed for (1) arrhythmia management strategy and (2) thromboembolic risk/need for systemic anticoagulation (**Fig. 4**).

Rhythm Management

The potential benefits of a proactive sinus rhythm-maintaining have been studied in a randomized trial of 695 patients with POAF after elective cardiac surgery treated with a rhythm versus rate-control strategy.[9] There was no difference between groups in terms of length of stay, rate and duration of anticoagulation, stroke, or sinus rhythm at discharge or 60 days postdischarge; fewer than 10% of patients were in AF at 60 days irrespective of treatment strategy.[9] Thus, rate-control strategy is a reasonable first-line approach for stable asymptomatic patients. Patients with hemodynamic instability, symptoms, or difficult rate control should be considered for sinus-rhythm restoration and adjunctive AADs, with amiodarone having advantages in the acute postsurgical period. Other antiarrhythmics may be considered after carefully weighing the risk/benefit ratio. POAF can be challenging to rate control because of enhanced adrenergic tone and risks of hemodynamically significant postconversion pauses and/or sinus bradycardia.

There are no published data to guide rhythm management for POAF after noncardiac surgery. The general principles shown in **Fig. 4** may be applied.

Thromboembolic Risk

There is evidence that POAF is associated with increased stroke risk, modulated by the type of surgery. However, there is no risk score to stratify individual patients. On the other hand, hemostatic considerations in the early postoperative period militate against exposing patients to systemic anticoagulation. Many patients may have concomitant indications for antiplatelet therapy, and adding an anticoagulant may significantly increase the risk of major bleeding.

Most guideline documents recommend anticoagulation for patients with POAF after cardiac surgery without guidance for thromboembolic risk stratification, AF burden/duration threshold to warrant treatment, timing of initiation, duration of treatment, and specific anticoagulant.[53–55] As a general principle, patients with AF more than 48 to 72 hours after surgery should probably be anticoagulated after discussing risks and benefits with the patient and surgical team. Until recently, warfarin was often chosen because of concern around lack of reversal agents for direct oral anticoagulants (DOACs); however, treatment practices are evolving toward greater use of DOACs. A pilot study of 65 patients with POAF after CABG surgery found similar complication rates for treatment with warfarin versus apixaban.[68] It is common practice to reassess the need for anticoagulation 3 months postsurgery and discontinue treatment if there is no evidence of recurrent AF. However, the evidence suggesting high AF-recurrence rates after POAF argues for reconsideration of this practice.

There is no literature to guide anticoagulation management for POAF after noncardiac surgery. Anticoagulation should be considered in patients with AF more than 48 to 72 hours after surgery and reassessed. Because of long-term AF-recurrence risks, follow-up is important.

FUTURE DIRECTIONS

In general, there is a dearth of data to guide management for POAF after noncardiac surgery and much further research is needed in this area. As perioperative management and surgical techniques evolve, the benefits of specific agents for prophylaxis need to be reevaluated (eg, beta-blockers for cardiac surgery). Whether POAF prophylaxis improves short- and/or long-term clinical outcomes needs to be better established.

The cellular and molecular determinants of POAF after noncardiac surgery need to be investigated. Conversely, in patients undergoing cardiac surgery at highest risk for POAF, should

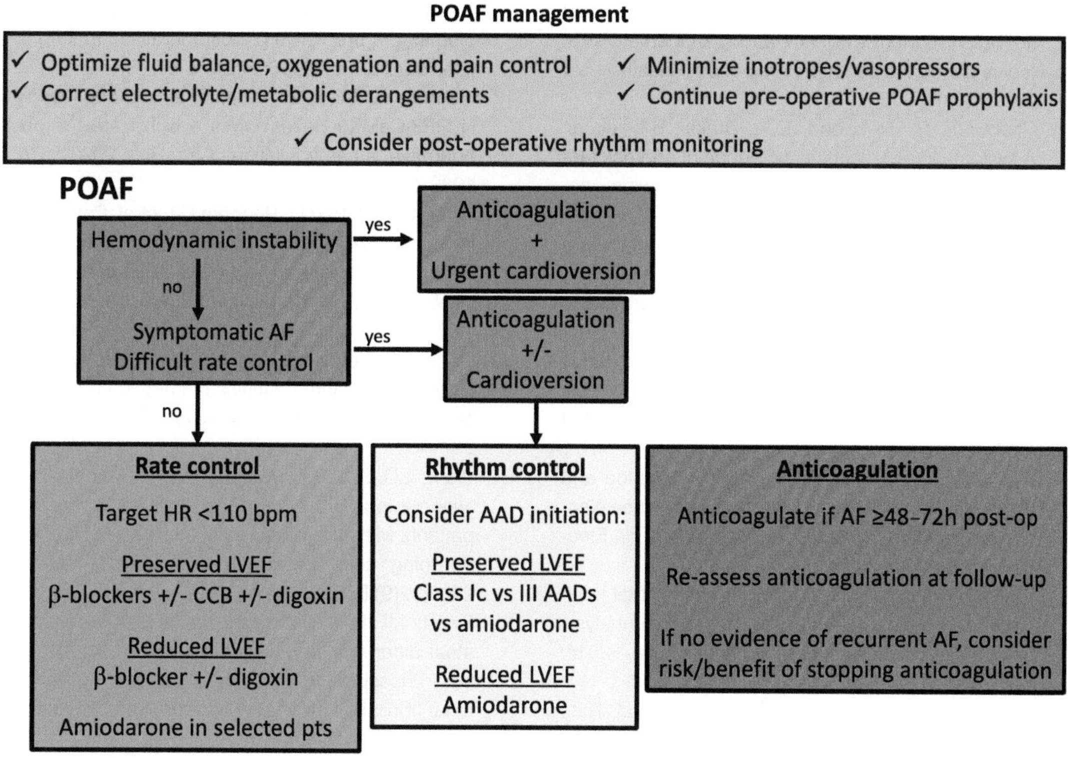

POAF management

Fig. 4. Principles of clinical management of POAF. AAD, antiarrhythmic drug; AF, atrial fibrillation; CCB, calcium-channel blocker; HR, heart rate; LVEF, left ventricular ejection fraction; OR, operating room; POAF, post-operative atrial fibrillation.

prophylactic intraoperative ablation be considered? Or left atrial appendage ligation?

Data are needed to refine the management of anticoagulation for POAF (timing, duration, threshold, agent). It is becoming increasingly evident that most patients with POAF after noncardiac surgery are asymptomatic. Should postoperative cardiac monitoring be routinely recommended in this population?

SUMMARY

There is growing evidence that POAF is an important postoperative diagnosis resulting from the interaction between a subclinical atrial substrate, surgery-induced substrate, and transient postoperative factors. Prophylaxis for POAF after cardiac surgery is well established but the indications for preoperative treatment in noncardiac surgery need further investigation. POAF should be managed with a rate-control approach in the absence of compelling indication, and anticoagulated if AF is present more than 48 to 72 hours after surgery. There is an important need for additional research to enable better evidence-based management of POAF.

FUNDING SOURCES

The authors' work was supported by the National Institutes of Health (R01-HL131517, R01-HL136389, and R01-HL089598 to D. Dobrev), the German Research Foundation (DFG, Do 769/4-1 to D. Dobrev), the Canadian Institutes of Health Research (1484011), and Heart and Stroke Foundation of Canada (18-22032) to S. Nattel.

DISCLOSURE

D. Dobrev is a member of the scientific advisory boards of OMEICOS Therapeutics GmbH and Acesion Pharma. The other authors have nothing to disclose.

REFERENCES

1. Dobrev D, Aguilar M, Heijman J, et al. Postoperative atrial fibrillation: mechanisms, manifestations and management. Nat Rev Cardiol 2019;16(7):417–36.
2. Koshy AN, Hamilton G, Theuerle J, et al. Postoperative atrial fibrillation following noncardiac surgery increases risk of stroke. Am J Med 2020;133(3):311–22.e5.

3. Karamchandani K, Khanna AK, Bose S, et al. Atrial fibrillation: current evidence and management strategies during the perioperative period. Anesth Analg 2020;130(1):2–13.

4. Chebbout R, Heywood EG, Drake TM, et al. A systematic review of the incidence of and risk factors for postoperative atrial fibrillation following general surgery. Anaesthesia 2018;73(4):490–8.

5. Shrivastava V, Nyawo B, Dunning J, et al. Is there a role for prophylaxis against atrial fibrillation for patients undergoing lung surgery? Interact Cardiovasc Thorac Surg 2004;3(4):656–62.

6. Bagheri R, Yousefi Y, Rezai R, et al. Atrial fibrillation after lung surgery: incidence, underlying factors, and predictors. Kardiochir Torakochirurgia Pol 2019;16(2):53–6.

7. Siu CW, Tung HM, Chu KW, et al. Prevalence and predictors of new-onset atrial fibrillation after elective surgery for colorectal cancer. Pacing Clin Electrophysiol 2005;28(Suppl 1):S120–3.

8. Ojima T, Iwahashi M, Nakamori M, et al. Atrial fibrillation after esophageal cancer surgery: an analysis of 207 consecutive patients. Surg Today 2014; 44(5):839–47.

9. Gillinov AM, Bagiella E, Moskowitz AJ, et al. Rate control versus rhythm control for atrial fibrillation after cardiac surgery. N Engl J Med 2016;374(20): 1911–21.

10. Kosmidou I, Chen S, Kappetein AP, et al. New-onset atrial fibrillation after PCI or CABG for left main disease: the EXCEL trial. J Am Coll Cardiol 2018; 71(7):739–48.

11. Chua SK, Shyu KG, Lu MJ, et al. Clinical utility of CHADS2 and CHA2DS2-VASc scoring systems for predicting postoperative atrial fibrillation after cardiac surgery. J Thorac Cardiovasc Surg 2013; 146(4):919–26.e1.

12. Cameron MJ, Tran DTT, Abboud J, et al. Prospective external validation of three preoperative risk scores for prediction of new onset atrial fibrillation after cardiac surgery. Anesth Analg 2018;126(1):33–8.

13. Pollock BD, Filardo G, da Graca B, et al. Predicting new-onset post-coronary artery bypass graft atrial fibrillation with existing risk scores. Ann Thorac Surg 2018;105(1):115–21.

14. Mariscalco G, Biancari F, Zanobini M, et al. Bedside tool for predicting the risk of postoperative atrial fibrillation after cardiac surgery: the POAF score. J Am Heart Assoc 2014;3(2):e000752.

15. Lee CT, Strauss DM, Stone LE, et al. Preoperative CHA2DS2-VASc score predicts postoperative atrial fibrillation after lobectomy. Thorac Cardiovasc Surg 2019;67(2):125–30.

16. Passman RS, Gingold DS, Amar D, et al. Prediction rule for atrial fibrillation after major noncardiac thoracic surgery. Ann Thorac Surg 2005;79(5): 1698–703.

17. Turagam MK, Mirza M, Werner PH, et al. Circulating biomarkers predictive of postoperative atrial fibrillation. Cardiol Rev 2016;24(2):76–87.

18. Heijman J, Muna AP, Veleva T, et al. Atrial Myocyte NLRP3/CaMKII nexus forms a substrate for postoperative atrial fibrillation. Circ Res 2020;127(8): 1036–55.

19. Workman AJ, Pau D, Redpath CJ, et al. Post-operative atrial fibrillation is influenced by beta-blocker therapy but not by pre-operative atrial cellular electrophysiology. J Cardiovasc Electrophysiol 2006; 17(11):1230–8.

20. Dobrev D, Wettwer E, Kortner A, et al. Human inward rectifier potassium channels in chronic and postoperative atrial fibrillation. Cardiovasc Res 2002;54(2): 397–404.

21. Wang GD, Shen LH, Wang L, et al. Relationship between integrated backscatter and atrial fibrosis in patients with and without atrial fibrillation who are undergoing coronary bypass surgery. Clin Cardiol 2009;32(9):E56–61.

22. Swartz MF, Fink GW, Lutz CJ, et al. Left versus right atrial difference in dominant frequency, K(+) channel transcripts, and fibrosis in patients developing atrial fibrillation after cardiac surgery. Heart Rhythm 2009;6(10):1415–22.

23. Swartz MF, Fink GW, Sarwar MF, et al. Elevated preoperative serum peptides for collagen I and III synthesis result in post-surgical atrial fibrillation. J Am Coll Cardiol 2012;60(18):1799–806.

24. Ishii Y, Schuessler RB, Gaynor SL, et al. Inflammation of atrium after cardiac surgery is associated with inhomogeneity of atrial conduction and atrial fibrillation. Circulation 2005;111(22):2881–8.

25. Zhang Z, Zhang C, Wang H, et al. n-3 polyunsaturated fatty acids prevents atrial fibrillation by inhibiting inflammation in a canine sterile pericarditis model. Int J Cardiol 2011;153(1):14–20.

26. Ryu K, Li L, Khrestian CM, et al. Effects of sterile pericarditis on connexins 40 and 43 in the atria: correlation with abnormal conduction and atrial arrhythmias. Am J Physiol Heart Circ Physiol 2007;293(2): H1231–41.

27. Fu XX, Zhao N, Dong Q, et al. Interleukin-17A contributes to the development of post-operative atrial fibrillation by regulating inflammation and fibrosis in rats with sterile pericarditis. Int J Mol Med 2015; 36(1):83–92.

28. Zhang Y, Wang YT, Shan ZL, et al. Role of inflammation in the initiation and maintenance of atrial fibrillation and the protective effect of atorvastatin in a goat model of aseptic pericarditis. Mol Med Rep 2015; 11(4):2615–23.

29. Huang Z, Chen XJ, Qian C, et al. Signal Transducer and Activator of Transcription 3/MicroRNA-21 feedback loop contributes to atrial fibrillation by

promoting atrial fibrosis in a rat sterile pericarditis model. Circ Arrhythm Electrophysiol 2016;9(7): e003396.

30. Jeong EM, Liu M, Sturdy M, et al. Metabolic stress, reactive oxygen species, and arrhythmia. J Mol Cell Cardiol 2012;52(2):454–63.

31. Aranki SF, Shaw DP, Adams DH, et al. Predictors of atrial fibrillation after coronary artery surgery. Current trends and impact on hospital resources. Circulation 1996;94(3):390–7.

32. Hravnak M, Hoffman LA, Saul MI, et al. Resource utilization related to atrial fibrillation after coronary artery bypass grafting. Am J Crit Care 2002;11(3): 228–38.

33. Lin MH, Kamel H, Singer DE, et al. Perioperative/postoperative atrial fibrillation and risk of subsequent stroke and/or mortality. Stroke 2019;50(6): 1364–71.

34. Megens MR, Churilov L, Thijs V. New-onset atrial fibrillation after coronary artery bypass graft and long-term risk of stroke: a meta-analysis. J Am Heart Assoc 2017;6(12):e007558.

35. Butt JH, Xian Y, Peterson ED, et al. Long-term thromboembolic risk in patients with postoperative atrial fibrillation after coronary artery bypass graft surgery and patients with nonvalvular atrial fibrillation. JAMA Cardiol 2018;3(5):417–24.

36. Butt JH, Olesen JB, Gundlund A, et al. Long-term thromboembolic risk in patients with postoperative atrial fibrillation after left-sided heart valve surgery. JAMA Cardiol 2019;4(11):1139–47.

37. Conen D, Alonso-Coello P, Douketis J, et al. Risk of stroke and other adverse outcomes in patients with perioperative atrial fibrillation 1 year after noncardiac surgery. Eur Heart J 2020;41(5):645–51.

38. Butt JH, Olesen JB, Havers-Borgersen E, et al. Risk of thromboembolism associated with atrial fibrillation following noncardiac surgery. J Am Coll Cardiol 2018;72(17):2027–36.

39. Tao L, Xiaodong X, Fan L, et al. Association between new-onset postoperative atrial fibrillation and 1-year mortality in elderly patients after hip arthroplasty. Aging Clin Exp Res 2020;32(5):921–4.

40. Rostagno C, Cartei A, Rubbieri G, et al. Postoperative atrial fibrillation is related to a worse outcome in patients undergoing surgery for hip fracture. Intern Emerg Med 2020. https://doi.org/10.1007/s11739-020-02372-6.

41. Ahlsson A, Fengsrud E, Bodin L, et al. Postoperative atrial fibrillation in patients undergoing aortocoronary bypass surgery carries an eightfold risk of future atrial fibrillation and a doubled cardiovascular mortality. Eur J Cardiothorac Surg 2010;37(6): 1353–9.

42. Lee SH, Kang DR, Uhm JS, et al. New-onset atrial fibrillation predicts long-term newly developed atrial fibrillation after coronary artery bypass graft. Am Heart J 2014;167(4):593–600 e1.

43. Park-Hansen J, Greve AM, Clausen J, et al. New-onset of postoperative atrial fibrillation is likely to recur in the absence of other triggers. Ther Clin Risk Manag 2018;14:1641–7.

44. Lubitz SA, Yin X, Rienstra M, et al. Long-term outcomes of secondary atrial fibrillation in the community: the Framingham Heart Study. Circulation 2015;131(19):1648–55.

45. Lomivorotov VV, Efremov SM, Pokushalov EA, et al. Randomized trial of fish oil infusion to prevent atrial fibrillation after cardiac surgery: data from an implantable continuous cardiac monitor. J Cardiothorac Vasc Anesth 2014;28(5):1278–84.

46. El-Chami MF, Merchant FM, Smith P, et al. Management of new-onset postoperative atrial fibrillation utilizing insertable cardiac monitor technology to observe recurrence of AF (MONITOR-AF). Pacing Clin Electrophysiol 2016;39(10):1083–9.

47. Higuchi S, Kabeya Y, Matsushita K, et al. Perioperative atrial fibrillation in noncardiac surgeries for malignancies and one-year recurrence. Can J Cardiol 2019;35(11):1449–56.

48. Kotecha D, Castella M. Is it time to treat postoperative atrial fibrillation just like regular atrial fibrillation? Eur Heart J 2020;41(5):652–654a.

49. Yao C, Veleva T, Scott L Jr, et al. Enhanced cardiomyocyte NLRP3 inflammasome signaling promotes atrial fibrillation. Circulation 2018;138(20):2227–42.

50. Voigt N, Li N, Wang Q, et al. Enhanced sarcoplasmic reticulum $Ca2+$ leak and increased $Na+-Ca2+$ exchanger function underlie delayed afterdepolarizations in patients with chronic atrial fibrillation. Circulation 2012;125(17):2059–70.

51. Voigt N, Heijman J, Wang Q, et al. Cellular and molecular mechanisms of atrial arrhythmogenesis in patients with paroxysmal atrial fibrillation. Circulation 2014;129(2):145–56.

52. Arsenault KA, Yusuf AM, Crystal E, et al. Interventions for preventing post-operative atrial fibrillation in patients undergoing heart surgery. Cochrane Database Syst Rev 2013;(1):CD003611.

53. Andrade JG, Verma A, Mitchell LB, et al. 2018 focused update of the canadian cardiovascular society guidelines for the management of atrial fibrillation. Can J Cardiol 2018;34(11):1371–92.

54. January CT, Wann LS, Calkins H, et al. 2019 AHA/ACC/HRS focused update of the 2014 AHA/ACC/HRS guideline for the management of patients with atrial fibrillation: a report of the American College of Cardiology/American Heart Association Task Force on Clinical Practice guidelines and the heart rhythm society. J Am Coll Cardiol 2019;74(1): 104–32.

55. Kirchhof P, Benussi S, Kotecha D, et al. 2016 ESC Guidelines for the management of atrial fibrillation

developed in collaboration with EACTS. Eur Heart J 2016;37(38):2893–962.

56. Wang L, Wang H, Hou X. Short-term effects of pre-operative beta-blocker use for isolated coronary artery bypass grafting: a systematic review and meta-analysis. J Thorac Cardiovasc Surg 2018; 155(2):620–629 e1.

57. Schubert SA, Hawkins RB, Mehaffey JH, et al. Pre-operative beta-blocker use correlates with worse outcomes in patients undergoing aortic valve replacement. J Thorac Cardiovasc Surg 2019; 158(6):1589–15897 e3.

58. Mitchell LB, Exner DV, Wyse DG, et al. Prophylactic oral amiodarone for the prevention of arrhythmias that begin early after revascularization, valve replacement, or repair: PAPABEAR: a randomized controlled trial. JAMA 2005;294(24):3093–100.

59. Cook RC, Yamashita MH, Kearns M, et al. Prophylactic magnesium does not prevent atrial fibrillation after cardiac surgery: a meta-analysis. Ann Thorac Surg 2013;95(2):533–41.

60. Burgess DC, Kilborn MJ, Keech AC. Interventions for prevention of post-operative atrial fibrillation and its complications after cardiac surgery: a meta-analysis. Eur Heart J 2006;27(23):2846–57.

61. Dieleman JM, Nierich AP, Rosseel PM, et al. Intraoperative high-dose dexamethasone for cardiac surgery: a randomized controlled trial. JAMA 2012; 308(17):1761–7.

62. Whitlock RP, Devereaux PJ, Teoh KH, et al. Methylprednisolone in patients undergoing cardiopulmonary bypass (SIRS): a randomised, double-blind, placebo-controlled trial. Lancet 2015;386(10000): 1243–53.

63. Zheng Z, Jayaram R, Jiang L, et al. Perioperative rosuvastatin in cardiac surgery. N Engl J Med 2016; 374(18):1744–53.

64. Lennerz C, Barman M, Tantawy M, et al. Colchicine for primary prevention of atrial fibrillation after open-heart surgery: systematic review and meta-analysis. Int J Cardiol 2017;249:127–37.

65. Wang H, Chen J, Zhao L. N-3 polyunsaturated fatty acids for prevention of postoperative atrial fibrillation: updated meta-analysis and systematic review. J Interv Card Electrophysiol 2018;51(2):105–15.

66. Zhao BC, Huang TY, Deng QW, et al. Prophylaxis against atrial fibrillation after general thoracic surgery: trial sequential analysis and network meta-analysis. Chest 2017;151(1):149–59.

67. Group PS, Devereaux PJ, Yang H, et al. Effects of extended-release metoprolol succinate in patients undergoing non-cardiac surgery (POISE trial): a randomised controlled trial. Lancet 2008; 371(9627):1839–47.

68. Chapin TW, Leedahl DD, Brown AB, et al. Comparison of anticoagulants for postoperative atrial fibrillation after coronary artery bypass grafting: a pilot study. J Cardiovasc Pharmacol Ther 2020;25(6): 523–30.

Post–Cardiac Surgery Atrial Fibrillation
Risks, Mechanisms, Prevention, and Management

Jason D. Matos, MD[a], Frank W. Sellke, MD[b], Peter Zimetbaum, MD[c,d],*

KEYWORDS

• Cardiac surgery • Atrial fibrillation • Coronary artery bypass grafting • Anticoagulation

KEY POINTS

- Post–cardiac surgery atrial fibrillation (PCSAF) is a common complication of cardiac surgery; age is the strongest risk factor followed by renal failure, left ventricular dysfunction, pulmonary disease, valve surgery, and need for a perioperative aortic balloon pump.
- The mechanism of PCSAF incidence is heterogeneous, triggered by inflammation and oxidative stress, leading to initiation through increased signal heterogeneity, shortened effective refractory periods, and calcium loading.
- Numerous therapies have been proposed for PCSAF prevention, but β-blockade and amiodarone have the most robust evidence; colchicine's role is potentially emerging.
- PCSAF is managed in the acute stages similar to nonsurgical atrial fibrillation—acute rate control and rhythm control based on other factors, including symptoms.
- There is clinical equipoise surrounding anticoagulation for PCSAF, although it is endorsed by major societal guidelines. AF after coronary artery bypass grafting appears to carry a lower thromboembolic risk than AF after valvular surgery.

INTRODUCTION

Atrial fibrillation (AF) is the most common complication of cardiac surgery (CS), with an incidence of 20% to 25% after coronary artery bypass graft (CABG) surgery and a higher 30% to 35% incidence after valve surgery.[1] The rhythm, although not imminently life threatening, poses numerous challenges to the clinician, including correct choice of pharmacotherapy, determining need for cardioversion (CV), and weighing the risk/benefit ratio of anticoagulation.

RISK FACTORS

Many clinical and operative factors heighten risk for post-CS AF (PCSAF). Most notable is advanced age; this relationship becomes logarithmic once a patient's age surpasses 55 years.[2] Male sex, history of heart failure, and chronic obstructive pulmonary disease also are clinical risk factors, although not as predictive as age.[3] Concurrent mitral valve surgery, use of an intra-aortic balloon pump (IABP), and withdrawal of β-blockade are intraoperative risk factors for

[a] Department of Medicine, Division of Cardiology, Beth Israel Deaconess Medical Center, Harvard Medical School, 185 Pilgrim Road, Baker Building 4th Floor, Boston, MA 02215, USA; [b] Division of Cardiothoracic Surgery, Department of Surgery, Cardiovascular Research Center, Rhode Island Hospital, Alpert Medical School of Brown University, 2 Dudley Street, MOC 360, Providence, RI 02905, USA; [c] Department of Medicine, Division of Cardiology, Beth Israel Deaconess Medical Center, Harvard Medical School, Boston, MA, USA; [d] Smith Center for Cardiovascular Outcomes Research, Beth Israel Deaconess Medical Center, Boston, MA, USA
* Corresponding author. 330 Brookline Avenue, Boston, MA 02215.
E-mail address: pzimetba@bidmc.harvard.edu

Card Electrophysiol Clin 13 (2021) 133–140
https://doi.org/10.1016/j.ccep.2020.11.011
1877-9182/21/© 2020 Elsevier Inc. All rights reserved.

PCSAF.[2,3] On-pump CABG once was postulated as a risk factor compared with off-pump CABG, but this was refuted by a well-done randomized trial.[4,5]

Using many of these risk factors, a postoperative AF score has been established to help predict PCSAF. This particular score incorporates age, renal function, preoperative use of an IABP, chronic obstructive lung disease, emergency status of surgery, valve surgery, and left ventricular ejection fraction less than 30%. In the study, patients with a score of 0 had a PCSAF rate of approximately 12%, whereas those with a score of greater than or equal to 3 had a rate of 42%.[6]

An additional original proposed intraoperative risk factor is poor left atrial appendage (LAA) mechanical function during transesophageal echocardiogram (TEE), as assessed through pulse wave doppler. In a prospective analysis of 107 patients without prior clinical history of AF undergoing CS, the presence of sinus rhythm on electrocardiogram (ECG) but mechanical fibrillation of the LAA on TEE was associated with a higher rate of PCSAF ($P = .08$). When assessing patients who underwent isolated CABG, this relationship reached statistical significance ($P = .03$).[7]

LENGTH OF STAY/FINANCIAL IMPLICATIONS

Not unexpectedly, development of PCSAF has been linked to poor patient outcomes, including length of stay, intensive care unit admission, stroke, heart failure, and mortality. Despite adjustment for confounders, however, association cannot be equated with proved causation; likely, many unmeasured confounders are involved.[8–10]

PCSAF appears to influence hospitalization costs and length of stay. Using hierarchical modeling, Mehaffey and colleagues[11] demonstrated that PCSAF, although nowhere near the most expensive post-CS complication, ranks as the second most costly across a population, due to its high incidence.

PROPOSED MECHANISMS

AF initiation is complex and not completely understood, but it is thought to initiate most often from pulmonary vein triggers and perpetuate in the vulnerable left atrium. Certain electrophysiologic settings promote this, including increased conduction heterogeneity across the atria; a shortened effective refractory period (ERP), which enhances the ability for a premature signal to propagate; and increased in calcium available to myocardial cells.[12]

The principle insults from CS include the pericardiotomy and the atriotomy, which create a hyperinflammatory state. Inflammation can decrease ERP of a myocardial cell and also increase signal heterogeneity by decreasing connexin 40/43 protein levels.[13–15] In addition, inflammation may decrease levels of the protein sarcolipin. Sarcolipin normally inhibits the SERCA protein. When SERCA is left to act unabated, calcium levels can increase substantially in the myocardium. High intracellular calcium promotes delayed after-depolarizations, which can serve as a nidus for AF initiation.[16]

Oxidative stress also is associated with PCSAF, which has led to several mechanistic hypotheses. Plasma and urine fatty acid–derived oxidative stress biomarker levels in the immediate postoperative period and at postoperative day 2 demonstrated an association with PCSAF.[17] A separate study showed a substantial difference in expression of prespecified genes associated with oxidative stress among those who went on to develop PCSAF.[18]

POST–CARDIAC SURGERY ATRIAL FIBRILLATION PREVENTION

Several medications and procedures have been evaluated for AF prophylaxis before, during, or after CS. The most notable are described and a summary of guideline recommendations can be found in **Fig. 1**.

β-Blockers

β-Blockers are among the most widely prescribed cardiac medications due to their favorable risk/benefit profile and confirmed benefits in systolic heart failure and angina. In addition, rate control of AF with β-blockade often precedes any attempt at rhythm control due to ease of use and proved symptomatic benefit.

Numerous small randomized trials in the 1990s and 2000s reported substantial decreases in new-onset PCSAF rates with preoperative β-blockade use. A meta-analysis of these trials noted that, although the reduction of PCSAF was significant (odds ratio [OR] 0.36; 95% CI, 0.28–0.47), the effect size withered when focusing on studies that did not mandate β-blocker withdrawal in the control arm (OR 0.69; 95% CI, 0.54–0.87).[19]

Both the Canadian and European cardiovascular societies provide strong recommendations for continuing β-blocker use through CS to help prevent PCSAF.[20,21]

	🇺🇸	🇨🇦	🇪🇺	Authors
PSCAF Prevention				
Preoperative β-blockers		Recomm	Ib	Continue β-blockers in all patients
Preoperative amiodarone	IIa	Recomm	IIa	Consider if protocol in place to discontinue after 6 wk.
Preoperative Colchicine	IIb			Consider– await further data.
Magnesium/Atrial Pacing		Suggest		
PCSAF Rate vs Rhythm				
β-Blocker/Calcium Channel Blocker	Ia/Ib	Suggest		β-Blocker recommended first line
Amiodarone/Cardioversion	IIa	Suggest	IIa	Amiodarone +/-cardioversion if symptoms/heart failure.
Anticoagulation				
Initiate perioperative anticoagulation for PCSAF	IIa	Suggest	IIa	Consider withholding in first month unless prior stroke/TIA history present.

☐ = Class I/Firm Recommendation   ☐ = Class II/Suggestion   ■ = No Recommendation

Fig. 1. Summary of guideline recommendations (American College of Cardiology, Canadian Cardiovascular Society, European Society of Cardiology) for medications and procedures that have been evaluated for AF prophylaxis before, during, or after CS. Authors, recommendations of the authors of this chapter; CS, cardiac Surgery; PCSAF, post cardiac surgery atrial fibrillation; Recomm= recommendation.

Amiodarone

A class III antiarrhythmic, amiodarone, is widely prescribed for rhythm control of AF. Similar to β-blockers, many small randomized controlled trials also have demonstrated its benefit for PCSAF prophylaxis,[22] The most notable, the PAPABEAR trial, randomized patients to placebo versus amiodarone for 6 days before and 6 days after CS. Atrial tachyarrhythmias occurred in fewer amiodarone patients than placebo patients (hazard ratio [HR] 0.52; 95% CI, 0.34–0.69).[23] A more recent observational database analysis demonstrated similar findings.[24]

Several concerns exist, however, for routine amiodarone use. For one, amiodarone increases rates of bradycardia and QT interval prolongation.[23] Side effects of amiodarone, such as nausea, often prompt discontinuation.[25] In addition, routine amiodarone use necessitates a robust protocol to ensure appropriate deprescription to prevent undue pulmonary, thyroid, or liver toxicity.[26] Finally, previous work suggests that pharmacologic CV, similar to electrical CV, can promote atrial stasis and therefore increase stroke risk after initiation.[27,28] As a result, many experts postulate that amiodarone initiation for ongoing AF necessitates concurrent anticoagulation use.

Despite these issues, all 3 major cardiovascular societies (American College of Cardiology, European Society of Cardiology, Canadian Cardiovascular Society) do endorse amiodarone use for AF prophylaxis.[21,29,30]

Statin Medications

A small randomized study suggested statin medications, through their pleiotropic anti-inflammatory effects, reduce PCSAF.[31] A subsequent larger randomized study, however, demonstrated no benefit. As a result, statins are not prescribed routinely for this indication.[32]

Steroids

Similarly, smaller observational and randomized studies demonstrated a reduction in PCSAF rates with preoperative steroid use. However, 2 recent large randomized studies of preoperative dexamethasone and methylprednisolone showed no benefit.[33,34]

Magnesium

Magnesium, through its potential to manage calcium handling, appears to reduce PCSAF. A meta-analysis described this benefit (HR 0.57; 95% CI, 0.42–0.77) but also cautioned that the significance fades when only evaluating trials where preoperative β-blockade was continued (HR 0.83; 95% CI, 0.60–1.16).[19] The Canadian Cardiovascular Society suggests a consideration of magnesium, particularly if serum levels are below normal.[29]

Colchicine

The COPPS trial, a small randomized clinical trial of colchicine, another anti-inflammatory therapy, when initiated on postoperative day 3, reduced rates of PCSAF.[35] Both American and Canadian societies suggest consideration of colchicine for PCSAF prevention.[29,30] Further randomized trials are under way to evaluate the benefit of preoperative colchicine administration for preventing PCSAF in both cardiac and thoracic surgeries.

Atrial Pacing

By suppressing atrial ectopy, rate smoothing via atrial pacing emerged as a possible prophylactic intervention for PCSAF. Despite encouraging data, biatrial pacing only, rather than single atrium pacing, appears to drive the clinical benefit.[19] This more complex pacing protocol often poses technical complications with sensing and capture issues; therefore, atrial pacing is not widely used for PCSAF prophylaxis. Canadian guidelines suggest consideration of this therapy at higher volume centers.

POST–CARDIAC SURGERY ATRIAL FIBRILLATION TREATMENT
Rate Control versus Rhythm Control

AF, no matter the clinical setting, requires management of symptoms along with limiting thromboembolic risk. A majority of patients with PCSAF require either rate control and/or rhythm control to help mitigate palpitations, shortness of breath, and other manifestations of heart failure. A randomized trial of more than 500 post-CS patients demonstrated no difference in rehospitalization rates at 60 days when comparing a primary rate control versus rhythm control strategy for AF. By postoperative day 7, the same number of patients in each clinical arm remained in AF, suggesting that PCSAF may be self-limiting entity for many patients. There was an approximately 25% crossover in both arms, primarily due to treatment failure in the rate control group and medication intolerance in the rhythm control group.[36]

Antiarrhythmic Choice

The most common antiarrhythmic drug used in the postoperative period is amiodarone. Within the initial 24 hours to 36 hours, amiodarone can help reduce ventricular rates, but its antiarrhythmic properties may not manifest for days until the drug reaches steady state. Class Ic antiarrhythmic agents, such as flecainide, are contraindicated for PCSAF, because all patients with PCSAF by definition have structural heart abnormalities that preclude use. Sotalol and dronedarone are available but are prescribed less often due to more significant QT prolongation and limited efficacy, respectively.

The American College of Cardiology recommends rate control as first-line; amiodarone and CV can be employed similar to the use in the nonsurgical population.[30] The Canadian Cardiovascular Society suggests either rate or rhythm control initially.[29] The European Society of Cardiology provides no specific guidance on rate control therapy but notes antiarrhythmic medications should be considered[21] (see **Fig. 1**).

THROMBOEMBOLIC PROPHYLAXIS
General Principles

Anticoagulation for AF in the nonsurgical setting is determined based on a patient's risk factors for thromboembolism. Most frequently, this is assessed via the congestive heart failure, hypertension, age, diabetes, prior stroke/transient ischemic attack (TIA), and vascular disease (CHA_2-DS_2-VASc) score, with a score of greater than 1 often triggering anticoagulation use whereas a score less than or equal to 1 favors withholding of therapy pending a thoughtful discussion with the patient. Anticoagulation is not recommended when the score is 1 from female gender alone.

Unfortunately, limited guidance exists regarding the approach to anticoagulation therapy for new AF in the perioperative setting. As for PCSAF, a large retrospective study of more than 16,000 patients demonstrated that, despite controlling for 32 variables, warfarin use for PCSAF was associated with a lower mortality compared with no anticoagulation use. This work, among others, prompted the American, Canadian, and European cardiology societies to provide a weak recommendation for anticoagulation for PCSAF[37] (see **Fig. 1**).

Cardiac versus Noncardiac Surgery

More recent work has challenged the blanket dogma that all patients with PCSAF, and more generally all postoperative AF patients, warrant anticoagulation similar to the nonoperative AF population. A California database evaluated differences in stroke rates among postsurgical patients who did and did not develop perioperative AF. Stroke rates, not surprisingly, were higher among those patients who developed AF. The net increase in thromboembolism rate, however, was significantly higher among the non-CS patents compared with those in the CS cohort ($P<.001$ for interaction).[38] Similarly, a large meta-analysis of 35 studies of postoperative AF with more than 2 million patients found a much stronger association with stroke in patients undergoing non-CS (HR 2.00; 95% CI, 1.70–2.35) versus CS (HR 1.20; 95% CI, 1.07–1.34).[39]

Coronary Artery Bypass Graft versus Valve Surgery

The studies, discussed previously, indicate a heterogeneity in thromboembolic risk with postoperative AF depending on the surgical type. Butt and colleagues,[40–42] utilizing a comprehensive Danish nationwide database, further explored these discrepancies through evaluation of thromboembolic risk for AF after isolated CABG, isolated valvular surgery, and non-CS. In each of their 3 publications, thromboembolism event rates were compared with matched patients with nonsurgical, nonvalvular AF (NVAF).[40–42]

Compared with age, sex, and CHA2DS2-VASc score matched patients in the database with NVAF, post-CABG AF patients had lower rates of thromboembolism (adjusted HR 0.55; 95% CI, 0.32–0.95),[42] whereas patients with AF after valvular surgery or after non-CS had similar rates of thromboembolism compared with matched NVAF cohorts (HR 1.22; 95% CI, 0.88–1.68, and HR 0.95; 95% CI, 0.85–1.07, respectively).[40,41] Patients who underwent aortic valve surgery had lower thromboembolic rates compared with patients post–mitral valve surgery.

Contemporary Use/Outcomes

Despite multiple national guideline recommendations for anticoagulation, a retrospective study of the Society of Thoracic Surgeons (STS) database found that only 26% of patients in the United States and Canada who develop PCSAF after isolated CABG are prescribed anticoagulation at discharge despite a mean CHA2DS2-VASc score of just above 3. This apparent disregard of guidelines may be warranted, at least in the short term,

because this same study found no association with anticoagulation and 30-day adjusted stroke readmissions (adjusted OR 0.87; 95% CI, 0.65–1.16). Furthermore, there was an increase in the 30-day bleeding readmission rate among anticoagulated patients (adjusted OR 4.30; 95% CI, 3.69–5.02).[43] Perhaps anticoagulation for post-CABG AF should be deferred until at least 30 days postoperatively, at a point where the potential for thromboembolic protection outweighs the bleeding risks.

Monitoring for Recurrence

PCSAF, once believed a short-lived entity, more recently has been described as a condition with a significant recurrence rate, documented as high as 30% to 60% by 1 year using various combinations of serial ECGs, Holter monitors, and implantable loop recorders.[44,45] In addition, multiple studies have noted a correlation between AF burden and thromboembolic risk.[46] Because post-CABG AF poses lower thromboembolic risk than AF after valvular surgery, the authors propose extended rhythm monitoring to determine whether anticoagulation is warranted in the long term (**Fig. 2**).

Direct Oral Anticoagulant Use

Direct anticoagulants have revolutionized treatment of AF. Their use in PCSAF, however, has a paucity of evidence. A small, randomized pilot study of warfarin versus apixaban in PCSAF showed a similar safety profile between the 2 drug classes.[47] The aforementioned analysis of the STS database, however, found a statistically significant signal for increased 30-day mortality

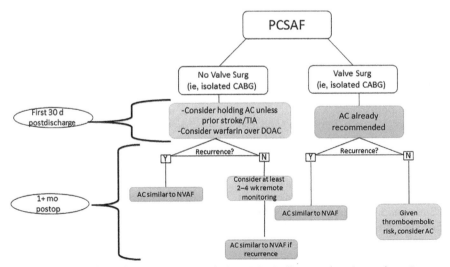

Fig. 2. PCSAF management algorithm. AC, anticoagulation; DOAC, direct oral anticoagulant; Surg, surgery.

among patients prescribed direct anticoagulants compared with no anticoagulant. The same signal was not seen with warfarin use.[43] As further evidence is awaited, direct oral anticoagulants, especially in the immediate 30 days postoperatively, should be used with caution.

PCSAF's mechanism of action is unique and the immediate perioperative period is one of high bleeding risk. In an era of more tailored medicine, deferring to traditional guidelines and risk scores for anticoagulation in this setting no longer should be the norm. Prospective randomized data are sorely needed to help better navigate these clinical crossroads.

Left Atrial Appendage Exclusion

The LAA is the site of a majority of thrombi in the setting of AF and also may serve as a nidus for AF initiation. In hopes of prevention of AF and/or eliminating the need for anticoagulation, LAA exclusion is a common procedure performed concurrently with CABG and valve surgery. Evaluating efficacy of this procedure is a challenge due to the numerous avenues that exist for LAA exclusion, including oversewing, excision, and the Atriclip (AtriCure, Mason, Ohio). One propensity score-matched analysis of more than 10,000 patients demonstrated no difference in stroke rates among patients who did or did not undergo oversewing/excision of the LAA.[48] Two upcoming randomized trials, LAAOS III and ATLAS, will investigate the efficacy of LAA occlusion for stroke prevention in CS patients with and without prior AF, respectively.[49,50]

SUMMARY

PCSAF is a common yet heterogeneous complication of CS. To mitigate the downstream morbidity of this arrhythmia, β-blockers and amiodarone often are prophylactically prescribed, and more data on colchicine are forthcoming. If PCSAF does develop, immediate clinical management regarding rate and rhythm control mirrors that of the nonsurgical AF population.

Despite major societies recommending anticoagulation, PCSAF appears to be associated with lower thromboembolic risk compared with non-CS AF and nonsurgical AF. CABG and valvular surgery must be considered separate entities when considering anticoagulation. Most clinicians in the United States and Canada defer anticoagulation in PCSAF despite guidelines, likely justifiably so given the disturbing bleeding risks seen in the first 30 days. Due to its unique mechanisms and risk/benefit profile, the decision to anticoagulate for PCSAF involves more nuance and requires more data.

CLINICS CARE POINTS

- There is no data to suggest first line rhythm control is superior to rate control with post-cardiac surgery atrial fibrillation (PCSAF).
- Amiodarone can supplement beta blockers for PCSAF prevention, but providers should recognize the drug's adverse effects and possibility that pharmacologic cardioversion can elicit atrial stasis similar to electrical cardioversion.
- Atrial fibrillation (AF) after isolated CABG appears to carry lower thromboembolic risk than AF after non-cardiac surgery or valvular surgery.

DISCLOSURE

The authors have no financial conflicts of interest to disclose.

REFERENCES

1. Echahidi N, Pibarot P, O'Hara G, et al. Mechanisms, prevention, and treatment of atrial fibrillation after cardiac surgery. J Am Coll Cardiol 2008;51: 793–801.
2. Shen J, Lall S, Zheng V, et al. The persistent problem of new-onset postoperative atrial fibrillation: a single-institution experience over two decades. J Thorac Cardiovasc Surg 2011;141:559–70.
3. Aranki SF, Shaw DP, Adams DH, et al. Predictors of atrial fibrillation after coronary artery surgery. Current trends and impact on hospital resources. Circulation 1996;94:390–7.
4. Legare JF, Buth KJ, King S, et al. Coronary bypass surgery performed off pump does not result in lower in-hospital morbidity than coronary artery bypass grafting performed on pump. Circulation 2004;109: 887–92.
5. Enc Y, Ketenci B, Ozsoy D, et al. Atrial fibrillation after surgical revascularization: is there any difference between on-pump and off-pump? Eur J Cardiothorac Surg 2004;26:1129–33.
6. Mariscalco G, Biancari F, Zanobini M, et al. Bedside tool for predicting the risk of postoperative atrial fibrillation after cardiac surgery: the POAF score. J Am Heart Assoc 2014;3:e000752.
7. Qizhe Cai AN, Matos JD, Mahmood F, et al. Discordance between electrocardiograph rhythm and atrial appendage Doppler wave form phenotype predicts post cardiac surgery atrial fibrillation: a prospective intraoperative study. American Heart Association Abstract; 2019. 11479.

8. Almassi GH, Schowalter T, Nicolosi AC, et al. Atrial fibrillation after cardiac surgery: a major morbid event? Ann Surg 1997;226:501–11 [discussion: 11–3].

9. Villareal RP, Hariharan R, Liu BC, et al. Postoperative atrial fibrillation and mortality after coronary artery bypass surgery. J Am Coll Cardiol 2004;43:742–8.

10. Kosmidou I, Chen S, Kappetein AP, et al. New-onset atrial fibrillation after PCI or CABG for left main disease: the EXCEL trial. J Am Coll Cardiol 2018;71:739–48.

11. Mehaffey JH, Hawkins RB, Byler M, et al. Cost of individual complications following coronary artery bypass grafting. J Thorac Cardiovasc Surg 2018;155:875–82.e1.

12. Dobrev D, Aguilar M, Heijman J, et al. Postoperative atrial fibrillation: mechanisms, manifestations and management. Nat Rev Cardiol 2019;16:417–36.

13. Ryu K, Li L, Khrestian CM, et al. Effects of sterile pericarditis on connexins 40 and 43 in the atria: correlation with abnormal conduction and atrial arrhythmias. Am J Physiol Heart Circ Physiol 2007;293:H1231–41.

14. Zhang Y, Wang YT, Shan ZL, et al. Role of inflammation in the initiation and maintenance of atrial fibrillation and the protective effect of atorvastatin in a goat model of aseptic pericarditis. Mol Med Rep 2015;11:2615–23.

15. Ishii Y, Schuessler RB, Gaynor SL, et al. Inflammation of atrium after cardiac surgery is associated with inhomogeneity of atrial conduction and atrial fibrillation. Circulation 2005;111:2881–8.

16. Zaman JA, Harling L, Ashrafian H, et al. Post-operative atrial fibrillation is associated with a pre-existing structural and electrical substrate in human right atrial myocardium. Int J Cardiol 2016;220:580–8.

17. Wu JH, Marchioli R, Silletta MG, et al. Oxidative stress biomarkers and incidence of postoperative atrial fibrillation in the omega-3 fatty acids for prevention of postoperative atrial fibrillation (OPERA) trial. J Am Heart Assoc 2015;4:e001886.

18. Ramlawi B, Otu H, Mieno S, et al. Oxidative stress and atrial fibrillation after cardiac surgery: a case-control study. Ann Thorac Surg 2007;84:1166–72 [discussion: 72–3].

19. Burgess DC, Kilborn MJ, Keech AC. Interventions for prevention of post-operative atrial fibrillation and its complications after cardiac surgery: a meta-analysis. Eur Heart J 2006;27:2846–57.

20. Mitchell LB, Committee CCSAFG. Canadian Cardiovascular Society atrial fibrillation guidelines 2010: prevention and treatment of atrial fibrillation following cardiac surgery. Can J Cardiol 2011;27:91–7.

21. Kirchhof P, Benussi S, Kotecha D, et al. 2016 ESC Guidelines for the management of atrial fibrillation developed in collaboration with EACTS. Europace 2016;18:1609–78.

22. Bagshaw SM, Galbraith PD, Mitchell LB, et al. Prophylactic amiodarone for prevention of atrial fibrillation after cardiac surgery: a meta-analysis. Ann Thorac Surg 2006;82:1927–37.

23. Mitchell LB, Exner DV, Wyse DG, et al. Prophylactic oral amiodarone for the prevention of arrhythmias that begin early after revascularization, valve replacement, or repair: PAPABEAR: a randomized controlled trial. JAMA 2005;294:3093–100.

24. Atreya AR, Priya A, Pack QR, et al. Use and outcomes associated with perioperative amiodarone in cardiac surgery. J Am Heart Assoc 2019;8:e009892.

25. Patel AA, White CM, Gillespie EL, et al. Safety of amiodarone in the prevention of postoperative atrial fibrillation: a meta-analysis. Am J Health Syst Pharm 2006;63:829–37.

26. Leelathanalerk A, Dongtai W, Huckleberry Y, et al. Evaluation of deprescribing amiodarone after new-onset atrial fibrillation in critical illness. Am J Med 2017;130:864–6.

27. Verhaert D, Puwanant S, Gillinov AM, et al. Atrial fibrillation after open heart surgery: how safe is early conversion without anticoagulation? J Am Soc Echocardiogr 2009;22:212.e1-3.

28. Jovic A, Troskot R. Recovery of atrial systolic function after pharmacological conversion of chronic atrial fibrillation to sinus rhythm: a Doppler echocardiographic study. Heart 1997;77:46–9.

29. Macle L, Cairns J, Leblanc K, et al. 2016 focused update of the canadian cardiovascular society guidelines for the management of atrial fibrillation. Can J Cardiol 2016;32:1170–85.

30. January CT, Wann LS, Calkins H, et al. 2019 AHA/ACC/HRS focused update of the 2014 AHA/ACC/HRS guideline for the management of patients with atrial fibrillation: a Report of the American College of Cardiology/American heart association Task Force on clinical Practice guidelines and the heart rhythm society. Heart Rhythm 2019;74(1):104–32.

31. Patti G, Chello M, Candura D, et al. Randomized trial of atorvastatin for reduction of postoperative atrial fibrillation in patients undergoing cardiac surgery: results of the ARMYDA-3 (Atorvastatin for Reduction of MYocardial Dysrhythmia after cardiac surgery) study. Circulation 2006;114:1455–61.

32. Zheng Z, Jayaram R, Jiang L, et al. Perioperative rosuvastatin in cardiac surgery. N Engl J Med 2016;374:1744–53.

33. Whitlock RP, Devereaux PJ, Teoh KH, et al. Methylprednisolone in patients undergoing cardiopulmonary bypass (SIRS): a randomised, double-blind, placebo-controlled trial. Lancet 2015;386:1243–53.

34. Dieleman JM, Nierich AP, Rosseel PM, et al. Intraoperative high-dose dexamethasone for cardiac surgery: a randomized controlled trial. JAMA 2012; 308:1761–7.

35. Imazio M, Brucato A, Ferrazzi P, et al. Colchicine reduces postoperative atrial fibrillation: results of the Colchicine for the Prevention of the Postpericardiotomy Syndrome (COPPS) atrial fibrillation substudy. Circulation 2011;124:2290–5.

36. Gillinov AM, Bagiella E, Moskowitz AJ, et al. Rate control versus rhythm control for atrial fibrillation after cardiac surgery. N Engl J Med 2016;374: 1911–21.

37. El-Chami MF, Kilgo P, Thourani V, et al. New-onset atrial fibrillation predicts long-term mortality after coronary artery bypass graft. J Am Coll Cardiol 2010;55:1370–6.

38. Gialdini G, Nearing K, Bhave PD, et al. Perioperative atrial fibrillation and the long-term risk of ischemic stroke. JAMA 2014;312:616–22.

39. Lin MH, Kamel H, Singer DE, et al. Perioperative/postoperative atrial fibrillation and risk of subsequent stroke and/or mortality. Stroke 2019;50: 1364–71.

40. Butt JH, Olesen JB, Gundlund A, et al. Long-term thromboembolic risk in patients with postoperative atrial fibrillation after left-sided heart valve surgery. JAMA Cardiol 2019;4:1139–47.

41. Butt JH, Olesen JB, Havers-Borgersen E, et al. Risk of thromboembolism associated with atrial fibrillation following noncardiac surgery. J Am Coll Cardiol 2018;72:2027–36.

42. Butt JH, Xian Y, Peterson ED, et al. Long-term thromboembolic risk in patients with postoperative atrial fibrillation after coronary artery bypass graft surgery and patients with nonvalvular atrial fibrillation. JAMA Cardiol 2018;3:417–24.

43. Matos JD, McIlvaine S, Grau-Sepulveda M, et al. Anticoagulation and amiodarone for new atrial fibrillation after coronary artery bypass grafting: prescription patterns and 30-day outcomes in the United States and Canada. J Thorac Cardiovasc Surg 2020. https://doi.org/10.1016/j.jtcvs.2020.01.077.

44. El-Chami MF, Merchant FM, Smith P, et al. Management of new-onset postoperative atrial fibrillation utilizing insertable cardiac monitor technology to observe recurrence of AF (MONITOR-AF). Pacing Clin Electrophysiol 2016;39:1083–9.

45. Lee SH, Kang DR, Uhm JS, et al. New-onset atrial fibrillation predicts long-term newly developed atrial fibrillation after coronary artery bypass graft. Am Heart J 2014;167:593–600 e1.

46. Matos JD, Waks JW, Zimetbaum PJ. Tailored anticoagulation for thromboembolic risk reduction in paroxysmal atrial fibrillation. J Innov Card Rhythm Manag 2018;9:3116–25.

47. Chapin TW, Leedahl DD, Brown AB, et al. Comparison of anticoagulants for postoperative atrial fibrillation after coronary artery bypass grafting: a pilot study. J Cardiovasc Pharmacol Ther 2020;25(6): 523–30.

48. Melduni RM, Schaff HV, Lee HC, et al. Impact of left atrial appendage closure during cardiac surgery on the occurrence of early postoperative atrial fibrillation, stroke, and mortality: a propensity score-matched analysis of 10 633 patients. Circulation 2017;135:366–78.

49. Left atrial appendage occlusion study III (LAAOS III). Available at: https://clinicaltrials.gov/ct2/show/NCT01561651. Accessed August 25, 2020.

50. AtriClip® left atrial appendage exclusion Concomitant to structural heart procedures (ATLAS) (ATLAS). Available at: https://clinicaltrials.gov/ct2/show/NCT02701062. Accessed August 25, 2020.

Pulmonary Disease, Pulmonary Hypertension and Atrial Fibrillation

Roddy Hiram, PhD[a],*, Steeve Provencher, MD, MSc[b,c]

KEYWORDS

- Chronic lung diseases • Pulmonary hypertension • Antiarrhythmic therapy • Atrial fibrillation
- Right heart disease • Right atrial remodeling

KEY POINTS

- Chronic diseases of the lungs and their vessels are important causes of atrial fibrillation.
- A central underlying pathophysiologic theme is increased pulmonary artery pressure, which exerts a pressure load on the right heart and causes right atrial remodeling.
- Atrial fibrillation ablation is an important treatment option for atrial fibrillation associated with right heart disease, but it is important to look for right atrial sources of arrhythmia.
- Effective treatment of the underlying pulmonary or pulmonary vascular disease is essential for optimal therapy of patients with atrial fibrillation in the setting of right heart disease.

INTRODUCTION

Atrial fibrillation (AF) is the most common sustained cardiac arrhythmia[1] and is associated with an increased risk of cardiovascular complications including stroke and heart failure. The prevalence of AF increases with aging and comorbid conditions like obesity, heart disease, diabetes, and/or hypertension.[2] Increasing data also suggest that parenchymal and vascular lung diseases are also AF risk factors.[3,4]

This review aims to discuss the pathophysiology and treatment challenges of AF in patients with right heart disease (RHD) induced by pulmonary diseases, pulmonary hypertension (PH) and pulmonary arterial hypertension.

EPIDEMIOLOGY OF ATRIAL FIBRILLATION IN RESPIRATORY DISEASES

Asthma

Asthma is a chronic inflammatory airway disease involving mucus hypersecretion and smooth muscle hypercontractility.[5] In asthmatic patients, inhalation of irritants or allergens leads to inflammatory cell infiltration and bronchial contractile responses, provoking airway obstruction.[6] The associated chronic airway remodeling is characterized by smooth muscle hypertrophy, inflammatory cell infiltration, collagen deposition, and epithelial desquamation.[7] During acute exacerbations, patients experience respiratory distress that can be associated with hypoxemia, cyanosis, and cardiovascular events.[8] The Norwegian Nord-Trøndelag Health Study (HUNT) revealed that patients who were diagnosed within 15 years with asthma had a 38% increased risk of developing AF compared with nonasthmatics.[9] Moreover, patients with uncontrolled asthma were 74% more likely to develop AF compared with patients with controlled asthma (**Table 1**).[9] The investigators suggested that the increased blood concentrations of inflammatory mediators or biomarkers in patients with asthma, together with the potential side

a Department of Medicine, Montreal Heart Institute (MHI), Université de Montréal, Montréal, Quebec, Canada; b Centre de Recherche de l'Institut Universitaire de Cardiologie et de Pneumologie de Quebec, Quebec, Canada; c Department of medicine, Université Laval, 2325 rue de l'Universite, Montréal, Quebec G1V 0A6, Canada
* Corresponding author. Montreal Heart Institute Research Center, 5000 Belanger Street, Montreal, Quebec H1T 1C8, Canada.
E-mail address: roddyhiram@gmail.com

Card Electrophysiol Clin 13 (2021) 141–153
https://doi.org/10.1016/j.ccep.2020.10.001
1877-9182/21/© 2020 Elsevier Inc. All rights reserved.

Table 1
Pulmonary disease, pulmonary hypertension, and AF

Respiratory Disease	Type of Study	Diseased Patients (n)	Atrial Arrhythmia (%)	Patients (Sex, Age)	References
Asthma	Prospective 6-mo cohort	5961	AF: 38%	Female: 54.5% Male: 45.5% Age: 46 ± 16.1	Cepelis et al,[9] 2018
Chronic obstructive pulmonary disease	Retrospective 11-y cohort	1,345,270	AF: 18%	Female: 50.7% Male: 59.1% Age: 76 ± 20	Xiao et al,[14] 2019
Sleep apnea	Prospective study	524	AF: 29%	Female: 74% Male: 26% Age: 69 ± 14.5	Gami et al,[22] 2004
Pneumonia	Retrospective 5-y cohort	32,689	AF:8%	Female: 2% Male: 98% Age: 75 ± 7	Soto-Gomez et al,[28] 2013
Lung cancer	Retrospective 1-y study	159,615	AF: 6%	Female: 44% Male: 56% Age: 73 ± 1.4	Bandyopadhyay et al,[38] 2019
Interstitial lung disease	Retrospective 6-y study	121	AF: 10%	Female: 23 Male: 77 Age: 67 ± 8	Hyldgaard et al,[40] 2014
Acute respiratory distress syndrome	Prospective study	282	AF: 10%	Female: 46% Male: 54% Age: 52 ± 16	Ambrus et al,[42] 2015
PH	Retrospective 6-y study	231	AF: 3% Other SVA: 12%	Female: 56% Male: 44% Age: 49 ± 13	Tongers et al,[47] 2007
Pulmonary arterial hypertension	Retrospective 13-y study	282	AF: 4% Other SVA: 20%	Female: 61% Male: 39% Age: 47.3 ± 4.3	Ruiz-Cano et al,[48] 2011
PH	Prospective 5-y study	157	AF: 20%	Female: 65% Male: 35% Age: 60 ± 10	Olsson et al,[49] 2013
PH	Retrospective 4-y study	225	AF: 31%	Female:63% Male:37% Age: 71.2 ± 1.1	Rottlaender et al,[50] 2012
Pulmonary arterial hypertension	Prospective 6-y study	280	AF: 6% Other SVA: 16%	Female: 72.5 Male: 27.5 Age: 39 ± 15	Wen et al,[51] 2014
Pulmonary arterial hypertension	Retrospective 7-y study	77	AF:16%	Female: 47% Male: 53% Age: 59 ± 10	Cannillo et al,[52] 2015

Review of clinical cohort studies reporting incidence of AF in various respiratory diseases.

effect of beta-agonist drugs commonly prescribed in asthma, may contribute to the development of AF. Data from other large cohorts suggest that the prevalence of hypertension, type 2 diabetes, heart failure and AF, is increased in patients with asthma, also predisposing to AF.[10]

Chronic Obstructive Pulmonary Disease

Chronic obstructive pulmonary disease (COPD) is a chronic lung disease characterized by persistent expiratory airflow obstruction.[11] COPD includes emphysema, typified by loss of alveolar structure; and chronic bronchitis, characterized by airway inflammation and mucus hypersecretion.[12] Chronic local inflammation leads to peripheral airway narrowing, limited airflow, and breakdown of alveoli and bronchioles. Damage to capillary vessels also contributes to impaired gas exchange.[3,13] As the disease worsens, it provokes dyspnea, hypoxemia, hypercapnia, and an increased risk of arrhythmia. A recent study of 1.3 million American patients with COPD revealed an 18% increased risk of AF (see **Table 1**).[14] COPD was independently associated with the occurrence of AF in other observational studies.[10] Although the mechanisms underlying the arrhythmic risk are unclear, COPD-induced hypoxia promotes pulmonary vasoconstriction and long-term excess pressure load on the right heart. Inflammation and hypoxic mediators like hypoxia-inducible factor 1, matrix metalloproteinases (MMPs), and transforming growth factor-β have also been described to be involved in atrial remodeling leading to AF. In addition, preclinical studies suggest that COPD is associated with heightened sympathetic activity, larger left atrium and greater fibrosis in the pulmonary veins and left atrium.[15] Similar to the case of asthma, treatment with beta-adrenergic agonist drugs and glucocorticoids lower potassium levels and have direct proarrhythmic properties,[16] increasing AF vulnerability. Among patients hospitalized for acute exacerbations of COPD, AF also remains an independent predictor for mortality.[17,18]

Sleep Apnea

Obstructive sleep apnea (OSA) is characterized by episodic nocturnal collapse of the oropharyngeal muscles, causing temporary breathing cessation. Manifestations include excessive snoring, oxygen desaturation, daytime sleepiness leading to reduced quality of life, and stress and anxiety disorders.[19] OSA-related hypoxia and upper airway closure also provoke systemic inflammation, potentially contributing to cardiovascular diseases.[20] Accordingly, OSA increases the risk of hypertension, stroke, and AF.[21] A prospective study showed that 29% of patients with OSA developed AF (see **Table 1**).[22] An experimental model of OSA showed a 56% increase in AF inducibility.[23] The mechanisms linking OSA to AF are multifactorial. Repeated OSA induces left-sided cardiac remodeling with left atrial dilation and fibrosis.[23] OSA-associated hypoxia and hypercapnia cause autonomic nervous system abnormalities and inflammation, leading to atrial arrhythmogenic electrophysiologic changes.[24]

Pneumonia

Pneumonia is an acute lung infection most commonly caused by bacteria or viruses and is a leading cause of death in adults greater than 65 years old.[25] Pneumonia leads to the filling of bronchioles and alveoli with pus and inflammatory fluid and causes high fever, cough, breathing difficulties, poor gas exchange, cyanosis, and tachycardia.[26,27] Little is known about the association between pneumonia and atrial arrhythmias. A retrospective study involving more than 100 hospitals reported that 8% of 32,689 patients with pneumonia developed AF (see **Table 1**).[28] Circulating inflammatory mediators have also been suggested to participate in the development of AF in patients with pneumonia.[29,30] Although disseminated infections rarely occur, the bacterial, fungal, or viral components of pneumonia can infect the endocardium or the pericardium and/or the myocardium adjacent to the pleura and damage cardiac tissue, leading to localized inflammation and fibrosis that can contribute to AF.

Lung Cancer

Lung cancer is the leading cancer worldwide.[31] People with a history of smoking and/or tobacco cigarette use are more at risk of contracting lung cancer, although it can occur in the absence of a smoking history.[32] Lung cancers can invade or metastasize to the pericardium, leading to AF.[33] Repeated tobacco exposure also leads to chronic inflammation, with interleukins (like IL-1, IL-6, IL-8), cyclo-oxygenase enzymes and metalloproteases (MMP1, MMP2, MMP3, MMP12) associated with lung cancer risk.[34] The same inflammatory effectors also contribute to atrial arrhythmogenicity. Systemic inflammation reflected by biomarkers like C-reactive protein is common in lung cancer and promotes AF risk.[35,36] Accordingly, the risk of AF is significantly increased in patients with lung cancer,[37] with 6% developing AF in 1 study (see **Table 1**).[38]

Interstitial Lung Disease

Interstitial lung disease characterizes pulmonary disorders causing scarring and severe fibrosis in the lung tissue.[39] Patients experience shortness of breath, decreased oxygen in the bloodstream, respiratory failure, and right-sided heart failure.[39] AF is frequently diagnosed in patients with interstitial lung disease. A retrospective 6-year study on 121 patients with interstitial lung disease reported that 10% had AF.[40]

Acute Respiratory Distress Syndrome

Acute respiratory distress syndrome (ARDS) is a lung condition that occurs when fluid builds up in the alveoli, leading to impaired oxygenation. ARDS can be caused by pneumonia, sepsis, pancreatitis, or other severe insults of the lung.[41] ARDS is characterized by acute inflammatory injury, hypoxemia, and severe shortness of breath. The syndrome is associated with an increased risk of sudden death and survivors experience cardiac complications, such as arrhythmias.[41] A recent study of 282 patients with ARDS has shown that 10% developed new-onset AF.[42]

Multiple respiratory diseases are associated with the development of increased pulmonary arterial resistance leading to PH. The second part of this review emphasizes the particular pathophysiology and treatment challenges of AF in PH-induced RHD.

PATHOPHYSIOLOGY OF ATRIAL FIBRILLATION IN PULMONARY HYPERTENSION AND RIGHT HEART DISEASE
Right Heart Remodeling Leading to Atrial Fibrillation

Pulmonary hypertension–induced right heart disease
Characteristics of pulmonary hypertension Primary PH is a chronic progressive disease characterized by increased pulmonary arterial pressures at rest.[43,44] PH is associated with high morbidity and mortality. Patients often report chronic fatigue, dyspnea at rest, chest pressure and palpitations, and can cause hemoptysis (which can be life threatening), right-sided heart enlargement, heart failure, and arrhythmias (see **Table 1**).[45]

Classification of pulmonary hypertension PH is classified into 5 groups according to the 6th World Symposia on Pulmonary Hypertension.[43,46] Although group 1 PH (or pulmonary arterial hypertension) and group 4 PH (chronic thromboembolic PH) received much attention in recent years, PH owing to left heart disease (group 2) and chronic lung disease (group 3) remain the most common types of PH (**Box 1**).

Clinical reports of atrial fibrillation in pulmonary hypertension Atrial arrhythmias are common in PH. A variety of studies study in patients with PH, most of which were retrospective, estimated AF incidences between 3% and 31%.[47–52] The general absence of left heart disease in patients with pulmonary arterial hypertension suggests that the chronic PH-induced right-sided heart

---

Box 1
Classification of pulmonary hypertension

Group 1. Pulmonary arterial hypertension

1.1. Idiopathic pulmonary arterial hypertension

1.2. Heritable pulmonary arterial hypertension

1.3. Drug- and toxin-induced pulmonary arterial hypertension

1.4. Pulmonary arterial hypertension long-term responders to calcium channel blockers

1.5. Pulmonary arterial hypertension with overt features of venous/capillaries

1.6. Persistent PH of the newborn syndrome

Group 2. PH owing to left heart disease

2.1. PH owing to heart failure with preserved LVEF

2.2. PH owing to heart failure with reduced LVEF

2.3. Valvular heart disease

2.4. Congenital/acquired cardiovascular conditions leading to postcapillary PH

Group 3. PH owing to lung diseases and/or hypoxia

3.1. Obstructive lung disease

3.2. Restrictive lung disease

3.3. Other lung disease with mixed restrictive/obstructive pattern

3.4. Hypoxia without lung disease

3.5. Developmental lung disorders

Group 4. PH owing to pulmonary artery obstructions

4.1. Chronic thromboembolic PH

4.2. Other pulmonary artery obstructions

Group 5. PH with unclear and/or multifactorial mechanisms

5.1. Hematologic disorders

5.2. Systemic and metabolic disorders

5.3. Complex congenital heart disease

5.4. Others

Updated classification of PH according to the 6th World Symposium on Pulmonary Hypertension. *Abbreviation*: LEVF, left ventricular ejection fraction.
Adapted from Simonneau G, Montani D, Celermajer DS, et al. Haemodynamic definitions and updated clinical classification of pulmonary hypertension. Eur Respir J 2019;53:180191. Reproduced with permission of the © ERS 2020; https://doi.org/10.1183/13993003.01913-2018 Published 24 January 2019.

remodeling may be the principal factor responsible for AF development.[53]

Cardiac remodeling leading to atrial fibrillation
Ventricular hypertrophy and dilation Chronic increases in pulmonary artery pressure at rest create a pressure load on the right heart,[53] initially resulting in adaptive right ventricular hypertrophy.[54] In many cases, however, the condition progresses inexorably toward a maladaptive phenotype with dilation, tricuspid regurgitation resulting from dilation of the annulus, and culminating in right ventricular failure and death. In patients with acute decompensated systolic heart failure, right ventricular dysfunction is an important predictor of AF vulnerability.[55] Consistently, in experimental monocrotaline–induced PH, extensive right atrial remodeling was seen, including dilation, conduction abnormalities, inflammation, and fibrosis, along with increased AF vulnerability (**Fig. 1**).[56]

Development of atrial fibrillation substrate in pulmonary hypertension Mechanical stretch generates an AF-promoting arrhythmogenic substrate.[57] In the animal model of PH-induced RHD, genes involved in cardiac hypertrophy (*Acta1*, *Myl3*, and *Myh7*) are overexpressed in the right atrium.[58] In addition, PH-induced right atrial remodeling alters atrial action potentials in potentially arrhythmogenic ways (**Fig. 2**).[58–60] Stretch-activated channels responsive to cardiac loading may constitute therapeutic antiarrhythmic targets.[61]

Conduction abnormalities and arrhythmogenicity Changes in the atrial structure associated with dilation and stretch increase the risk of ectopy and arrhythmogenicity.[4] Conduction slows with lateralization, dephosphorylation and deregulated expression of connexins (Cxs) like Cx40 and Cx43 (see **Fig. 2**).[62] The expression of genes involved in Ca^{2+} handling (*Ryr2*, *Sln*, *Plb*, *Serca*, and *Scn5a*) is also perturbated with RHD, possibly leading to afterdepolarization-induced ectopic activity.[56]

Inflammation and fibrosis Inflammation may be the common final pathway of stress-induced

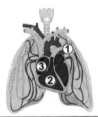

Fig. 1. Mechanistic cascade from pulmonary hypertension to AF. Increased pressures in the pulmonary arteries leads to pulmonary hypertension and right-sided heart disease that contributes to the arrhythmogenic substrate in the right atrium as shown.

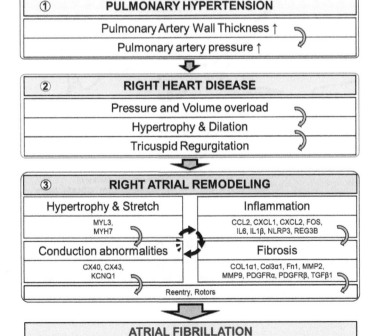

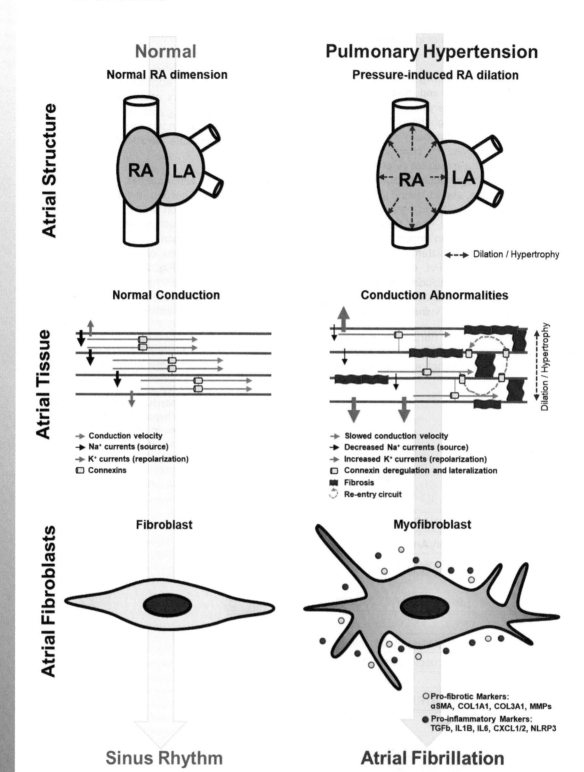

Fig. 2. Pulmonary hypertension-induced right atrial remodeling leading to AF. Pressure-induced right atrial remodeling involves right atrial dilation, conduction abnormalities, and proinflammatory- and profibrotic-triggered myofibroblast proliferation leading to arrhythmogenesis.

dysfunction.[63] There is extensive evidence suggesting a contribution of inflammation to the development of the AF substrate.[30] Long-term atrial pressure overload, along with volume overload owing to secondary tricuspid regurgitation, lead to local and systemic inflammation associated with an increased expression of interleukins and cytokines such as transforming growth factor-β, tumor necrosis factor-α, vascular endothelial growth factor, connective tissue growth factor, IL6, and IL-1β.[23,43,46] These molecules activate profibrotic signaling pathways, leading to overexpression of genes like *αSma*, *Col1*, *Col3*, *Mmp2*, and *Mmp9*. Fibroblast proliferation and differentiation to myofibroblasts increases the production of fibrous tissue (see **Fig. 2**),[56,59] promoting conduction slowing and the occurrence and maintenance of AF.

Other Arrhythmogenic Mechanisms Associated with Pulmonary Hypertension and Lung Disease

Besides the pressure and volume loads on the right heart that can be caused by pulmonary disease, a variety of other associated features might be involved in AF-promoting arrhythmogenesis. These include acid–base abnormalities, hypoxia, electrolyte disturbances, and changes in endocrine function.[63]

Autonomic system disorders, like enhanced sympathetic nervous system activity, and consequences of therapeutic interventions like beta-adrenergic agonists and glucocorticoids, might contribute to atrial arrhythmogenesis.[64] Such effects may be both direct, like the calcium-handling changes that promote arrhythmogenic afterdepolarizations owing to beta-adrenergic stimulation, and indirect, like the left heart remodeling owing to hypertension and salt/water retention caused by glucocorticoids.[65–69]

TREATMENT CHALLENGES OF ATRIAL FIBRILLATION IN PATIENTS WITH PULMONARY HYPERTENSION AND PULMONARY ARTERIAL HYPERTENSION
Sinus Rhythm Control

A recent article reviewed the current clinical management of atrial arrhythmias, including AF, in patients with PH.[70] Because patients with PH often show fragile right ventricular function, rate control agents like beta-blockers or calcium channel blockers are difficult to use safely and effectively. Digitalis may improve right ventricular contractility in PH,[71,72] and might therefore be of interest for rate control. In contrast, the potential ventricular proarrhythmic risk of digitalis needs to be considered. The approach recommended by the European Society of Cardiology and the European Respiratory Society is prompt rhythm control whenever possible.[44]

Antiarrhythmic Medications

Antiarrhythmic drugs must be used carefully, and any possible interactions with concomitant anti-PH medications must be considered. Amiodarone use requires increased caution in patients with parenchymal lung disease. Amiodarone can inhibit cytochrome P450 (CYP)2C9, potentially increasing the plasma concentrations of bosentan, an endothelin receptor antagonist often used to relax pulmonary vascular smooth muscle in patients with PH.[47] Furthermore, amiodarone-induced pulmonary toxicity can be a major problem in the face of compromised pulmonary function.[73]

Anticoagulation

Anticoagulant drugs are often used in patients with PH and those with AF. Clinicians must be mindful of potential drug interactions with anticoagulants.[74] Dabigatran, rivaroxaban, and apixaban must be used cautiously in combination with other medications like bosentan, amiodarone or aspirin, that interact with cytochrome P450 (CYP)3A or the permeability glycoprotein efflux transporter.[74]

Catheter Ablation and Anesthesia

Catheter ablation across the cavotricuspid isthmus is a successful technique with relatively low complication rates for typical atrial flutter. However, the right-sided cardiac remodeling, including tricuspid regurgitation and right atrial dilation that facilitate the occurrence of atrial flutter, can present technical challenges to catheter ablation.[75] Pulmonary veins are targeted for catheter ablation in patients with PH with AF as in other conditions, but it is important to consider non–pulmonary vein triggers in the right atrium.[76] Moreover, catheter ablation usually requires general anesthesia, which is more complex in patients with pulmonary disease and/or PH.[77] A possible algorithm for AF management in patients with PH is presented in **Fig. 3**.

POTENTIAL TARGETS FOR NOVEL THERAPEUTIC RESEARCH AND DEVELOPMENT

A pathophysiologic approach might help to identify novel therapeutic targets for AF associated with RHD.

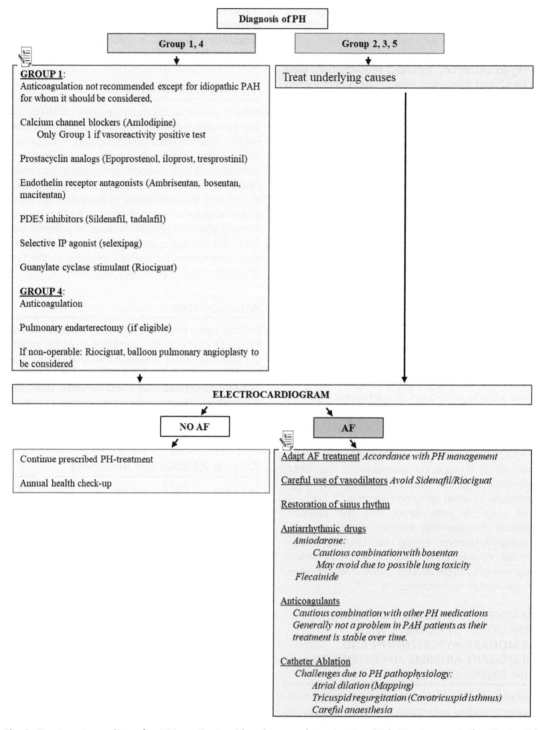

Fig. 3. Treatment paradigms for AF in patients with pulmonary hypertension (PH). Management of patients with PH diagnosed with AF is a complex approach, which involves the careful use of combined medications to avoid pharmacologic incompatibility and toxicity.

Prevent Right-Sided Cardiac Hypertrophy

Right ventricular hypertrophy leads to right atrial remodeling is an important contributor to arrhythmogenicity in pulmonary disease. To the extent possible, the underlying lung and/or pulmonary vascular disease should be controlled to prevent right ventricular hypertrophy. Histone deacetylases modulate gene-expression and are dysregulated in heart disease, including that associated with PH.[57] Recently, histone deacetylases 6 inhibition has been shown to prevent pressure overload-induced right ventricular hypertrophy in PH.[78] Thus, it may be possible to target the molecular signaling leading to right ventricular hypertrophy and thereby prevent right atrial remodeling and AF.

Correct Contraction and Conduction Abnormalities

Gap junctions are crucial in contractile tissues to ensure signal conduction and contractility. Recently, it was shown that reduced Cx43 activity could contribute to pulmonary vascular dysfunction in PH.[79] It has been demonstrated that Cx40 and Cx43 remodeling also contributes to AF.[80] Restoring normal gap junction function might improve both AF-related remodeling and the PH that causes it.

Sodium and potassium channels play an important role in cardiac electrophysiology. Heritable SCN5A defects are associated with increased AF vulnerability.[81] Increased activity of the potassium channel KCNA5 has been suspected to increase AF vulnerability in human.[82] In contrast, abnormal SCN5A expression has been observed in patients with PH and right ventricular hypertrophy.[83] In addition, altered expression or function of KCNA5 has been reported in patients with PH.[84] These studies suggest that the underlying mechanisms leading to SNC5A and KCNA5 malfunction may contribute to the pathogenesis of both PH and associated AF and therefore constitute therapeutic targets (**Table 2**).

Resolve or Suppress Inflammation

Chronic and unresolved inflammation has been described to play a crucial role in the genesis and maintenance of both PH and AF.[85,86] Among proinflammatory components, the NLRP3 inflammasome plays an important role in the development of lung injury and PH.[87] NLRP3 signaling has also been described to play a central role in AF.[88] NLRP3 mediates activation of other

Table 2
Relevant targets for future therapy

Molecules	Mechanism of Action	References
Cardiac hypertrophy		
Histone deacetylases	Load-induced cardiac hypertrophy	Boucherat et al,[78] 2017
Contraction and conduction		
CX43	Gap junction, intercellular communication	Htet et al,[79] 2018; Jennings & Donahue,[80] 2013
SCN5A	Voltage-dependent sodium channel	Olson et al,[81] 2005; Banerjee et al,[83] 2020
KCNA5	Voltage-gated potassium current	Christophersen et al,[82] 2013; Remillard et al,[84] 2007
Inflammation and fibrosis		
NLRP3 inflammasome	Inflammatory response to cellular damages, stress	Tang et al,[87] 2015; Yao et al,[88] 2018
IL1β, IL6, CCL2, tumor necrosis factor-α, transforming growth factor-β	Proinflammatory cytokines and chemoattractants	Price et al,[91] 2012; Huertas et al,[92] 2020; Hiram et al,[93] 2020
Bromodomain-containing protein 4, connective tissue growth factor, collagen I and III	Vascular and cardiac fibrosis	Song et al,[95] 2019; Van der Feen et al,[96] 2019

Review of key molecular pathways that contribute commonly to the severity of PH and to atrial arrhythmogenicity.

proinflammatory mediators like IL-1β, inhibition of which has shown beneficial effects in an animal model of PH.[89] Plasma IL-1β concentrations are increased in patients with AF.[90] Blood levels of other proinflammatory interleukins and cytokines such as IL6, CCL2, tumor necrosis factor-α, transforming growth factor-β, are elevated in patients with PH.[91,92] Expression of the same mediators is increased in AF, both in animal models and patients.[56,86] Anti-inflammatory therapy may help to prevent PH or AF via inhibition of expression of these mediators; however, no treatment to date specifically and effectively targets PH and/or AF by targeting inflammatory mediators.[86,92] Recently, it has been shown that daily injections of low-doses of a mediator that promotes the resolution of inflammation, resolvin-D1, suppresses proinflammatory signaling molecule production while increasing levels of anti-inflammatory effectors such as IL10, M2-macrophage, soc3, and Reg3B in a rat model of RHD-associated AF.[93] In parallel, adverse right atrial remodeling was prevented and AF promotion was suppressed.

Inflammation participates in the activation of profibrotic pathways. It is well known that atrial fibrosis promotes conduction abnormalities and reentry associated with increased AF vulnerability.[94] Inhibition of bromodomain-containing protein 4 decreases the development of cardiac hypertrophy and overexpression of fibrotic markers like connective tissue growth factor and collagens I and III.[95] A recent study that led to the initiation of a clinical trial, demonstrated that inhibition of bromodomain-containing protein 4 using RVX208 attenuates right ventricular and pulmonary vascular remodeling in rat models of hypoxia- and monocrotaline-induced PH96 (see **Table 2**).

SUMMARY

A significant number of patients with diseases of the lungs and their vasculature develop AF. The mechanisms linking lung disease to AF are incompletely understood, but substantial progress has been made in understanding them. Careful consideration of the specific pathophysiologic features of RHD-associated AF is helpful to optimize management and develop new therapeutic approaches.

CLINICS CARE POINTS

- Lung diseases, especially pulmonary hypertension should be considered as risk factors of AF.
- Management of AF patients with pulmonary hypertension may include prompt rhythm control when possible.

- Pharmacological treatment approaches must consider careful use of antiarrhythmic drugs in interaction with anti-PH and anticoagulant medications.
- Future therapeutic strategies may involve the prevention of chronic right-sided cardiac hypertrophy, amelioration of atrial conduction and contractile properties, and suppression of chronic and unresolved inflammation.

REFERENCES

1. Saad MN, Morin DP, Khatib S. Atrial fibrillation: current perspective. Ochsner J 2009;9(4):241–7.
2. Andrade J, Khairy P, Dobrev D, et al. The clinical profile and pathophysiology of atrial fibrillation: relationships among clinical features, epidemiology, and mechanisms. Circ Res 2014;114(9):1453–68.
3. Goudis CA, Ketikoglou DG. Obstructive sleep and atrial fibrillation: pathophysiological mechanisms and therapeutic implications. Int J Cardiol 2017; 230:293–300.
4. Rajdev A, Garan H, Biviano A. Arrhythmias in pulmonary arterial hypertension. Prog Cardiovasc Dis 2012;55(2):180–6.
5. Mims JW. Asthma: definitions and pathophysiology. Int Forum Allergy Rhinol 2015;5 Suppl 1:S2–6.
6. Liu MC, Hubbard WC, Proud D, et al. Immediate and late inflammatory responses to ragweed antigen challenge of the peripheral airways in allergic asthmatics. Cellular, mediator, and permeability changes. Am Rev Respir Dis 1991;144(1):51–8.
7. Doeing DC, Solway J. Airway smooth muscle in the pathophysiology and treatment of asthma. J Appl Physiol 2013;114(7):834–43.
8. Tattersall MC, Guo M, Korcarz CE, et al. Asthma predicts cardiovascular disease events: the multi-ethnic study of atherosclerosis. Arterioscler Thromb Vasc Biol 2015;35(6):1520–5.
9. Cepelis A, Brumpton BM, Malmo V, et al. Associations of asthma and asthma control with atrial fibrillation risk: results from the Nord-Trøndelag health study (HUNT). JAMA Cardiol 2018;3(8):721–8.
10. Carter P, Lagan J, Fortune C, et al. Association of cardiovascular disease with respiratory disease. J Am Coll Cardiol 2019;73(17):2166–77.
11. Singh D, Agusti A, Anzueto A, et al. Global strategy for the diagnosis, management, and prevention of chronic obstructive lung disease: the GOLD science committee report 2019. Eur Respir J 2019;53(5): 1900164.
12. Decramer M, Janssens W, Miravitlles M. Chronic obstructive pulmonary disease. Lancet 2012; 379(9823):1341–51.
13. King PT. Inflammation in chronic obstructive pulmonary disease and its role in cardiovascular disease and lung cancer. Clin Transl Med 2015;4(1):68.

14. Xiao X, Han H, Wu C, et al. Prevalence of atrial fibrillation in hospital encounters with end-stage COPD on home oxygen: national trends in the United States. Chest 2019;155(5):918–27.
15. Chan CS, Lin YS, Lin YK, et al. Atrial arrhythmogenesis in a rabbit model of chronic obstructive pulmonary disease. Transl Res 2020;223:25–39.
16. Matarese A, Sardu C, Shu J, et al. Why is chronic obstructive pulmonary disease linked to atrial fibrillation? A systematic overview of the underlying mechanisms. Int J Cardiol 2019;276:149–51.
17. Abdullah AS, Eigbire G, Ali M, et al. Relationship of atrial fibrillation to outcomes in patients hospitalized for chronic obstructive pulmonary disease exacerbation. J Atr Fibrillation 2019;12(2):2117.
18. Echevarria C, Steer J, Bourke SC. Comparison of early warning scores in patients with COPD exacerbation: DECAF and NEWS score. Thorax 2019;74(10):941–6.
19. Devine JF. Chronic obstructive pulmonary disease: an overview. Am Health Drug Benefits 2008;1(7):34–42.
20. Jordan AS, McSharry DG, Malhotra A. Adult obstructive sleep apnoea. Lancet 2014;383(9918):736–47.
21. Redline S, Yenokyan G, Gottlieb DJ, et al. Obstructive sleep apnea-hypopnea and incident stroke: the sleep heart health study. Am J Respir Crit Care Med 2010;182(2):269–77.
22. Gami AS, Pressman G, Caples SM, et al. Association of atrial fibrillation and obstructive sleep apnea. Circulation 2004;110:364–7.
23. Iwasaki YK, Kato T, Xiong F, et al. Atrial fibrillation promotion with long-term repetitive obstructive sleep apnea in a rat model. J Am Coll Cardiol 2014;64(19):2013–23.
24. Stevenson IH, Roberts-Thomson KC, Kistler PM, et al. Atrial electrophysiology is altered by acute hypercapnia but not hypoxemia: implications for promotion of atrial fibrillation in pulmonary disease and sleep apnea. Heart Rhythm 2010;7(9):1263–70.
25. Mandell LA, Wunderink RG, Anzueto A, et al. Infectious Diseases Society of America/American Thoracic Society consensus guidelines on the management of community-acquired pneumonia in adults. Clin Infect Dis 2007;44(Suppl 2):S27–72.
26. Stadie WC. The oxygen of the arterial and venous blood in pneumonia and its relation to cyanosis. J Exp Med 1919;30(3):215–40.
27. Stone WJ. Pericarditis as a complication in pneumonia: based on three hundred necropsies. JAMA 1919;73(4):254–8.
28. Soto-Gomez N, Anzueto A, Waterer GW, et al. Pneumonia: an arrhythmogenic disease? Am J Med 2013;126:43–8.
29. Kellum JA, Kong L, Fink MP, et al. Understanding the inflammatory cytokine response in pneumonia and sepsis: results of the genetic and inflammatory markers of sepsis (GenIMS) study. Arch Intern Med 2007;167(15):1655–63.
30. Harada M, Van Wagoner DR, Nattel S. Role of inflammation in atrial fibrillation pathophysiology and management. Circ J 2015;79(3):495–502.
31. Siegel RL, Miller KD, Jemal A. Cancer statistics, 2020. CA Cancer J Clin 2020;70(1):7–30.
32. Burns DM. Primary prevention, smoking, and smoking cessation: implications for future trends in lung cancer prevention. Cancer 2000;89(11 Suppl):2506–9.
33. Cates CU, Virmani R, Vaughn WK, et al. Electrocardiographic markers of cardiac metastasis. Am Heart J 1986;112(6):1297–303.
34. Dela Cruz CS, Tanoue LT, Matthay RA. Lung cancer: epidemiology, etiology, and prevention. Clin Chest Med 2011;32(4):605–44.
35. Issac TT, Dokainish H, Lakkis NM. Role of inflammation in initiation and perpetuation of atrial fibrillation: a systematic review of the published data. J Am Coll Cardiol 2007;50(21):2021–8.
36. Chung MK, Martin DO, Sprecher D, et al. C-reactive protein elevation in patients with atrial arrhythmias: inflammatory mechanisms and persistence of atrial fibrillation. Circulation 2001;104(24):2886–91.
37. Jakobsen CB, Lamberts M, Carlson N, et al. Incidence of atrial fibrillation in different major cancer subtypes: a nationwide population-based 12 year follow up study. BMC Cancer 2019;19(1):1105.
38. Bandyopadhyay D, Ball S, Hajra A, et al. Impact of atrial fibrillation in patients with lung cancer: insights from National Inpatient Sample. Int J Cardiol Heart Vasc 2019;22:216–7.
39. Kolb M, Vašáková M. The natural history of progressive fibrosing interstitial lung diseases. Respir Res 2019;20(1):57.
40. Hyldgaard C, Hilberg O, Bendstrup E. How does comorbidity influence survival in idiopathic pulmonary fibrosis? Respir Med 2014;108(4):647–53.
41. Fan E, Brodie D, Slutsky AS. Acute respiratory distress syndrome: advances in diagnosis and treatment. JAMA 2018;319(7):698–710.
42. Ambrus DB, Benjamin EJ, Bajwa EK, et al. Risk factors and outcomes associated with new-onset atrial fibrillation during acute respiratory distress syndrome. J Crit Care 2015;30(5):994–7.
43. Simonneau G, Montani D, Celermajer DS, et al. Haemodynamic definitions and updated clinical classification of pulmonary hypertension. Eur Respir J 2019;53:1801913.
44. Galiè N, Humbert M, Vachiery JL, et al. 2015 ESC/ERS Guidelines for the diagnosis and treatment of pulmonary hypertension. Eur Heart J 2016;37(1):67–119.
45. Frost A, Badesch D, Gibbs JSR, et al. Diagnosis of pulmonary hypertension. Eur Respir J 2019;53(1):1801904.

46. Galiè N, McLaughlin VV, Rubin LJ, et al. An overview of the 6th World Symposium on pulmonary hypertension. Eur Respir J 2019;53(1):1802148.

47. Tongers J, Schwerdtfeger B, Klein G, et al. Incidence and clinical relevance of supraventricular tachyarrhythmias in pulmonary hypertension. Am Heart J 2007;153(1):127–32.

48. Ruiz-Cano MJ, Gonzalez-Mansilla A, Escribano P, et al. Clinical implications of supraventricular arrhythmias in patients with severe pulmonary arterial hypertension. Int J Cardiol 2011;146:105–6.

49. Olsson KM, Nickel NP, Tongers J, et al. Atrial flutter and fibrillation in patients with pulmonary hypertension. Int J Cardiol 2013;167(5):2300–5.

50. Rottlaender D, Motloch LJ, Schmidt D, et al. Clinical impact of atrial fibrillation in patients with pulmonary hypertension. PLoS One 2012;7(3):e33902.

51. Wen L, Sun ML, An P, et al. Frequency of supraventricular arrhythmias in patients with idiopathic pulmonary arterial hypertension. Am J Cardiol 2014; 114(9):1420–5.

52. Cannillo M, Grosso Marra W, Gili S, et al. Supraventricular arrhythmias in patients with pulmonary arterial hypertension. Am J Cardiol 2015;116(12): 1883–9.

53. Humbert M, Morrell NW, Archer SL, et al. Cellular and molecular pathobiology of pulmonary arterial hypertension. J Am Coll Cardiol 2004;43(12 Suppl S):13S–24S.

54. Lambert M, Boet A, Rucker-Martin C, et al. Loss of KCNK3 is a hallmark of RV hypertrophy/dysfunction associated with pulmonary hypertension. Cardiovasc Res 2018;114:880–93.

55. Aziz EF, Kukin M, Javed F, et al. Right ventricular dysfunction is a strong predictor of developing atrial fibrillation in acutely decompensated heart failure patients, ACAP-HF data analysis. J Card Fail 2010; 16(10):827–34.

56. Hiram R, Naud P, Xiong F, et al. Right atrial mechanisms of atrial fibrillation in a rat model of right heart disease. J Am Coll Cardiol 2019;74(10):1332–47.

57. Janse MJ. Why does atrial fibrillation occur? Eur Heart J 1997;18(Suppl C):C12–8.

58. Nazir SA, Lab MJ. Mechanoelectric feedback in the atrium of the isolated Guinea-pig heart. Cardiovasc Res 1996;32(1):112–9.

59. Kalifa J, Jalife J, Zaitsev AV, et al. Intra-atrial pressure increases rate and organization of waves emanating from the superior pulmonary veins during atrial fibrillation. Circulation 2003;108(6): 668–71.

60. Nattel S, Dobrev D. Deciphering the fundamental mechanisms of atrial fibrillation: a quest for over a century. Cardiovasc Res 2016;109(4):465–6.

61. Bode F, Katchman A, Woosley RL, et al. Gadolinium decreases stretch-induced vulnerability to atrial fibrillation. Circulation 2000;101(18):2200–5.

62. Nattel S, Burstein B, Dobrev D. Atrial remodeling and atrial fibrillation: mechanisms and implications. Circ Arrhythm Electrophysiol 2008;1(1):62–73.

63. Liu YZ, Wang YX, Jiang CL. Inflammation: the common pathway of stress-related diseases. Front Hum Neurosci 2017;11:316.

64. Liu L, Zhao M, Yu X, et al. Pharmacological modulation of vagal nerve activity in cardiovascular diseases. Neurosci Bull 2019;35(1):156–66.

65. Undem BJ, Kollarik M. The role of vagal afferent nerves in chronic obstructive pulmonary disease. Proc Am Thorac Soc 2005;2(4):355–72.

66. Thomsen M, Nordestgaard BG, Sethi AA, et al. β2-adrenergic receptor polymorphisms, asthma and COPD: two large population-based studies. Eur Respir J 2012;39(3):558–66.

67. Bratel T, Wennlund A, Carlström K. Impact of hypoxaemia on neuroendocrine function and catecholamine secretion in chronic obstructive pulmonary disease (COPD). Effects of long-term oxygen treatment. Respir Med 2000;94(12):1221–8.

68. Olsson SB. Atrial fibrillation–Where do we stand today? J Intern Med 2001;250(1):19–28.

69. Buch P, Friberg J, Scharling H, et al. Reduced lung function and risk of atrial fibrillation in the Copenhagen City Heart Study. Eur Respir J 2003;21(6): 1012–6.

70. Wanamaker B, Cascino T, McLaughlin V, et al. Atrial arrhythmias in pulmonary hypertension: pathogenesis, prognosis and management. Arrhythm Electrophysiol Rev 2018;7(1):43–8.

71. Rich S, Seidlitz M, Dodin E, et al. The short-term effects of digoxin in patients with right ventricular dysfunction from pulmonary hypertension. Chest 1998;114(3):787–92.

72. Mathur PN, Powles AC, Pugsley SO, et al. Effect of long-term administration of digoxin on exercise performance in chronic airflow obstruction. Eur J Respir Dis 1985;66(4):273–83.

73. Siu C, Wong MP, Ho C, et al. Fatal lung toxic effects related to Dronedarone use. Arch Intern Med 2012; 172(6):516–7.

74. Hellwig T, Gulseth M. Pharmacokinetic and pharmacodynamic drug interactions with new oral anticoagulants: what do they mean for patients with atrial fibrillation? Ann Pharmacother 2013;47(11): 1478–87.

75. Luesebrink U, Fischer D, Gezgin F, et al. Ablation of typical right atrial flutter in patients with pulmonary hypertension. Heart Lung Circ 2012;21(11): 695–9.

76. Anter E, Di Biase L, Contreras-Valdes FM, et al. Atrial substrate and triggers of Paroxysmal atrial fibrillation in patients with obstructive sleep apnea. Circ Arrhythm Electrophysiol 2017;10(11):e005407.

77. Pilkington SA, Taboada D, Martinez G. Pulmonary hypertension and its management in patients

undergoing non-cardiac surgery. Anaesthesia 2015; 70(1):56–70.

78. Boucherat O, Chabot S, Paulin R, et al. HDAC6: a novel histone deacetylase implicated in pulmonary arterial hypertension. Sci Rep 2017;7(1):4546.

79. Htet M, Nally JE, Shaw A, et al. Connexin 43 plays a role in pulmonary vascular reactivity in mice. Int J Mol Sci 2018;19(7):1891.

80. Jennings MM, Donahue JK. Connexin remodeling contributes to atrial fibrillation. J Atr Fibrillation 2013;6(2):839.

81. Olson TM, Michels VV, Ballew JD, et al. Sodium channel mutations and susceptibility to heart failure and atrial fibrillation. JAMA 2005;293(4):447–54.

82. Christophersen IE, Olesen MS, Liang B, et al. Genetic variation in KCNA5: impact on the atrial-specific potassium current IKur in patients with lone atrial fibrillation. Eur Heart J 2013;34(20): 1517–25.

83. Banerjee D, Grammatopoulos TN, Palmisciano A, et al. Alternative splicing of the cardiac sodium channel in pulmonary arterial hypertension [published online ahead of print, 2020]. Chest 2020; 158(2):735–8.

84. Remillard CV, Tigno DD, Platoshyn O, et al. Function of Kv1.5 channels and genetic variations of KCNA5 in patients with idiopathic pulmonary arterial hypertension. Am J Physiol Cell Physiol 2007;292(5): C1837–53.

85. Hassoun PM. Inflammation in pulmonary arterial hypertension: is it time to quell the fire? Eur Respir J 2014;43(3):685–8.

86. Hu YF, Chen YJ, Lin YJ, et al. Inflammation and the pathogenesis of atrial fibrillation. Nat Rev Cardiol 2015;12(4):230–43.

87. Tang B, Chen GX, Liang MY, et al. Ellagic acid prevents monocrotaline-induced pulmonary artery hypertension via inhibiting NLRP3 inflammasome activation in rats. Int J Cardiol 2015;180:134–41.

88. Yao C, Veleva T, Scott L Jr, et al. Enhanced cardiomyocyte NLRP3 inflammasome signaling promotes atrial fibrillation [published correction appears in Circulation. 2019;139(17):e889]. Circulation 2018; 138(20):2227–42.

89. Voelkel NF, Tuder RM, Bridges J, et al. Interleukin-1 receptor antagonist treatment reduces pulmonary hypertension generated in rats by monocrotaline. Am J Respir Cell Mol Biol 1994;11(6):664–75.

90. Sazonova SI, Ilushenkova JN, Batalov RE, et al. Plasma markers of myocardial inflammation at isolated atrial fibrillation. J Arrhythm 2018;34(5): 493–500.

91. Price LC, Wort SJ, Perros F, et al. Inflammation in pulmonary arterial hypertension. Chest 2012; 141(1):210–21.

92. Huertas A, Tu L, Humbert M, et al. Chronic inflammation within the vascular wall in pulmonary arterial hypertension: more than a spectator. Cardiovasc Res 2020;116(5):885–93.

93. Hiram R, Xiong F, Naud P, et al. The inflammation resolution promoting molecule resolvin-D1 prevents atrial proarrhythmic remodeling in experimental right heart disease. [published online ahead of print] Cardiovasc Res 2020. cvaa186.

94. Nattel S. Molecular and cellular mechanisms of atrial fibrosis in atrial fibrillation. JACC Clin Electrophysiol 2017;3(5):425–35.

95. Song S, Liu L, Yu Y, et al. Inhibition of BRD4 attenuates transverse aortic constriction- and TGF-β-induced endothelial-mesenchymal transition and cardiac fibrosis. J Mol Cell Cardiol 2019;127:83–96.

96. Van der Feen DE, Kurakula K, Tremblay E, et al. Multicenter preclinical validation of BET inhibition for the treatment of pulmonary arterial hypertension. Am J Respir Crit Care Med 2019;200(7):910–20.

Atrial Fibrillation in Inherited Channelopathies

Baha'a Al-Azaam, MD[a,b], Dawood Darbar, MBChB, MD[a,b,c],*

KEYWORDS

- Atrial fibrillation • Brugada syndrome • Channelopathies • Long QT syndrome • Short QT syndrome
- Early repolarizations

KEY POINTS

- Improved understanding of the cause and pathogenesis of atrial fibrillation (AF) in inherited arrhythmia syndromes (Brugada syndrome; long QT syndrome; short QT syndrome; and early repolarization) has provided important insights into the underlying pathophysiological mechanisms of this common arrhythmia and identified potential mechanism-based therapies.
- The incidence of AF in inherited channelopathies is highly variable, often underdiagnosed, and to a large part depends on the pathophysiological mechanisms of the underlying condition.
- A diagnosis of AF has major impact on the clinical assessment and management of patients with inherited channelopathies.
- The underlying pathophysiological mechanisms for AF in patients with inherited channelopathies include both reentry and enhanced automaticity.

FAMILIAL ATRIAL FIBRILLATION

Background

Atrial fibrillation (AF), the common sustained arrhythmia in clinical practice, has major public health implications due to its associated morbidity and increased mortality, with an expected increase in the prevalence of AF from 12.1 to 15.9 million by 2050 in the United States alone.[1] The epidemic of AF is due to the burgeoning elderly population and the identification of novel risk factors, for example, genetics.[2] Until recently, AF was considered to be a sporadic, nongenetic disorder but studies at multiple centers have identified both common and rare genetic variants contributing to AF susceptibility. Although the underlying pathophysiology remains unclear, the authors and others have shown that AF is a genetic disease with variable age-dependent penetrance determined by diverse genetic and acquired arrhythmogenic mechanisms.

Genetics of Familial Atrial Fibrillation

A significant proportion of patients lack traditional risk factors for AF and present at a young age, and although this type was previously called "lone," it is now better termed "familial or early onset" (EO) AF. Linkage analysis, candidate gene, and next generation sequencing (NGS) have identified mutations in cardiac ion channels, transcription factors, and myocardial structural proteins linked with EOAF (**Table 1**). Conversely, genome-wide association studies have identified more than 100 common genetic variants associated with the arrhythmia.[3]

Funding sources: This work is in part supported by NIH T32 HL139439 and NIH R01 HL138737 grants to Dr D. Darbar.

a Division of Cardiology, Department of Medicine, University of Illinois at Chicago, 820 S Wood Street, Suite 920S, Chicago, IL 60612, USA; b Division of Cardiology, Department of Pharmacology, University of Illinois at Chicago, 820 S Wood Street, Suite 920S, Chicago, IL 60612, USA; c Department of Medicine, Jesse Brown Veterans Administration, 820 S Wood Street, Suite 920S, Chicago, IL 60612, USA
* Corresponding author. Division of Cardiology, University of Illinois at Chicago, 840 South Wood Street, 920S (MC 715), Chicago, IL 60612.
E-mail address: Darbar@uic.edu

Card Electrophysiol Clin 13 (2021) 155–163
https://doi.org/10.1016/j.ccep.2020.10.004

Table 1
Characterization of inherited channelopathies associated with atrial fibrillation

Inherited Channelopathy	Prevalence of AF	Clinical Impact	Genes	Mechanisms of AF	Implications for Treatment
Familial (early onset) AF	11%–22%	• Increased risk of cardioembolic stroke • Vascular dementia • Atrial and ventricular cardiomyopathy	• Ion channels/transporters (K^+, Na^+, Ca^{2+}) • Transcription factors/signaling molecules (*NKX2.5, NPPA, PITX2, TBX5*) • Myocardial structural proteins (*ANK2, CAV1, GJA5/A1, MYH6, TTN*)	• *Reentry:* modulation of APD, cell-cell coupling, and conduction heterogeneity • *Automaticity:* APD prolongation triggering EADs	AADs PVI
Brugada syndrome (BrS)	6%–53%	• Increased risk of cardioembolic stroke • Increased risk of inappropriate ICD shocks	*CACNA1C* and *CACNB2b* (LOF) *SCN5A* and *SCN10A* (LOF)	• *Reentry:* phase 2 reentry; delayed sinoatrial node recovery time and conduction heterogeneity • *Automaticity:* autonomic modulation	Quinidine PVI
Congenital long QT syndrome (LQTS)	0.5%–2%	Increased risk of inappropriate ICD shocks	*KCNQ1 (LOF)* *SCN5A (GOF)*	• *Reentry:* Increased TDR • *Automaticity:* enhanced late sodium current triggering EADs	Flecainide (LQT3)
Short QT syndrome (SQTS)	15%–24%	Inappropriate ICD shocks due to: • Rapid AF • Tall and peaked T waves causing "double" counting	*KCNH2 GOF* *KCNQ1 GOF* *KCNJ2 GOF* *CACNA2D1, CACNA1C,* and *CACNB2* (LOF)	*Reentry:* prolonged TDR with prolonged T_{peak}-T_{end} as a surrogate index	Quinidine flecainide
Early repolarization syndrome (ERS)	25%	Increased risk of inappropriate ICD shocks	*KCNJ8 (GOF)*	*Reentry:* increased TDR	Quinidine PVI

Abbreviations: AADs, antiarrhythmic drugs; APD, action potential duration; EAD, early after-depolarization; ECG, electrocardiogram; GOF, gain-of-function; ICD, implantable cardioverter defibrillator; LOF, loss-of-function; PVI, pulmonary vein isolation; TdP, torsades de pointes; TDR, transmural dispersion of repolarization; VF, ventricular fibrillation.

Genetic approaches to AF have provided important insights into underlying pathophysiology, but direct impact of these discoveries to the bedside care of patients has been limited because of the challenges of adequately recapitulating human AF in cellular models.[4] Although in vitro models for assessing AF variants have been used by many,[5,6] cardiomyocytes (CMs) have very distinct electrophysiologic (EP) properties, and heterologous expression systems cannot capture the full spectrum of functional changes. Furthermore, as ion channels are species specific, murine models cannot replicate human AF.[7,8] Ideally, deciphering the cellular mechanisms of AF-causing mutations requires using human atrial CMs, which are rarely available. Conversely, abundant and patient-specific atrial-induced pluripotent stem cell–derived (iPSC) CMs not only possess the complex array of cardiac ion channels that make up the atrial action potential (AP) but can be electrically coupled to model electrical impulse propagation and elucidate AF mechanisms.[9,10] Thus, modeling AF-linked mutations using atrial iPSC-CMs offers a naturally integrated system with distinct advantages over heterologous systems and transgenic murine models.

BRUGADA SYNDROME AND ATRIAL FIBRILLATION
Epidemiology

AF is the most common sustained atrial arrhythmia in BrS with incidence of 6% to 53%.[11] One of the largest retrospective studies of 560 patients with BrS showed 9% incidence of AF with other studies reporting similar rates.[12,13] The varying incidence is related to whether the study was prospective or retrospective; sample size; frequency and intensity of AF monitoring; duration of follow-up; and if the study was single versus multicenter.[11,12]

Clinical Impact

Because AF is common in BrS and can go undetected with routine detection methods, unrecognized AF may lead to higher risk of thromboembolic events, with one study showing 14% rate of cardioembolic stroke.[13] In addition, one study reported that patients with BrS with AF have worse prognosis when compared with patients without AF. Importantly, AF is not a risk factor for sudden cardiac death (SCD) but rather seems to be a marker of more advanced disease.[12]

Several studies have reported inappropriate implantable cardioverter defibrillator (ICD) shocks due to rapid AF in 30% to 39% of patients with BrS.[13,14] A meta-analysis of more than 1700 patients found that there is a significant association between AF and an increased risk of major arrhythmic events including SCD, ventricular fibrillation (VF), supraventricular tachycardia (SVT), or appropriate shock in patients with BrS.[15]

GENETIC BASIS OF ATRIAL FIBRILLATION IN BRUGADA SYNDROME
Pathophysiology

Many studies have reported an association between genetic variants/genes common to both EOAF and BrS including α1- (CACNA1C) and β-subunits (CACNB2b) of the L-type cardiac calcium channel (Cav1.2)[16] and SCN5A and SCN10A encoding the cardiac voltage-gated sodium channels Nav1.5 and Nav1.8, respectively.[17,18] However, SCN5A loss-of-function (LOF) mutations have the strongest association with both EOAF and BrS, with the variants reducing sodium channel membrane surface channel expression, accelerating inactivation, or altering channel gating (see Table 1).

Epicardial CMs exhibit spike-and-dome APs with a characteristic notch due to a prominent transient outward current (I_{to}). Ventricular arrhythmias are thought to be due to heterogeneity in phase 1 of the AP across epicardial, midmyocardial ("M"), and endocardial CMs from either decrease in the inward sodium current (I_{Na}) and/or calcium currents (I_{Ca}) or I_{to} increase causing a shift in balance and loss-of-dome transitions. Heterogeneity in spike-and-dome and loss-of-dome provides a substrate for shorter APs and transmural dispersion of repolarization (TDR), leading to transition of electrotonic current from phase 2 AP sites to already recovered loss-of-dome sites resulting in abnormal reexcitation known as phase-2 reentry. This coupled extrasystole if captured during the vulnerable window will trigger ventricular tachycardia (VT)/VF. In the atria with abundant I_{to} an AF episode may also be triggered by closely coupled extrasystoles, implicating a common mechanism for both atrial and ventricular arrhythmias in patients with BrS.[11,19]

A second potential reentrant mechanism of AF in patients with BrS relates to cardiac conduction disease associated with SCN5A LOF mutations. Studies have shown that patients carrying an SCN5A BrS-causing mutation have significantly prolonged His ventricular (HV) intervals and are more likely to develop atrial arrhythmias.[20,21] Kusano and colleagues[22] showed that delayed sinoatrial (SA) node recovery time and intraatrial electrical conduction creates a reentrant AF substrate in patients harboring SCN5A mutations with data showing a greater induction of AF. There is also a diurnal variation in ventricular arrhythmias and AF in patients with BrS, with most arrhythmias occurring between midnight and early morning.[22] This circadian pattern suggests that nocturnal vagal activity and withdrawal of sympathetic activity may play an important role in arrhythmogenesis in both VT/VF and AF in BrS. Structural changes characterized by epicardial surface and interstitial fibrosis, increased collagen throughout the heart, and reduced gap junction expression in the right ventricular outflow tract seen in BrS are also thought to play a role in creating reentrant circuits, abnormal potentials, and induction of arrhythmias.[22,23]

Implications for Treatment

A pharmacologic approach with the goal of rebalancing the epicardial AP in the right ventricle and restoring the dome may decrease arrhythmogenesis in BrS.[12] However, such an approach is challenging patients with BrS with AF because sodium channel blocking (class I) antiarrhythmic drugs (AAD) including amiodarone are proarrhythmic precipitate ventricular arrhythmias.[14,24] Quinidine is the exception because it blocks I_{to} normalizing the epicardial AP dome, preventing phase-2 reentry and polymorphic VT in experimental models of BrS.[25] When hydroquinidine was given to patients with BrS and AF, there was no recurrence of atrial arrhythmias over a 2-year follow-up.[12] Studies have also shown that pulmonary vein isolation (PVI) is a highly effective treatment of AF in patients with BrS with freedom from recurrence of atrial arrhythmias without AADs in 83%,[26] to 91.8%[14] on long-term follow-up.

LONG QT SYNDROME AND ATRIAL FIBRILLATION
Epidemiology

Congenital long QT syndrome (LQTS), characterized by a prolonged QT interval on the ECG, is associated with increased risk for SCD due to life-threatening arrhythmia. With more than 15 different forms of the syndrome, LQT1, LQT2, and LQT3 are by far the most common in clinical practice, accounting for 85% to 95% of cases.[27] The incidence of AF in LQTS is 0.5% to 2% and much higher than age-matched general population.[28,29] Furthermore, AF is more common in LQT1 and likely underdetected, as paroxysmal can be asymptomatic.[30]

Clinical Impact

The major clinical impact of AF in patients with LQTS is the risk for inappropriate shocks due to

rapid AF, with studies reporting that 27% of patients received ICD shocks[31] with other studies reporting multiple device mode switches due to atrial tachyarrhythmias.[30]

Pathophysiology

A prolonged QT interval results either from a decrease in repolarizing outward potassium currents (I_K) or from an increase in depolarizing inward I_{Na}/I_{Ca}, creating a pathophysiological substrate for LQTS.[32] Almost 75% of patients with LQTS harbor mutations in KCNQ1 (LQT1; LOF),[33] KCNH2 (LQT2; LOF),[34] and SCN5A (LQT3; gain-of-function [GOF]),[35] which encode the major pore-forming α-subunits of the macromolecular channel complexes Kv7.1 (I_{Ks}), Kv11.1 (I_{Kr}), and Nav1.5 (I_{Na}), respectively. Multiple studies have linked patients with genotype-positive LQTS and AF to LOF mutations in KCNQ1[27,36] and GOF SCN5A mutations.[37]

The canonical Nav1.5 channel encoded by SCN5A mediates the inward I_{Na} composed of the peak and late sodium currents ($I_{Na,L}$), with GOF mutations modulating both currents and triggering torsades de pointes (TdP) and AF. These mutations augment the peak amplitude of I_{Na}, cause negative shifts in the voltage-dependence of activation, and accelerate recovery from inactivation. Similarly, an increase in I_{Na-L}, along with increased sarcoplasmic reticulum calcium release, generates early after-depolarization (EADs) and delayed afterdepolarizations (DAD).[38] Increased $I_{Na,L}$, which occurs mostly in M cells than endocardial or epicardial cells, leads to increased TDR and refractoriness causing reentrant excitation and TdP.[39] Because the ionic channels responsible for both ventricular and atrial repolarization are similar but nonidentical, any potential delay in atrial repolarization in patients with LQTS may predispose to AF by a similar mechanism to TdP. The increased I_{Na-L} can prolong the atrial action potential duration (APD) and trigger EADs and AF. Kirchhof and colleagues[40] reported that APD was longer in patients with LQTS than in controls at all 3 repolarization levels, and patients with altered atrial electrical conduction were at increased risk for polymorphic atrial tachyarrhythmias. Satoh and Zipes, the first to describe atrial TdP, showed that blocking potassium channels using cesium generated atrial EADs with polymorphic atrial tachycardia that subsequently degenerated into AF.[41]

Implications for Treatment

Management of AF in patients with LQTS is challenging, as many of the AADs used to treat the arrhythmia are contraindicated due to their proar-rhythmic risk. However, recent guidelines recommend flecainide as a suitable option for patients with LQT3.[42]

SHORT QT SYNDROME AND ATRIAL FIBRILLATION
Epidemiology

Patients with SQTS, a hereditary channelopathy characterized by short QT intervals (QT<360 or QTc<370 msec), present with syncope, paroxysmal AF, VT/VF, and SCD.[43] The reported incidence of AF in SQTS is 15% to 24%,[44,45] with one study finding a higher incidence of the arrhythmia in genotype-positive (19%) versus genotype-negative patients (0%),[46] and the highest prevalence of AF was in SQT2 patients.[47]

Clinical Impact

Patients with SQTS are at risk for inappropriate ICD shocks due to rapid AF and "double counting" of the tall peaked T waves (Fig. 1).[48] However, inappropriate shocks resulting from rapid atrial arrhythmias and double counting can be prevented by reprogramming device therapies for heart rates exceeding 210 beats/min and adjusting sensitivity parameters.[44,48]

Pathophysiology of Atrial Fibrillation in Short QT Syndrome

The 6 subtypes of SQTS consist of GOF mutations in KCNH2 (SQT1), KCNQ1 (SQT2), and KCNJ2 (SQT3) and LOF mutations in CACNA2D1 (SQT4), CACNA1C (SQT5), and CACNB2 (SQT6).[49,50] One study reported no difference in the genetic profiles and clinical presentation with SQTS genotype-positive patients having no higher risk of cardiac events than genotype-negative patients.[46]

The SQTS, characterized by accelerated cellular repolarization, is due to either enhanced outward repolarizing I_K or a reduced inward depolarizing I_{Ca}. The transmural voltage gradient between the different layers of the ventricular myocardium generates varying repolarization time contributing to T-wave formation on the ECG. Although under normal conditions the repolarization disparities are minimal, patients with SQTS, characterized by tall, peaked, and symmetric T waves (see Fig. 1), have prolonged T_{peak}-T_{end}, with the difference in this interval providing a surrogate index of TDR. Infusing pinacidil, an I_{K-ATP} activator, in canine arterially perfused wedge preparation not only shortened the QT interval and prolonged T_{peak}–T_{end} interval but also augmented TDR creating a reentrant substrate for ventricular tachyarrhythmias.[51,52] Extramiana and Antzelevitch also reported that programmed electrical stimulation induced VT/VF after pinacidil with QT shortening versus controls with normal QT time and reduced T_{peak}–T_{end}. Because ion channel mutations are distributed in both ventricles and atria, the mechanism by which atrial arrhythmias arise may be similar to those in the ventricles.[51]

Implications of Treatment

Quinidine is the only AAD tested for the treatment of SQTS, with several studies reporting therapeutic efficacy in reducing the incidence of ventricular arrhythmias.[53] However, it remains unclear if it is efficacious for the prevention of AF in pediatric

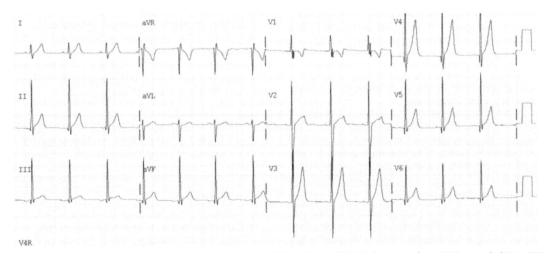

V4R

Fig. 1. An electrocardiogram from a patient with short QT syndrome (SQTS) showing short QT intervals (QTc <370 msec) and tall peaked T waves in the precordial leads, which can lead to "double" counting and inappropriate ICD shocks.

patients with SQTS.[44] Flecainide, a class I AAD that also blocks I_{Kr} and I_{to}, increases ventricular effective refractory period but acute administration of the drug did cause prolongation of refractoriness but only slight prolongation of QT interval.[54] Drugs such as ibutilide, sotalol, propafenone, carvedilol, metoprolol, and amiodarone have not undergone clinical testing because of scarcity of patients and the low event rate in patients with SQTS suitable for clinical trials.

EARLY REPOLARIZATION SYNDROME AND ATRIAL FIBRILLATION
Epidemiology

The ECG finding of ER, common in the general population with a prevalence of 1% to 2%, is characterized by elevation of the J point in the inferior and/or lateral leads and has generally been considered benign for decades. However, recent studies showed that certain patterns of ER are not benign and associated with increased risk for idiopathic VF and SCD.[55] The association between ERS and AF is less clear, with one study reporting a 25% prevalence of ER pattern in patients with EOAF as compared with 10% in age- and sex-matched healthy controls.[55] Conversely, other studies found no difference in the prevalence of ER pattern in patients with AF, even limiting analysis to those younger than 50 years.[56]

Clinical Impact

Patients with ERS and AF are prone to inappropriate ICD shocks due to rapid AF with ~20% incidence rate.[57] Reprogramming ICDs with higher detection rates (>200–240 bpm) and prolonged detection intervals may prevent shocks.[57] Dual-chamber ICDs are also helpful in reducing inappropriate shocks due to atrial arrhythmias but can be associated with higher complication rates at implantation.[58]

Pathophysiology of Atrial Fibrillation in Early Repolarization Syndrome

A *KCNJ8*GOF mutation, encoding the I_{K-ATP} (Kir6.1) has been associated with both AF and ERS with a *KCNJ8*-S422L variant shortening ventricular repolarization and increasing susceptibility to VT/VF. Because I_{K-ATP} channels are found in both the atria and ventricles, a *KCNJ8* mutation could shorten the AP in the atria and induce AF. Similar to BrS, the shortened effective refractory period induces ventricular arrhythmias by alteration in the outward shift in AP repolarizing currents due to a decrease in I_{Na} or I_{Ca} or an increase in I_{to}, I_{K-ATP}, or I_{K-Ach} giving rise to

transmural voltage gradient between endocardium and epicardium together with accentuation of the epicardial notch in different regions of the heart. Theoretically, diminished I_{Na} and slowed conduction velocity present in atria increases susceptibility to reentrant AF.[59]

Implications of Treatment

Many case reports suggest quinidine is the most effective AAD to reduce VF episodes and prevent AF.[60] However, adverse effects and a narrow therapeutic index necessitate monitoring quinidine levels.[61] Another therapeutic option to treat AF in patients with ERS is PVI, which can eliminate the trigger and/or modify the substrate, but this option is only suitable for patients with ICDs. However, the success rate is unclear due to limited numbers of patients and the genetic defect causing an atrial CM.[57]

CLINICS CARE POINTS

- Atrial Fibrillation (AF) is common in Brugada syndrome (BrS) and can go undetected with routine detection methods, unrecognized AF may lead to higher risk of thromboembolic events.
- There is a significant association between AF and an increased risk of major arrhythmic events including sudden cardiac death (SCD), ventricular fibrillation (VF), supraventricular tachycardia (SVT), or inappropriate shocks in patients with BrS.
- Pulmonary vein isolation (PVI) is a highly effective treatment of AF in patients with BrS.
- The major clinical impact of AF in patients with long QT syndrome (LQTS) is the risk for inappropriate shocks due to rapid AF. Recent guidelines recommend flecainide as a suitable option for patients with LQTS type 3.
- The reported incidence of AF in short QT syndrome (SQTS) is 15% to 24%; with the highest prevalence in SQT2 patients. Patients with SQTS are at risk for inappropriate ICD shocks due to rapid AF and "double counting" of the tall peaked T waves.
- Patients with early repolarization syndrome (ERS) and AF are prone to inappropriate ICD shocks due to rapid AF with an incidence of 20%. Reprogramming implantable cardioverter defibrillators (ICD) with higher detection rates (>200–240 bpm) and prolonged detection intervals may prevent shocks.
- Quinidine is the most effective antiarrhythmic drug (AAD) to reduce VF episodes and prevent AF. However, adverse effects and a narrow therapeutic index necessitate frequent monitoring of quinidine levels.

DISCLOSURES

None.

REFERENCES

1. Miyasaka Y, Barnes ME, Gersh BJ, et al. Secular trends in incidence of atrial fibrillation in Olmsted County, Minnesota, 1980 to 2000, and implications on the projections for future prevalence. Circulation 2006;114(2):119–25.
2. Kavousi M. Differences in epidemiology and risk factors for atrial fibrillation between women and men. Front Cardiovasc Med 2020;7:3.
3. Roselli C, Chaffin MD, Weng LC, et al. Multi-ethnic genome-wide association study for atrial fibrillation. Nat Genet 2018;50(9):1225–33.
4. Darbar D, Roden DM. Genetic mechanisms of atrial fibrillation: impact on response to treatment. Nat Rev Cardiol 2013;10(6):317–29.
5. Darbar D, Kannankeril PJ, Donahue BS, et al. Cardiac sodium channel (SCN5A) variants associated with atrial fibrillation. Circulation 2008;117(15): 1927–35.
6. Abraham RL, Yang T, Blair M, et al. Augmented potassium current is a shared phenotype for two genetic defects associated with familial atrial fibrillation. J Mol Cell Cardiol 2010;48(1):181–90.
7. Li Y, Sallam K, Schwartz PJ, et al. Patient-specific induced pluripotent stem cell-based disease model for pathogenesis studies and clinical pharmacotherapy. Circ Arrhythm Electrophysiol 2017;10(6): e005398.
8. Shi Y, Inoue H, Wu JC, et al. Induced pluripotent stem cell technology: a decade of progress. Nat Rev Drug Discov 2017;16(2):115–30.
9. Herron TJ, Rocha AM, Campbell KF, et al. Extracellular matrix-mediated maturation of human pluripotent stem cell-derived cardiac monolayer structure and electrophysiological function. Circ Arrhythm Electrophysiol 2016;9(4):e003638.
10. da Rocha AM, Campbell K, Mironov S, et al. hiPSC-CM monolayer maturation state determines drug responsiveness in high throughput pro-arrhythmia screen. Sci Rep 2017;7(1):13834.
11. Francis J, Antzelevitch C. Atrial fibrillation and Brugada syndrome. J Am Coll Cardiol 2008;51(12): 1149–53.
12. Giustetto C, Cerrato N, Gribaudo E, et al. Atrial fibrillation in a large population with Brugada electrocardiographic pattern: prevalence, management, and correlation with prognosis. Heart Rhythm 2014; 11(2):259–65.
13. de Asmundis C, Mugnai G, Chierchia GB, et al. Abnormally high risk of stroke in Brugada syndrome. J Cardiovasc Med (Hagerstown) 2019;20(2):59–65.
14. Rodríguez-Mañero M, Kreidieh B, Valderrábano M, et al. Ablation of atrial fibrillation in patients with Brugada syndrome: a systematic review of the literature. J Arrhythm 2019;35(1):18–24.
15. Kewcharoen J, Rattanawong P, Kanitsoraphan C, et al. Atrial fibrillation and risk of major arrhythmic events in Brugada syndrome: a meta-analysis. Ann Noninvasive Electrocardiol 2019;24(6):e12676.
16. Burashnikov E, Pfeiffer R, Barajas-Martinez H, et al. Mutations in the cardiac L-type calcium channel associated with inherited J-wave syndromes and sudden cardiac death. Heart Rhythm 2010;7(12):1872–82.
17. Hu D, Barajas-Martínez H, Pfeiffer R, et al. Mutations in SCN10A are responsible for a large fraction of cases of Brugada syndrome. J Am Coll Cardiol 2014;64(1):66–79.
18. Yagihara N, Watanabe H, Barnett P, et al. Variants in the SCN5A promoter associated with various arrhythmia phenotypes. J Am Heart Assoc 2016; 5(9):e003644.
19. Maoz A, Christini DJ, Krogh-Madsen T. Dependence of phase-2 reentry and repolarization dispersion on epicardial and transmural ionic heterogeneity: a simulation study. Europace 2014;16(3):458–65.
20. Smits JP, Eckardt L, Probst V, et al. Genotype-phenotype relationship in Brugada syndrome: electrocardiographic features differentiate SCN5A-related patients from non-SCN5A-related patients. J Am Coll Cardiol 2002;40(2):350–6.
21. Bordachar P, Reuter S, Garrigue S, et al. Incidence, clinical implications and prognosis of atrial arrhythmias in Brugada syndrome. Eur Heart J 2004; 25(10):879–84.
22. Kusano KF, Taniyama M, Nakamura K, et al. Atrial fibrillation in patients with Brugada syndrome relationships of gene mutation, electrophysiology, and clinical backgrounds. J Am Coll Cardiol 2008; 51(12):1169–75.
23. Toh N, Morita H, Nagase S, et al. Atrial electrophysiological and structural remodeling in high-risk patients with Brugada syndrome: assessment with electrophysiology and echocardiography. Heart Rhythm 2010;7(2):218–24.
24. Paul G, Yusuf S, Sharma S. Unmasking of the Brugada syndrome phenotype during the acute phase of amiodarone infusion. Circulation 2006;114(11): e489–91.
25. Antzelevitch C, Patocskai B. Brugada syndrome: clinical, genetic, molecular, cellular, and ionic aspects. Curr Probl Cardiol 2016;41(1):7–57.
26. Yamada T, Yoshida Y, Tsuboi N, et al. Efficacy of pulmonary vein isolation in paroxysmal atrial fibrillation patients with a Brugada electrocardiogram. Circ J 2008;72(2):281–6.
27. Priori SG, Schwartz PJ, Napolitano C, et al. Risk stratification in the long-QT syndrome. N Engl J Med 2003;348(19):1866–74.

28. Johnson JN, Tester DJ, Perry J, et al. Prevalence of early-onset atrial fibrillation in congenital long QT syndrome. Heart Rhythm 2008;5(5):704–9.

29. Mohler PJ, Splawski I, Napolitano C, et al. A cardiac arrhythmia syndrome caused by loss of ankyrin-B function. Proc Natl Acad Sci U S A 2004;101(24): 9137–42.

30. Zellerhoff S, Pistulli R, Mönnig G, et al. Atrial arrhythmias in long-QT syndrome under daily life conditions: a nested case control study. J Cardiovasc Electrophysiol 2009;20(4):401–7.

31. Horner JM, Kinoshita M, Webster TL, et al. Implantable cardioverter defibrillator therapy for congenital long QT syndrome: a single-center experience. Heart Rhythm 2010;7(11):1616–22.

32. Schwartz PJ, Crotti L, Insolia R. Long-QT syndrome: from genetics to management. Circ Arrhythm Electrophysiol 2012;5(4):868–77.

33. Wang Q, Curran ME, Splawski I, et al. Positional cloning of a novel potassium channel gene: KVLQT1 mutations cause cardiac arrhythmias. Nat Genet 1996;12(1):17–23.

34. Curran ME, Splawski I, Timothy KW, et al. A molecular basis for cardiac arrhythmia: HERG mutations cause long QT syndrome. Cell 1995;80(5): 795–803.

35. Wang Q, Shen J, Splawski I, et al. SCN5A mutations associated with an inherited cardiac arrhythmia, long QT syndrome. Cell 1995;80(5): 805–11.

36. Bartos DC, Anderson JB, Bastiaenen R, et al. A KCNQ1 mutation causes a high penetrance for familial atrial fibrillation. J Cardiovasc Electrophysiol 2013;24(5):562–9.

37. Benito B, Brugada R, Perich RM, et al. A mutation in the sodium channel is responsible for the association of long QT syndrome and familial atrial fibrillation. Heart Rhythm 2008;5(10):1434–40.

38. Han D, Tan H, Sun C, et al. Dysfunctional Nav1.5 channels due to SCN5A mutations. Exp Biol Med (Maywood) 2018;243(10):852–63.

39. el-Sherif N, Caref EB, Yin H, et al. The electrophysiological mechanism of ventricular arrhythmias in the long QT syndrome. Tridimensional mapping of activation and recovery patterns. Circ Res 1996;79(3): 474–92.

40. Kirchhof P, Eckardt L, Franz MR, et al. Prolonged atrial action potential durations and polymorphic atrial tachyarrhythmias in patients with long QT syndrome. J Cardiovasc Electrophysiol 2003;14(10): 1027–33.

41. Satoh T, Zipes DP. Cesium-induced atrial tachycardia degenerating into atrial fibrillation in dogs: atrial torsades de pointes? J Cardiovasc Electrophysiol 1998;9(9):970–5.

42. Al-Khatib SM, Stevenson WG, Ackerman MJ, et al. 2017 AHA/ACC/HRS guideline for management of patients with ventricular arrhythmias and the prevention of sudden cardiac death: executive summary: a report of the American college of cardiology/American heart association task force on clinical practice guidelines and the heart rhythm society. Heart Rhythm 2018;15(10):e190–252.

43. Gaita F, Giustetto C, Bianchi F, et al. Short QT Syndrome: a familial cause of sudden death. Circulation 2003;108(8):965–70.

44. Villafañe J, Atallah J, Gollob MH, et al. Long-term follow-up of a pediatric cohort with short QT syndrome. J Am Coll Cardiol 2013;61(11):1183–91.

45. Giustetto C, Di Monte F, Wolpert C, et al. Short QT syndrome: clinical findings and diagnostic-therapeutic implications. Eur Heart J 2006;27(20):2440–7.

46. Raschwitz LS, El-Battrawy I, Schlentrich K, et al. Differences in short QT syndrome subtypes: a systematic literature review and pooled analysis. Front Genet 2019;10:1312.

47. Harrell DT, Ashihara T, Ishikawa T, et al. Genotype-dependent differences in age of manifestation and arrhythmia complications in short QT syndrome. Int J Cardiol 2015;190:393–402.

48. Borggrefe M, Wolpert C, Antzelevitch C, et al. Short QT syndrome. Genotype-phenotype correlations. J Electrocardiol 2005;38(4 Suppl):75–80.

49. Pérez Riera AR, Paixão-Almeida A, Barbosa-Barros R, et al. Congenital short QT syndrome: landmarks of the newest arrhythmogenic cardiac channelopathy. Cardiol J 2013;20(5):464–71.

50. Gollob MH, Redpath CJ, Roberts JD. The short QT syndrome: proposed diagnostic criteria. J Am Coll Cardiol 2011;57(7):802–12.

51. Extramiana F, Antzelevitch C. Amplified transmural dispersion of repolarization as the basis for arrhythmogenesis in a canine ventricular-wedge model of short-QT syndrome. Circulation 2004;110(24): 3661–6.

52. Schimpf R, Borggrefe M, Wolpert C. Clinical and molecular genetics of the short QT syndrome. Curr Opin Cardiol 2008;23(3):192–8.

53. Mazzanti A, Maragna R, Vacanti G, et al. Hydroquinidine prevents life-threatening arrhythmic events in patients with short QT syndrome. J Am Coll Cardiol 2017;70(24):3010–5.

54. Gaita F, Giustetto C, Bianchi F, et al. Short QT syndrome: pharmacological treatment. J Am Coll Cardiol 2004;43(8):1494–9.

55. Hasegawa Y, Watanabe H, Ikami Y, et al. Early repolarization and risk of lone atrial fibrillation. J Cardiovasc Electrophysiol 2019;30(4):565–8.

56. McNair PW, Benenson DM, Ip JE, et al. Prevalence of early repolarization pattern in patients with lone atrial fibrillation. J Electrocardiol 2017;50(5):545–50.

57. Hwang KW, Nam GB, Han J, et al. Incidence of atrial tachyarrhythmias in patients with early repolarization syndrome. Int Heart J 2017;58(1):43–9.

58. Takahashi T, Bhandari AK, Watanuki M, et al. High incidence of device-related and lead-related complications in the dual-chamber implantable cardioverter defibrillator compared with the single-chamber version. Circ J 2002;66(8): 746–50.

59. Delaney JT, Muhammad R, Blair MA, et al. A KCNJ8 mutation associated with early repolarization and atrial fibrillation. Europace 2012;14(10):1428–32.

60. Voskoboinik A, Hsia H, Moss J, et al. The many faces of early repolarization syndrome: a single-center case series. Heart Rhythm 2020;17(2):273–81.

61. Squire A, Goldman ME, Kupersmith J, et al. Long-term antiarrhythmic therapy. Problem of low drug levels and patient noncompliance. Am J Med 1984;77(6):1035–8.

Social Risk Factors and Atrial Fibrillation

Andres Klein, MD[a], Mohammad Shenasa, MD[b], Adrian Baranchuk, MD, FRCPC, FCCS[c],*

KEYWORDS

• Atrial fibrillation • Prevention • Social risk factors

KEY POINTS

• Modifiable risk factor management is becoming one of the 3 treatment pillars in atrial fibrillation.
• Factors, such as alcohol intake, tobacco smoking, caffeine, chocolate, cannabis use, air pollution, and others, are grouped in the social risk factors category because they are closely related with lifestyle habits and customs.
• Early identification of these factors could help prevent atrial fibrillation.

INTRODUCTION

During the past decades, attention has been focused on new techniques and technologies to help patients with atrial fibrillation (AF), whereas disease prevention has received significantly less attention. Currently, modifiable risk factors are becoming 1 of the 3 treatment pillars in AF management along with anticoagulation as well as conventional rate and rhythm control strategies with either antiarrhythmic drugs or invasive procedures to prevent cryptogenic stroke.[1] Despite established associations between AF and other cardiovascular disease (CVD) processes, such as coronary artery disease, type 2 diabetes mellitus, hypertension, heart failure, and valvular heart disease, in some patients, the underlying etiology remains unknown.[2] In these instances, the condition is termed *lone AF* and is present in approximately 3% to 11% of all patients with AF.[3] Moreover, between 11% and 30% of AF patients have none of the well-known traditional risk factors[4,5] and, therefore, cannot be helped by preventive therapies, such as reducing blood pressure or treating obstructive sleep apnea. Therefore, this population potentially could benefit from the identification (and correction) of novel (or recently described) modifiable risk factors.

Factors, such as alcohol intake, tobacco smoking, caffeine and chocolate intake, cannabis use, air pollution, and others (**Fig. 1**), are grouped in the social risk factor category because they are closely related with lifestyle habits (**Table 1**). Some of these factors can be modified relatively easily at a personal level (despite the complexity of addictions) by implementing lifestyle changes, but others, such as air pollution, may require more complex solutions, including social-demographic changes, legislation and other complex modifications.

The mechanisms proposed for these social factors to be associated with AF development are variable but include autonomic dysfunction, atrial inflammation, myocardial fibrosis, oxidative stress, and even direct toxicity with consequent atrial remodeling. Most of these changes could be subtle, remaining undiscovered under the traditional AF work-up.

[a] Arrhythmia Service, Division of Cardiology, Department of Medicine, University of Ottawa Heart Institute, 40 Ruskin Street, Ottawa, ON K1Y 4W7, Canada; [b] Department of Cardiovascular Services, Heart and Rhythm Medical Group, 18324 Twin Creeks Road, Monte Sereno, CA 95030, USA; [c] Division of Cardiology, Queen's University, Kingston, Ontario, Canada
* Corresponding author. Cardiac Electrophysiology and Pacing, Kingston General Hospital, Queen's University, 76 Stuart Street, Kingston, Ontario K7L 2V7, Canada. ,
E-mail addresses: Adrian.Baranchuk@kingstonhsc.ca; barancha@kgh.kari.net

Card Electrophysiol Clin 13 (2021) 165–172
https://doi.org/10.1016/j.ccep.2020.10.008
1877-9182/21/© 2020 Elsevier Inc. All rights reserved.

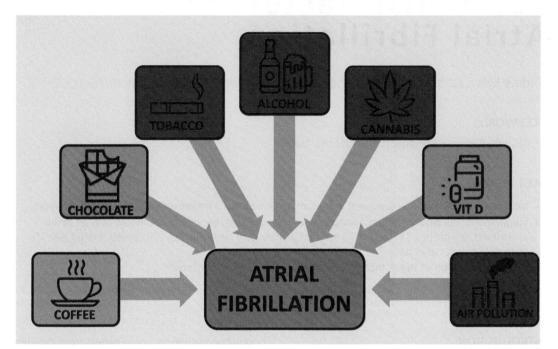

Fig. 1. Social risk factors for AF. Red, evidence suggests increased AF risk; yellow, no association or more evidence is needed; and green, likely protective effect.

This article aims to summarize those social risk factors that are linked somehow and in different degrees with AF. Early identification of these factors not only could help prevent AF but also decrease the burden of the disease.

ALCOHOL

Alcohol may be the most socially accepted substance that has such a strong impact on AF and cardiovascular health in general. Half of adults regularly consume alcohol.[6,7]

Several studies support a strong relationship between increased incidence of AF and alcohol intake despite other benefits to the cardiovascular system when taken in moderation, according to current guidelines.[6]

It was more than 4 decades ago when the term, *holiday heart syndrome*, was used to describe the association between acute alcohol intoxication and increased risk of transient AF, which is common during weekends and holidays.[8,9] In 2 out of 3 patients hospitalized for paroxysmal AF, acute alcohol consumption was the triggering factor for the arrhythmia event.[10–12]

Binge drinking is defined as consuming more than 4 standard drinks (10–14 g of alcohol per drink) over a 2-hour period.[6] One in 6 adults is exposed to binge drinking on a monthly basis, and the prevalence of binge drinking is twice as high in men than in women.[6,11]

AF occurs in up to 60% of binge drinkers with or without an underlying alcoholic cardiomyopathy[7] Patients with a history of binge drinking have a 21% increased risk of future hospitalization for AF.[10] The Copenhagen City Heart Study showed that a weekly alcohol intake of 35 or more drinks was associated with a 45% increase in the relative risk (RR) of incident AF among men.[13] The Framingham Study, among 1055 AF cases occurring during long-term follow-up, found an increased risk (RR 1.34; 95% CI, 1.01–1.78) with consumption of more than 36 g per day (approximately >3 drinks/d).[14] Several studies support a linear dose-response relationship between amount of chronic alcohol intake and AF risk.[15–18]

Larsson and colleagues[15] found, in a meta-analysis of 7 prospective studies, including 12,554 AF cases, that, with each standard drink increase in daily alcohol consumption, there was an association with an 8% increase risk of new-onset AF.

Gallagher and colleagues[16] showed, in a more recent meta-analysis, including 249,496 patients, that a low alcohol intake (up to 1 standard drink/d) was not associated with AF development. Additionally, moderate levels of alcohol intake were associated with a heightened AF risk in men (HR 1.26) but not in women (HR 1.03).[16]

In individuals who already had an episode of AF, appropriate modification of drinking habits improved clinical course of recurrent AF.[19–23]

Table 1
Novel social risk factors, impacts on atrial fibrillation, and suggested modifications and lifestyle changes

Risk Factors	Mechanisms for Triggering Atrial Fibrillation	Suggested Lifestyle Modifications
Alcohol	• ↓ Vagal tone • ↑ Adrenergic tone • Direct cardiotoxicity • ↓ Conduction • ↓ ERP • Inflammation • Fibrosis	• Avoid binge drinking (4 drinks over 2 h) • Up to 1 drink/d not associated with risk
Caffeine	• Favor conversion into sinus rhythm • Fibrosis	• 1–3 cups/d could have a protective effect.
Smoking	• ↑ Plasma catecholamines • ↑ HR and BP • Nicotine induced ↑ ERP • Inflammation • Fibrosis • ↑Transforming growth factor β/collagen	• Never smoking showed lower risk than former smokers. • Earlier quitting
Chocolate	• ↑ Endothelial function • ↓ BP • Less impact on AF	• No significant risk or benefits shown
Cannabis	• CB2 detected in cardiac myocyte • Effect is not clear • Autonomic imbalance	• Avoid high doses. • Avoid synthetic forms.
Air pollution	• Oxidative stress • Inflammation • Autonomic imbalance	• Complex multilevel solutions. • PM2.5 mask wearing should prevent its effect.
Vit D levels	• Deficiency is associated with electromechanical effects in the left atrium and leads to left atrial fibrosis.	• Maintain levels in the normal range. • Avoid unnecessary supplements

Abbreviations: BP, blood pressure; ERP, effective refractory period; HR, heart rate.

Symptomatic recurrence was documented more often in regular drinkers than in those who did not consume alcohol (50% vs 24%, respectively) and daily alcohol intake was an independent predictor of AF recurrence.[19]

Moreover, moderate to high alcohol consumption is an independent risk factor for progression of paroxysmal AF toward persistent and permanent AF (odds ratio 2.7).[20]

An improvement in AF ablation outcomes after alcohol abstinence postprocedure also was shown in several studies,[21–23] reporting also that abstainers when compared with former or current drinkers had a significantly lower AF recurrence rate after the first ablation (34.1% vs 41.9%, respectively).[21]

Avoiding alcohol consumption probably is the best strategy to prevent AF.[17] Given that a longer duration of abstinence was associated with a decreased risk of AF, earlier modification of alcohol use may have a greater influence on AF prevention. Every decade abstinence from alcohol intake was associated with an approximate 20% lower rate of incident AF.[24]

CAFFEINE

Coffee is the most popular drink in many parts of the word. Americans drink more coffee than soda, juice, and tea (combined). It has, together with other products containing caffeine (such us energy drinks), a bad reputation when it comes to inducing heart palpitations and triggering any kind of arrhythmias, including AF. Despite the theoretic relationship between caffeine and arrhythmogenesis, however, there is no evidence in humans that ingestion of caffeine, in doses typically consumed by a regular individual, can provoke AF.[25]

A review and meta-analysis, including mainly studies from Italy, the Nordic countries, and the United States, conducted by Caldeira and colleagues,[26] suggested that caffeine actually protected against cardiac arrhythmias. Moreover,

Casiglia and colleagues[27] observed for 12 years, in a population cohort of 1475 unselected men and women on liberalization to intake food or beverages containing caffeine, that the incidence of AF was significantly lower in the third tertile (2.2%) than in the first tertile (10.2%) or second tertile (5.7%) of caffeine intake ($P<.001$).

After genotyping for the $-163C>A$ polymorphism of the CYP1A2 gene, which regulates caffeine metabolism, they observed the same trend in all genotypes. In this study, a higher caffeine intake (>320 mg/d) was associated with lower incidence of AF.[27]

In a more recent study, Bodar and colleagues[28] prospectively studied men who participated in the Physicians' Health Study (N = 18,960). Their data suggested a lower risk of AF among men who reported coffee consumption of 1 cup/d to 3 cups/d.

It has been suggested that caffeine could favor the AF conversion into sinus rhythm. Also, some caffeine-induced changes in the cardiac remodeling and fibrosis process were thought to be linked with some resistance to AF.[29]

SMOKING

Cigarette smoking has been identified as a major modifiable risk factor for coronary artery disease, leading to preventable causes of death.[30,31] Smoking affects all phases of atherosclerosis, from endothelial dysfunction[32] to acute clinical events.[33] The role of cigarette smoking on cardiac arrhythmia, however, is defined less clearly.

Several mechanisms have been suggested as linking smoking to AF, including oxidative stress,[34,35] inflammation and atrial electrical alterations (remodeling),[36] and fibrosis.[37,38] Smoking-induced oxidative stress and increased carbon monoxide in smokers also could contribute to the development of cardiac arrhythmias.[39]

Epidemiologic studies have investigated the effects of smoking on AF; however, they showed some conflicting results. Findings from the Rotterdam Study showed that current and former smokers had an increased risk of AF compared with individuals who have never smoked (RR 1.51 and RR 1.49, respectively). No differences were found between men and women. AF incidence was related directly to years of previous smoking exposure and to number of cigarettes.[10] Results from the Atherosclerosis Risk in Communities study showed that current smokers had twice the risk of developing AF over up to 16 years of follow-up compared with never smokers. Unlike the Rotterdam Study, this study presented more encouraging conclusions for former smokers, reporting a significantly lower HR for incident AF

in former smokers compared with current smokers (1.32 vs 2.05, respectively).[40] Nevertheless, former smokers remained at increased risk for AF development compared with nonsmokers.[41] Therefore, to never start smoking seems the best strategy to avoid AF.

In a more recent meta-analysis by Zhu and colleagues,[41] including 286,217 participants, the investigators showed that active smoking increased the risk of incident AF by 23%. They also estimated that 6.7% of the total AF risk in men and 1.4% in women was attributable to smoking worldwide.

It was shown that even early exposure to secondhand smoke during gestational development and childhood could increase the risk of AF later in life by 37% and 40%, respectively.[42]

Findings from the previously discussed studies were based on self-reported smoking, which may be prone to inaccuracy and misclassification, resulting in a biased estimation. A more recent study registered plasma level of nicotine metabolite, cotinine, which was strongly associated with AF occurrence. Cotinine rises steeply with consumption of first 10 cigarettes per day but then reaches a plateau.[43] Among patients with recurrent AF, the risk of recurrence at 1 year after cardioversion was independently associated with the baseline smoking status in elderly women (vs nonsmokers; hazard ratio [HR] 1.71) but not in men.[44] Similar findings were shown after pulmonary vein isolation. Smokers had a significantly higher AF recurrence rate than nonsmokers (43% vs 14%, respectively) after 1-year follow up.[45] Also, some data suggest that the smoking cessation does not improve outcome of rhythm control strategies in patients with recurrent AF. The 1-year AF recurrence rate after cardioversion of persistent AF and catheter ablation was similar among current (58% vs 61%, respectively) and former smokers (47% and 40%, respectively).[44,45]

CHOCOLATE

Chocolate and cocoa products consumption has been shown to modestly lower blood pressure and to have favorable effects on CVD.[46,47] Evidence accumulated over the past few years has indicated that chocolate consumption is associated with reduced risk of total CVD,[48] ischemic heart disease,[49] and heart failure.[50]

Chocolate consumption, however, has been associated inconsistently with the risk of AF.

The Danish Diet, Cancer, and Health study was a large population-based prospective cohort study based on 55,502 participants who had provided information on chocolate intake at baseline.

Participants with higher levels of chocolate intake had a lower rate of clinically incident AF or flutter during a median of 13.5 years. Patients consuming 2 to 6 servings of chocolate per week had 20% less AF compared with those with a chocolate intake of less than 1 serving per month.[51]

In contrast, data from the Physicians' Health Study showed no significant association between chocolate consumption and incidental AF. In a secondary analysis, neither adiposity nor age modified the relation between chocolate consumption and AF.[52]

More recently, in 2 Swedish cohorts, chocolate consumption was not associated with risk of AF after adjustment for other risk factors. The lack of association was confirmed in a subsequent meta-analysis, including 5 cohort studies (180,454 participants).[53]

CANNABIS

Marijuana has become one of the most commonly abused substance in many countries. Also, more adverse events are being reported with the introduction of more potent marijuana products over the years. Delta-9-tetrahydrocannabinol (THC) is the active psychotropic component of marijuana, which acts mainly on G-protein cannabinoid receptors CB1 and CB2. CB2 was detected in cardiac myocyte and in the smooth muscles of blood vessels. The exact mechanism of the various vascular effect of marijuana is not clear, likely due to the paucity of laboratory data and to the complexity of the drug.[54]

Marijuana has clear electrophysiologic effects on the heart. Beaconsfield and colleagues[55] initially showed a decreased amplitude of the P waves in volunteers who smoked marijuana, suggesting electrical atrial abnormality (remodeling). Later, Miller and colleagues[56] investigated the effects of parenteral administration of THC, showing a significant decrease in sinoatrial conduction time, A-H interval, and atrioventricular nodal refractory periods following parenteral THC administration. The authors' group reported a case of symptomatic sinus arrest during acute consumption of cannabis.[57]

A scoping study of a total of 27 cases of arrhythmia associated with marijuana found that most cases were reported in young men (81%), with a mean age of 28 years ± 10.6 years, and AF represented 26% of all cases.[58]

An underestimation of AF is possible because patients could tend to be more asymptomatic and reluctant to seek medical care while under the influence of the drug.

Contrarily, in patients with congestive heart failure, a recent study suggested that cannabis users have lower odds of AF compared with nonusers, which was not explained by comorbid conditions, age, insurance type, and socioeconomic status.[59] There are case reports, however, of cannabis triggering lethal arrhythmias in patients with preexistent cardiomyopathies.[60]

Finally, synthetic cannabinoids also were associated with AF, and the effect of those drugs appears more potent than that of natural plants.[61]

AIR POLLUTION

Few studies suggest that air pollution exposure, even within hours, increases oxidative stress, inflammation,[62] and autonomic imbalance.[63] There is some evidence to support that autonomic tone responses and oxidative stress[64] increase the risk of triggering AF. Particulate matter (PM), also called particle pollution, is a general term for extremely small particles and liquid droplets in the atmosphere. PM2.5 (fine particles) have a diameter less than or equal to 2.5 μm and PM10 (coarse particles) a diameter less than or equal to 10 μm.

Liao and colleagues[65] demonstrated associations between ambient PM2.5 levels and important electrocardiogram (ECG) predictors of AF, such as P-wave morphology changes and PR duration, in participants equipped with personal PM2.5 and ECG recorders. This adds some additional support for the biological plausibility of an association between air pollution and AF, but, despite this, the evidence still is limited.

In a study conducted in Italy, air pollution levels were associated with increased AF emergency room visits within 24 hours of exposure. Effect estimates ranged between 1.4% for a 10-μg/m^3 increase of PM10 to 3% for a 10-μg/m^3 increase of PM2.5 at lag day 0 to 1.[66]

Similarly, in a nationwide cohort from the Korean general population, it was seen that a 10-μg/m^3 increase in ambient PM2.5 significantly increased emergency room admissions by 4.5% at lag day 3. No other pollutants showed a significant relationship with emergency room AF admission in this study and long-term exposure to air pollution had no significant impact on AF occurrence.[67]

Moreover, a recent population-based study found a statistically significant association between a moving average of 12-hour to 24-hour ambient levels of PM10 and AF episodes in a population of 75 year olds and 76 year olds undergoing ambulatory ECG monitoring in Stockholm. Positive but no significant associations were observed for PM2.5 and O$_3$. In subgroup analysis, stronger risk estimates were observed for PM2.5 exposure in participants with hypertension, and significant associations were observed for both PM10 and

O_3 exposure in participants with diabetes and participants with BMI greater than 25, in comparison with other participants.[68]

VITAMIN D LEVELS

Vitamin D (Vit D) deficiency has been shown not only to increase the risk of skeletal system diseases but also to have adverse effects on the cardiovascular system and inflammatory process, which are thought to be responsible for a high risk of AF. Moreover, Vit D deficiency has been shown to be associated with some electromechanical effects in the left atrium[69] and lead to left atrial fibrosis, with an increased risk of AF recurrence after cardioversion[70] and ablation.[71]

Despite these findings, the current literature shows inconsistent results about the association between Vit D and risk of AF.[72,73]

In 2930 Framingham Heart Study participants without prevalent AF, Vit D status was assessed by measuring 25-hydroxy (25-OH) Vit D levels. The investigators observed that 25-OH Vit D levels were not associated with the development of AF.[73]

In the other hand, excess of Vit D supplement also could be associated with AF. A large system-wide population study, including patients without a prior diagnosis of AF who received 25-OH Vit D as part of their clinical care, found that Vit D excess was associated with a significant independent risk of incident AF. Further studies should validate this observation and define safety margins for 25-OH Vit D supplement use.[74]

SUMMARY

In summary, several social risk factors have been shown to be linked somehow with AF. Some habits, such us heavy alcohol consumption and smoking or cannabis use, showed increasing the risk of AF, and, therefore, their withdrawal could have a potential benefit. As happens with other risk factors, the degree of exposure seems to play a crucial role. For example, the risk of developing AF in binge drinkers was significant.

Contrarily, other habits, like coffee drinking, could confer some protection when consumed in moderate doses (1–3 cups/d).

There likely is no association between chocolate consumption and AF; and, although some data suggest that excess of Vit D supplements could increase AF risk, it seems early to make any conclusion.

Air pollution is shown to play a role in triggering AF, but avoiding this factor unfortunately could require complex solutions.

Lifestyle modification place an increasingly important role in not only preventing AF but also improving outcomes after AF therapies, such as cardioversion or catheter ablation. Thus, early identification of this factors and intervention should be incorporated in clinical practice.

DISCLOSURE

The authors have nothing to disclose.

CLINICS CARE POINTS

- Acute alcohol consumption was the triggering factor for paroxysmal AF in 1 out of 3 cases.
- Despite its bad reputation, there is evidence showing a protective effect of caffeine against atrial fibrillation.
- Although some studies suggest that former smokers had a significantly risk of AF compared with current smokers, the risk of AF recurrence after ablation and cardioversion was similar.
- There is no evidence that chocolate consumption could be beneficial to prevent AF.

REFERENCES

1. Lau DH, Nattel S, Kalman JM, et al. Modifiable risk factors and atrial fibrillation. Circulation 2017;136:583–96.
2. Rosiak M, Dziuba M, Chudzik M, et al. Risk factors for atrial fibrillation: not always severe heart disease, not always so "lonely. Cardiol J 2010;17(5):437–42.
3. Gutierrez C, Blanchard DG. Atrial fibrillation: diagnosis and treatment. Am Fam Physician 2011;83(1):61–8.
4. Wyse DG, Van Gelder IC, Ellinor PT, et al. Lone atrial fibrillation: does it exist? J Am Coll Cardiol 2014;63:1715–23.
5. Brand FN, Abbott RD, Kannel WB, et al. Characteristics and prognosis of lone atrial fibrillation. 30-year follow-up in the Framingham Study. JAMA 1985;254:3449–53.
6. Courtney KE, Polich J. Binge drinking in young adults: data, definitions, and determinants. Psychol Bull 2009;135:142–56.
7. Waskiewicz A, Sygnowska E. Alcohol intake and cardiovascular risk factor profile in men participating in the WOBASZ study. Kardiol Pol 2013;71:359–65.
8. Ettinger PO, Wu CF. Regan TJ Arrhythmias and the "Holiday Heart": alcohol-associated cardiac rhythm disorders. Am Heart J 1978;95(5):555.
9. Tonelo D, Providencia R, Goncalves L. Holiday heart syndrome revisited after 34 years. Arq Bras Cardiol 2013;101:183–9.
10. Wilhelmsen L, Rosengren A, Lappas G. Hospitalizations for atrial fibrillation in the general male population: morbidity and risk factors. J Intern Med 2001;250:382–9.
11. Haseeb S, Alexander B, Baranchuk A. Wine and cardiovascular health: a comprehensive review. Circulation 2017;136:1434–48.

12. Voskoboinik A, Prabhu S. Ling LH alcohol and atrial fibrillation: a sobering review. J Am Coll Cardiol 2016;68:2567–76.

13. Mukamal KJ, Tolstrup JS, Friberg J, et al. Alcohol consumption and risk of atrial fibrillation in men and women: the Copenhagen city heart study. Circulation 2005;112:1736–42.

14. Djoussé L, Levy D, Ellison RC. Long-term alcohol consumption and the risk of atrial fibrillation in the Framingham Study. Am J Cardiol 2004;93(6):710.

15. Larsson SC, Drca N, Wolk A. Alcohol consumption and risk of atrial fibrillation: a prospective study and dose-response meta-analysis. J Am Coll Cardiol 2014;64:281–9.

16. Gallagher C, Hendriks JML, Elliott AD, et al. Alcohol and incident atrial fibrillation– a systematic review and meta-analysis. Int J Cardiol 2017;246:46–52.

17. Kodama S, Saito K, Tanaka S, et al. Alcohol consumption and risk of atrial fibrillation: a meta-analysis. J Am Coll Cardiol 2011;57:427–36.

18. Samokhvalov AV, Irving HM, Rehm J. Alcohol consumption as a risk factor for atrial fibrillation: a systematic review and meta-analysis. Eur J Cardiovasc Prev Rehabil 2010;17:706–12.

19. Planas F, Romero-Menor C, Vazquez-Oliva G, et al. Natural history of and risk factors for idiopathic atrial fibrillation recurrence (FAP Registry). Rev Esp Cardiol 2006;59:1106–12.

20. Ruigomez A, Johansson S, Wallander MA, et al. Predictors and prognosis of paroxysmal atrial fibrillation in general practice in the UK. BMC Cardiovasc Disord 2005;5:20.

21. Takigawa M, Takahashi A, Kuwahara T, et al. Impact of alcohol consumption on the outcome of catheter ablation in patients with paroxysmal atrial fibrillation. J Am Heart Assoc 2016;5:e004149.

22. Qiao Y, Shi R, Hou B, et al. Impact of alcohol consumption on substrate remodeling and ablation outcome of paroxysmal atrial fibrillation. J Am Heart Assoc 2015;4:e002349.

23. Barham WY, Sauer WH, Fleeman B, et al. Impact of alcohol consumption on atrial fibrillation outcomes following pulmonary vein isolation. J Atr Fibrillation 2016;9:1505.

24. Dixit S, Alonso A, Vittinghoff E, et al. Past alcohol consumption and incident atrial fibrillation: the atherosclerosis risk in communities (ARIC) study. PLoS One 2017;12:e0185228.

25. AU Dixit S, Stein PK, Marcus GMSO. Consumption of caffeinated products and cardiac ectopy. J Am Heart Assoc 2016;5(1):e002503.

26. Caldeira D, Martins C, Alves LB, et al. Caffeine does not increase the risk of atrial fibrillation: a systematic review and meta-analysis of observational studies. Heart 2013;99:1383–9.

27. Casiglia E, Tikhonoff V, Albertini F, et al. Caffeine intake reduces incident atrial fibrillation at a population level. Eur J Prev Cardiol 2018;25(10):1055–62.

28. Bodar D, Chen J, Djoussé L, et al. Coffee consumption and risk of atrial fibrillation in the physicians'health study. J Am Heart Assoc 2019;8:e011346.

29. Mattioli AV, Farinetti A, Miloro C, et al. Influence of coffee and caffeine consumption on atrial fibrillation in hypertensive patients. Nutr Metab Cardiovasc Dis 2011;21:412–7.

30. Ezzati M, Lopez AD. Estimates of global mortality attributable 847 to smoking in 2000. Lancet 2003;362:52.

31. Mons U, Muezzinler A, Gellert C, et al. Impact of smoking and smoking cessation on cardiovascular events and mortality among older adults: meta-analysis of individual participant data from prospective cohort studies of the CHANCES consortium. BMJ 2015;350:h1551.

32. Messner B, Bernhard D. Smoking and cardiovascular disease: mechanisms of endothelial dysfunction and early atherogenesis. Arterioscler Thromb Vasc Biol 2014;34:15.

33. Ambrose JA, Barua RS. The pathophysiology of cigarette smoking and cardiovascular disease: an update. J Am Coll Cardiol 2004;43:7.

34. Levitzky YS, Guo CY, Rong J, et al. Relation of smoking status to a panel of inflammatory markers: the framingham offspring. Atherosclerosis 2008;201:217–24.

35. Donohue JF. Ageing, smoking and oxidative stress. Thorax 2006;61:461–2.

36. Hayashi H, Omichi C, Miyauchi Y, et al. Age-related sensitivity to nicotine for inducible atrial tachycardia and atrial fibrillation. Am J Physiol Heart Circ Physiol 2003;285:H2091–8.

37. Goette A. Nicotine, atrial fibrosis, and atrial fibrillation: do microRNAs help to clear the smoke? Cardiovasc Res 2009;83:421–2.

38. Goette A, Lendeckel U, Kuchenbecker A, et al. Cigarette smoking induces atrial fibrosis in humans via nicotine. Heart 2007;93:1056–63.

39. Heeringa J, Kors JA, Hofman A, et al. Cigarette smoking and risk of atrial fibrillation: the Rotterdam study. Am Heart J 2008;156:1163–9.

40. Chamberlain AM, Agarwal SK, Folsom AR, et al. Smoking and incidence of atrial fibrillation: results from the atherosclerosis risk in communities (ARIC) study. Heart Rhythm 2011;8:1160–6.

41. Zhu W, Yuan P, Shen Y, et al. Association of smoking with the risk of incident atrial fibrillation: a meta-analysis of prospective studies. Int J Cardiol 2016;218:259–66.

42. Dixit S, Pletcher MJ, Vittinghoff E, et al. Secondhand smoke and atrial fibrillation: data from the Health eHeart Study. Heart Rhythm 2016;13:3–9.

43. Zuo H, Nygard O, Vollset SE, et al. Smoking, plasma cotinine and risk of atrial fibrillation: the Hordaland Health Study. J Intern Med 2018;283:73–82.

44. Kinoshita M, Herges RM, Hodge DO, et al. Role of smoking in the recurrence of atrial arrhythmias after cardioversion. Am J Cardiol 2009;104:678–82.

45. Fukamizu S, Sakurada H, Hiraoka M, et al. Effect of Cigarette Smoking on the Risk of Atrial Fibrillation Recurrence after Pulmonary Vein Isolation. Journal of Arrhythmia,2010 26: 21-29

46. Hooper L, Kay C, Abdelhamid A, et al. Effects of chocolate, cocoa, and flavan-3-ols on cardiovascular health: a systematic review and meta-analysis of randomized trials. Am J Clin Nutr 2012;95(3):740–51.

47. Ried K, Fakler P, Stocks NP. Effect of cocoa on blood pressure. Cochrane Database Syst Rev 2017;4: CD008893.

48. Kwok CS, Boekholdt SM, Lentjes MA, et al. Habitual chocolate consumption and risk of cardiovascular disease among healthy men and women. Heart 2015;101(16):1279–87.

49. Larsson SC, Akesson A, Gigante B, et al. Chocolate consumption and risk of myocardial infarction: a prospective study and meta-analysis. Heart 2016; 102(13):1017–22.

50. Gong F, Yao S, Wan J, et al. Chocolate consumption and risk of heart failure: a meta-analysis of prospective studies. Nutrients 2017;9(4). https://doi.org/10.3390/nu9040402.

51. Mostofsky E, Johansen MB, Tjønneland A, et al. Chocolate intake and risk of clinically apparent atrial fibrillation: the Danish Diet, Cancer, and Health Study. Heart 2017;103(15):1163–7.

52. Khawaja O, Petrone AB, Kanjwal Y, et al. Chocolate consumption and risk of atrial fibrillation (from the physicians' health study). Am J Cardiol 2015; 116(4):563–6.

53. Larsson SC, Drca N, Wolk A, et al. Chocolate consumption and risk of atrial fibrillation: two cohort studies and a meta-analysis. Am Heart J 2018;195: 86–90.

54. Vettor R, Pagotto U, Pagano C, et al. Here, there and everywhere: the endocannabinoid system. J Neuroendocrinol 2008;20(Suppl 1):iv–vi.

55. Beaconsfield P, Ginsburg J, Rainsbury R. Marihuana smoking. Cardiovascular effects in man and possible mechanisms. N Engl J Med 1972;287: 209–12.

56. Miller RH, Dhingra RC, Kanakis C Jr, et al. The electrophysiological effects of delta-9-tetrahydrocannabinol (cannabis) on cardiac conduction in man. Am Heart J 1977;94:740–7.

57. Grieve-Eglin L, Haseeb S, Wamboldt R, et al. Symptomatic sinus arrest induced by acute marijuana use. J Thorac Dis 2018;10(2):1121–3.

58. Korantzopoulos P, Liu T, Papaioannides D, et al. Atrial fibrillation and marijuana smoking. Int J Clin Pract 2008 Feb;62(2):308–13.

59. Adegbala O, Adejumo AC, Olakanmi O, et al. Relation of cannabis use and atrial fibrillation among

60. Baranchuk A, Johri AM, Simpson CS, et al. Ventricular fibrillation triggered by marijuana use in a patient with ischemic cardiomyopathy: a case report. Cases J 2008;1(1):373.

61. Efe TH, Felekoglu MA, Çimen T, et al. Atrial fibrillation following synthetic cannabinoid abuse. Turk Kardiyol Dern Ars 2017;45:362–4.

62. Feng S, Gao D, Liao F, et al. The health effects of ambient PM2.5 and potential mechanisms. Ecotoxicol Environ Saf 2016;128:67–74.

63. He F, Shaffer ML, Rodriguez-Colon S, et al. Acute effects of fine particulate air pollution on cardiac arrhythmia: the APACR study. Environ Health Perspect 2011;119(7):927–32.

64. Violi F, Carnevale R, Calvieri C, et al. Nox2 upregulation is associated with an enhanced risk of atrial fibrillation in patients with pneumonia. Thorax 2015;70(10):961–6.

65. Liao D, Shaffer ML, Cascio WE, et al. Fine particulate air pollution is associated with higher vulnerability to atrial fibrillation—the APACR study. J Toxicol Environ Health A 2011;74(11):693–705.

66. Solimini AG, Renzi M. Association between air pollution and emergency room visits for atrial fibrillation. Int J Environ Res Public Health 2017;14(6):661.

67. Kwon OK, Kim SH, Kang SH, et al. Association of short- and long-term exposure to air pollution with atrial fibrillation. Eur J Prev Cardiol 2019;26(11): 1208–16.

68. Dahlquist M, Frykman V, Kemp-Gudmunsdottir K, et al. Short-term associations between ambient air pollution and acute atrial fibrillation episodes. Environ Int 2020;141:105765.

69. Hanafy DA, Chang SL, Lu YY, et al. Electromechanical effects of 1,25-dihydroxyvitamin d with antiatrial fibrillation activities. J Cardiovasc Electrophysiol 2014;25(3):317–23.

70. Yaman B, Cerit L, Günsel HK, et al. Is there any link between Vitamin D and recurrence of atrial fibrillation after cardioversion? Braz J Cardiovasc Surg 2020;35(2):191–7.

71. Canpolat U, Aytemir K, Hazirolan T, et al. Relationship between vitamin D level and left atrial fibrosis in patients with lone paroxysmal atrial fibrillation undergoing cryoballoon-based catheter ablation. J Cardiol 2017;69(1):16–23.

72. Demir M, Uyan U, Melek M. The effects of vitamin D deficiency on atrial fibrillation. Clin Appl Thromb Hemost 2014;20(1):98–103.

73. Rienstra M, Cheng S, Larson MG, et al. Vitamin D status is not related to development of atrial fibrillation in the community. Am Heart J 2011;162(3):538–41.

74. Smith MB, May HT, Blair TL, et al. Vitamin D excess is significantly associated with risk of atrial fibrillation. Circulation 2011;124:A14699.

patients hospitalized for heart failure. Am J Cardiol 2018;122(1):129–34.

Exercise and Athletic Activity in Atrial Fibrillation

Alec Kherlopian, MD, MPH[a], Shayna Weinshel, BS, MS[b],
Christopher Madias, MD[c], N.A. Mark Estes III, MD[d],*

KEYWORDS

• Atrial fibrillation • Cardiac arrhythmia • Athlete • Endurance sports • Chronic exercise

KEY POINTS

• Low-to-moderate intensity exercise is associated with multiple favorable outcomes, including reduced cardiovascular disease and all-cause mortality.
• Clinical evidence suggests a paradoxic J-shaped curve in which chronic high-intensity training predisposes male and veteran athletes to an increased risk of atrial fibrillation (AF), a risk that is not observed across both genders.
• AF in the athlete is not associated with increased mortality; however, quality of life, exercise capacity, and athletic performance are hampered among athletes with AF.
• Additional research is needed to fill current gaps in knowledge pertaining to the natural history, pathophysiologic mechanisms, and management strategies to effectively prevent and treat athletes with AF.

INTRODUCTION

Peak athletic performance is often considered the epitome of physical fitness and optimal health. However, there is evidence that high-level endurance training and competition can result in an increased risk of atrial fibrillation (AF) in men.[1] Contemporary American Heart Association/American College of Cardiology (AHA/ACC) guideline documents define the competitive athlete as "one who participates in an organized team or individual sport that requires regular competition against others as a central component, places a high premium on excellence and achievement, and requires some form of systematic (and usually intense) training."[2] Emphasizing a component of organized, sanctioned competition, this population largely consists of students and professional athletes and excludes individuals involved in purely recreational, albeit high-intensity physical activities.[2]

Epidemiologic data have demonstrated a significantly higher risk of AF in male athletes participating in endurance sports compared with nonathletes.[3] However, competitive athletes typically lack common predisposing risk factors of AF seen within the general population, such as obesity, hypertension, diabetes, and sleep apnea.[4] Proposed pathophysiologic mechanisms of AF in the athlete include autonomic, structural, and electrophysiologic remodeling, in which high exercise volume (a product of exercise frequency and duration) is a prominent component.[5] Although individuals engaging in long-term recreational high-intensity exercise are excluded from

[a] Division of Cardiology, Tufts Medical Center, 800 Washington Street, Boston, MA 02111, USA; [b] University of Central Florida College of Medicine, 6850 Lake Nona Boulevard Orlando, FL 32827, USA; [c] Division of Cardiology, New England Cardiac Arrhythmia Center, Tufts Medical Center, 800 Washington Street, Boston, MA 02111, USA; [d] Heart and Vascular Institute, University of Pittsburgh Medical Center, South Tower 3rd Floor E352.2, 200 Lothrop Street, Pittsburgh, PA 15213, USA
* Corresponding author.
E-mail address: estesna@upmc.edu

Card Electrophysiol Clin 13 (2021) 173–182
https://doi.org/10.1016/j.ccep.2020.10.005
1877-9182/21/© 2020 Elsevier Inc. All rights reserved.

AHA/ACC's definition of an athlete, this review also describes important concepts from studies of nonathlete, intense exercisers.

The benefits of exercise are well established in the nonathlete population. Current available evidence supports a curvilinear dose-response relationship between regular physical activity and positive health outcomes, for example, reduced risk for all-cause mortality, cardiovascular disease mortality, all-cancer mortality, hypertension, diabetes, stroke, heart disease, and cancers.[6,7] Greatest relative risk reductions within nonathletes are observed at lower levels of physical activity with an attenuated benefit at higher exercise intensity.[6] Identification of an optimal exercise dose, above which there is minimal return or even detrimental effects, depends on the clinical outcome of interest.[8]

Contemporary evidence suggests low-to-moderate intensity exercise is also protective against the development of AF and may even reduce AF-related symptoms, morbidity, and mortality in patients with AF.[7,9–11] However, long-term, higher intensity exercise seems to be paradoxically associated with an increased risk of AF in men.[11] These findings support the concept of a J-shaped curve, in which individuals leading a sedentary lifestyle as well as those with extreme exercise volume seem to have an increased risk of AF.

EPIDEMIOLOGY

The literature describing incidence or prevalence of AF in athletes is limited to observational studies, including subjects who generally fit the AHA/ACC definition of the athlete; these studies demonstrate the influence of sex, age, endurance sports, and/or volume of training on risk of AF among athletes. Randomized controlled trials (RCTs) providing evidence of causation of these variables with the risk of AF are lacking. Although observational studies cannot confirm causality, there is a preponderance of evidence demonstrating an increase in AF risk among athletes across the globe. One of the earliest publications on this subject demonstrated increased incidence of AF among male Finnish orienteers relative to controls.[12] Subsequent publications led to a meta-analysis of additional case-control studies, showing the risk of AF increased greater than 5-fold in mostly male athletes within Finland, Switzerland, Spain, or Belgium compared with nonathlete controls (odds ratio [OR] 5.3 (3.6–7.9, 95% confidence interval)).[3,13] Some of these case-control studies performed in Spain demonstrated a threshold exercise volume of 1500 to 2000 lifetime training hours above which a greater

proportion of athletes had AF.[14,15] Moreover, a dose-response curve of AF prevalence versus lifetime training hours demonstrated a J-shaped curve wherein the lowest and highest lifetime training hours were associated with the greatest prevalence of AF.[15] Limitations of these studies include recall bias, as sports activity was defined based on self-reported questionnaires and poor generalizability given small sample size, limitation to European countries, and mostly male representation. Broadening the data to the United States, a prospective, questionnaire-based US Physicians' Health Study of 16,921 healthy men demonstrated an increased risk of AF among vigorous exercisers younger than 50 years relative to nonexercisers throughout the follow-up period.[14] Vigorous jogging was associated with an increased risk of AF as opposed to other activities including swimming, cycling, or racquet sports.[16] Although the participants of this study would not meet the AHA/ACC definition of a competitive athlete, the frequency of vigorous exercise was similar to athletes in the abovementioned case-control studies.[2,16]

Gender Differences

As studies were published that included larger proportions of women, it became clear that a greater incidence of AF in athletes was not an all-or-none concept. A large Norwegian (n = 309,540) prospective study, of which 52% were women, showed that men partaking in "hard training or sports competition regularly" relative to sedentary activity had an increased incidence of AF, which was defined by first use of flecainide or sotalol.[17] However, there was no significant difference among women with more intense physical activity relative to sedentary activity.[17] A major drawback of the study is that the outcome of measure may underestimate the incidence of AF and thus affect the gender differences observed.[17] Another large observational study of long-distance cross-country skiers in Sweden who competed in the *Vasaloppet* race showed an increased risk of AF among male skiers completing 3 or more races or achieving the fastest time relative to male nonskiers when controlling for confounding variables.[18] Interestingly, women skiers were at decreased risk of AF relative to female nonskiers.[18] Moreover, in a pooled analysis of multiple studies including men and women partaking in intense physical activity, women had a reduced risk of AF (OR 0.72, $P<.001$), whereas men had a significantly greater risk of AF (OR 3.29, $P = .0002$).[11] When considering different levels of physical activity (sedentary, moderate, and intense) and their association with AF incidence, the same pooled analysis demonstrated a J-shape relationship of AF incidence in men and a nearly inverted J-shape in women (**Fig. 1**).[11] Although all the participants within the *intense physical activity* category do not meet the AHA/ACC definition of an athlete, the concept of exercise discordantly affecting the incidence of AF among men versus women is highlighted. Current available data suggest a protective or neutral effect of intense exercise on the development of AF among women and an apparent increased risk among men.[11,13,14]

Differences of Age

In the general population, older age increases the risk of developing AF with a greater incidence among those older than 65 years.[19] However, among athletes the available data suggest there is a greater predilection for development of AF in those who are "middle aged," commonly defined as aged 40 to 60 years.[19,20] A large observational study among athletes from Spain demonstrated a significantly greater incidence of AF among athletes closer to middle age.[21] Moreover, a meta-analysis of 8 observational studies with mean age ranging between 39 and 69 years found an age threshold of 54 years, above which athletes no longer had a significant risk of developing AF.[19] The meta-analysis is limited by its significant heterogeneity and poor generalizability given mostly male athlete representation.

Type of Sport

The literature lacks sufficient data on the correlation between type of sport and the incidence of AF. Only one observational study suggests those participating in individualized endurance sports have increased risk of AF relative to team sports.[15] Most of the observational studies reviewing AF risk among athletes analyzed *endurance athletes* (ie, runners, joggers, cyclists, skiers, or soccer players) without particular attention to athletes performing nonaerobic training (ie, weightlifters).[3,9,11,12,14–16,22,23]

Morbidity and Mortality

Among the observational studies on AF incidence in athletes discussed earlier, only 2 assessed mortality as an outcome. From the limited data available, the greater risk of AF does not seem to confer an association with increased mortality in the athlete.[3,18] Among Swedish nonskiers and competitive skiers with AF, competitive skiers had a lower mortality after being diagnosed with AF.[18] Moreover, orienteers had lower mortality relative to controls even though the orienteers demonstrated an increased risk of AF.[12] The lower mortality among athletes may be related to the favorable effects of exercising on cardiometabolic risk factors.[12,18] Small observational studies have also shown male athletes with AF can develop a decrease in quality of life, sports activity, and exercise capacity.[9,24]

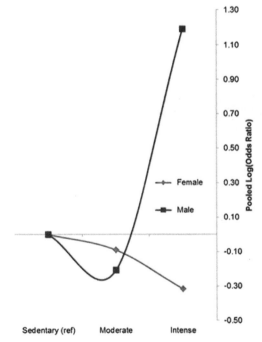

Fig. 1. Association between level of physical activity and risk of AF in men and women. High-intensity exercise seems to increase risk of AF in men and conversely reduce the risk in women. Sedentary lifestyle is known to increase the risk of AF among men and women, whereas moderate-intensity exercise reduces the risk of AF indifferent of sex.[11] (*From* Mohanty S, Mohanty P, Tamaki M, et al. Differential Association of Exercise Intensity With Risk of Atrial Fibrillation in Men and Women: Evidence from a Meta-Analysis. *J Cardiovasc Electrophysiol.* 2016;27(9):1021-1029; with permission.)

PATHOPHYSIOLOGY

Although the precise pathophysiologic mechanisms promoting AF in the athlete are incompletely understood, current evidence suggests a multifactorial interplay between autonomic tone, electrical remodeling, inflammation, and myocardial structural changes. Over time, these elements likely predispose to the substrate for reentry within atrial tissue and contribute to the generation of arrhythmogenic triggers, including pulmonary vein foci.

Genetic predisposition for AF among athletes is unknown but is evident among nonathletes.[25] The proposed pathophysiologic mechanisms are illustrated in **Fig. 2**.

Autonomic Mechanisms

The role of endurance training on enhanced vagal tone in athletes is well established.[4,26–29] Two studies demonstrated most of the athletes with lone AF exhibit characteristics of predominantly vagal AF, for example, nocturnal or postprandial episodes with rare occurrences during exercise.[4,26,27] Among endurance athletes, sinus bradycardia and atrioventricular block often occurred during sleep, demonstrating a substrate for vagal AF.[27] The association of low resting heart rate and increased risk of AF was evident in a meta-analysis of the general population across different countries, clinically demonstrating heightened vagal tone may potentially initiate or perpetuate AF.[30] Several recent studies also associate vagally mediated bradycardia with AF in athletes.[22,31]

Enhanced vagal activity shortens action potential duration and effective atrial refractory period via the G-protein gated potassium channel.[32]

This allows myocytes to readily accept premature impulses and contributes to the substrate for reentry.[33,34] Superimposing abrupt increases in sympathetic tone from intermittent high-intensity exercise among athletes with characteristic vagal predominance might further predispose to AF.[28]

Interestingly, early repolarization pattern (eg, J-point elevation), a common electrocardiographic finding in athletes, might be a marker for increased vagal tone.[35] A small-scale analysis of athletes suggests elevated vagal tone, evidenced by early repolarization pattern, contributes to increased left atrial filling pressures and left atrial enlargement (LAE). Atrial remodeling over time may ensue and predispose to AF.[35]

Structural and Electrophysiologic Mechanisms

Historically believed to be physiologic adaptation to high-intensity exercise, characteristic cardiac structural changes in the well-trained athlete include atrial enlargement and increased ventricular mass with diastolic dysfunction.[36] Larger atrial volumes allow for lower atrial deformation necessary to produce similar stroke volumes, which results in acute improvement in performance and reserve.[37]

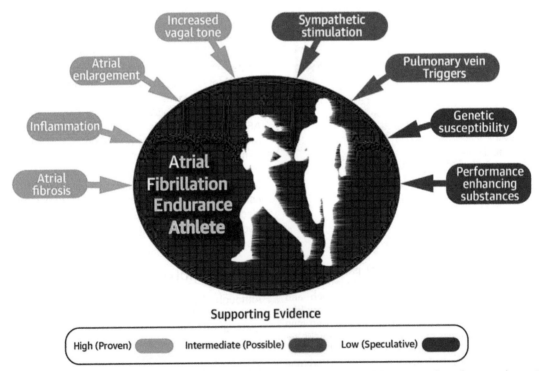

Fig. 2. Proposed pathophysiologic mechanisms of AF in the endurance athlete. Interplay of many elements contributing to AF development with intense endurance exercise are shown with color coding based on the level of supporting evidence.[52] (*From* Estes NAM, 3rd, Madias C. Atrial Fibrillation in Athletes: A Lesson in the Virtue of Moderation. *JACC Clin Electrophysiol.* 2017;3(9):921-928; with permission.)

LAE has been described as an independent risk factor for developing AF in the general population and may predispose to AF in the athlete.[26,38] A large-scale study demonstrated 20% of athletes have echocardiographic evidence of LAE, and several other studies corroborate the association of LAE with endurance training.[35,39,40] A small prospective study showed higher LA volume index in highly trained marathon runners relative to less active runners.[41] Elite handball players had greater LA size relative to sedentary controls.[37,41] Among athletes with LAE, the long-term myocardial damage from increased stroke volume reserve accompanied by increased wall stress might predispose to AF.[37] Ultimately, these findings implicate elevated wall stress in the development of AF in athletes by way of structural atrial remodeling.[37]

In a clinical trial, previously sedentary middle-aged adults randomized to 10 months of high-intensity exercise training showed remodeling of LA structure and function.[42] However, the degree of LA volume postexercise was less compared with that in endurance athletes with at least 5 years of training, which is consistent with the dose-response relationship of greater accumulated training on LAE seen in other studies.[42]

Based on the premise that slow conduction facilitates reentry and in turn AF, electrophysiologic remodeling has been assessed in studies analyzing delayed atrial activation on electrocardiography (ECG) via P-wave signal averaging.[43] Nonathletes showed no significant difference in the filtered P-wave duration after 2 years of intense training but did demonstrate increased LAE.[43] A Swiss study of middle-aged, nonelite endurance athletes showed those with greater than 4500 lifetime training hours had the most prolonged signal-averaged P-wave duration and those with lower training hours had less prolonged P-wave durations, suggesting training duration influences electrophysiologic remodeling.[44] There was no correlation between LA volume and electrophysiologic remodeling, bringing into question when LAE is truly pathologic.[44] In the same study, atrial ectopy burden was assessed because it has been proposed in the pathogenesis of AF in the athlete; premature atrial contractions (PAC) potentially trigger the initiation of paroxysmal AF.[44] The study demonstrated higher PAC burden with greater lifetime training.[44] However, conflicting data exist regarding PAC burden observed in nonathlete exercisers, as there was no statistical difference in PAC burden between low (<3000 hours), medium (3000–5999 hours), and high (>6000 hours) lifetime training, and overall PAC burden was low, thereby suggesting

endurance training does not significantly promote a high atrial ectopic burden.[45]

Inflammation and Fibrosis

High circulating levels of the proinflammatory cytokine, interleukin-6, is associated with increased LA size.[35] Atrial tissue signaling pathways potentially contributing to proliferation, hypertrophy, and collagen synthesis predisposing to AF include those involving transforming growth factor β, the renin-angiotensin-aldosterone system, oxidative stress, and tumor necrosis factor.[46] Electrical remodeling predisposing to calcium release within atrial myocytes via altered function of ryanodine receptors has been associated with AF in humans and mice models and is thought to occur via inflammatory pathways.[47]

Animal studies associate exercise-induced anatomic atrial remodeling with the development of AF in intensely exercised mice. Increased fibroblasts, hypertrophy, and inflammatory cell infiltration in atria of exercised mice were associated with slow conduction velocities and long P-wave durations, increasing the risk of reentry; tumor necrosis factor alpha (TNFα) has been proposed as the downstream influencer of inflammatory and fibrotic changes.[47] Exercise-induced elevation in diastolic atrial pressure is an important component, as stretch is capable of activating TNFα in fibroblasts and cardiac myocytes resulting in collagen deposition and in turn promoting AF. Interestingly, the pathophysiology behind the paradoxic J-shaped curve may partly be due to chronic systemic inflammation associated with both long-term high intensity exercise and an unhealthy sedentary lifestyle, whereas decreased inflammatory markers are observed in moderate physical activity.[48,49]

CLINICAL EVALUATION AND MANAGEMENT

The goal of AF management in athletes is similar to the general population: identify and treat reversible AF risk factors, address debilitating symptoms, prevent AF progression, and prevent stroke.[50–52]

Diagnostic Approach to Atrial Fibrillation in Athletes

The diagnostic approach and clinical management of AF in athletes are based on extrapolation from literature of nonathletes, observational studies, and expert consensus.[50,52,53] No recommendation exists for AF screening among asymptomatic athletes.[21] AF is suspected among athletes if palpitations, dizziness, or hampered physical performance exist.[54] As in nonathletes, AF is confirmed with ECG, ambulatory rhythm monitoring, or implanted loop recorder.[55] Athletes with AF should undergo a complete history emphasizing an association between AF-related symptoms and exercise; inquiry into use of performance-enhancing agents, illicit drugs, and alcohol; as well as physical examination.[50,51,55] Predisposing risk factors, such as hypertension and thyroid disease, should be routinely excluded. Exercise stress testing may be performed to assess for ischemia, exercise tolerance, and ventricular response during physical activity, when clinically indicated.[51,55] Echocardiography should be performed to evaluate for underlying structural heart disease, as patients with valvular disease and inherited cardiomyopathies have increased predilection for AF.[50,51] Thereafter, cardiac MRI may be considered if clinically appropriate. In select clinical presentations, arrhythmogenic channelopathies and bypass tracts should be assessed given their association with AF.[51] During management of AF, ambulatory rhythm monitoring is a useful tool to evaluate the AF burden, to assess efficacy of rate control at rest and during athlete-specific exercise, and to qualify suspected AF-related symptoms.[50,52] Ambulatory rhythm monitoring with over-the-counter wearable devices may be considered to detect AF in symptomatic athletes. Among such devices, those that have been approved by the Food and Drug Administration to distinguish AF from sinus rhythm should be preferred.[56] Notably, these devices are not programmed to identify other tachyarrhythmias.[56] Studies on clinical application of such wearable devices among athletes are necessary to determine their clinical benefit.

Exercise Recommendations in Athletes with Atrial Fibrillation

As excessive exercise can contribute to AF, deconditioning has been hypothesized to decrease recurrence of AF.[57] Although, there are no published prospective studies to substantiate this hypothesis, one observational study demonstrated a decrease in AF with detraining and another showed improved AF symptoms when decreasing sports activity.[57–59] Expert opinion and anecdotal evidence imply up to 3 months of deconditioning is reasonable in athletes with recurrent exercise-induced symptomatic paroxysms of AF as initial therapy.[23,57] Such detraining may also be diagnostic, potentially revealing an association between AF and exercise volume. The most recent AHA/ACC Task Force suggests considering deconditioning in certain cases without specific guidance.[50] Overall, substantial AF burden reduction in response to training

restriction is a clinical indicator for the safe resumption of less intense exercise.[23,57]

Symptomatic athletes who are not amenable to detraining or who fail an exercise restriction trial are treated with either a rate control or rhythm control strategy.

Pharmacologic Intervention

Pursuing a rate versus rhythm control strategy is largely guided by symptoms.[50,52,53] Dominance of vagal tone in athletes at rest, potentially ineffective rate control during intense training and/or competitions, and poor side-effect profile (eg, fatigue, depressed athletic performance) of beta-blockers and calcium channel blockers (CCB) hinder the utility of rate control in athletes.[50,52,53] Furthermore, beta-blocker therapy may be impractical given its categorization as a prohibited substance in certain sports.[60] Digoxin's negative dromotropic effect via enhancement of vagal tone lengthens the nodal refractory period, thereby slowing ventricular response; however, it is ineffective during exercise as adrenergic drive predominates.[23,61] Although a less practical option, rate control with either beta-blockers or CCB may be considered in asymptomatic or minimally symptomatic athletes.[50,52,53] Without universally accepted target resting and peak exercise heart rates in the athlete, a resting rate less than or equal to 90 beats/minute and peak exercise rate less than the maximum age-predicted rate while in sinus rhythm are frequently used as clinical target rates.[52]

Rhythm control is often preferred for symptomatic athletes in whom deconditioning is ineffective or prohibitive to competitive goals. In absence of RCTs on rhythm control in athletes, antiarrhythmic strategy should be extrapolated from evidence-based data of nonathletes with AF and take into consideration any underlying structural heart disease.[50,52,53,55] Disopyramide, a class I antiarrhythmic agent with anticholinergic effects, may be theoretically effective in vagally mediated AF, but with only anecdotal evidence.[55,62] Monotherapy with class I antiarrhythmics may slow conduction in the atrial tissue leading to 1:1 conduction of atrial flutter during high sympathetic tone with exercise, and thus a beta-blocker or CCB should be used as an adjunct.[23] Proarrhythmic side effects, bradycardia, and intolerance of AV nodal blocking agents or antiarrhythmic agents commonly limit their use in athletes.[48,55]

Anticoagulation for stroke prophylaxis relies on the clinical situation (periablation or pericardioversion) and objective evaluation of the individual stroke risk using CHA_2DS_2-VASc score.[50,52,53] A

CHA_2DS_2-VASc score greater than or equal to 2 in men and greater than or equal to 3 in women justifies anticoagulation, extrapolated from risk of stroke in the general population. Given the younger age of this patient population without many comorbidities, most of the athletes will not require anticoagulation.[50] Stroke risk has been analyzed among observational studies of competitive skiers, demonstrating skiers with AF have greater risk of stroke relative to skiers without AF, supporting the use of anticoagulating athletes when indicated and when benefits exceed the risks.[9,18] After catheter ablation, anticoagulation for a minimum of 2 months is recommended, and thereafter may be continued based on clinical judgment.[55]

Catheter Ablation in Athletes with Atrial Fibillation

Data assessing the efficacy of catheter ablation are limited in athletes.[48,63] Two small studies find catheter ablation to be effective; however, larger prospective RCTs are needed to validate these findings.[64,65] Invasive catheter ablation is reserved for symptomatic athletes who have failed antiarrhythmic therapy or for selected symptomatic athletes unwilling to attempt an initial medical therapy trial and/or unwilling to reduce/cease sports participation.[50,52,53] Given the limitations of pharmacologic therapy and current available data, the most recent guidelines establish catheter ablation as a reasonable first-line therapy in athletes with AF (class IIa indication).[48]

Athletic Participation and Restrictions

No competitive sports restrictions are indicated in athletes with well-tolerated and self-terminating AF.[50] Athletes with AF in the presence of structural heart disease who maintain appropriate ventricular rate during physical activity can participate in sports consistent with limitations dictated by their underlying structural heart disease.[66] The bleeding risk in athletes with AF undergoing anticoagulation therapy depends on a sport-specific risk of bodily collision, and participation in high-impact contact sports should be restricted.[50,67] Otherwise healthy athletes with AF who have undergone successful catheter ablation without arrhythmia recurrence after 4 to 6 weeks may participate in all competitive sports.[66]

SUMMARY

Substantial gaps remain in our understanding of the natural history, pathophysiology, and clinical management of AF in athletes. In the absence of robust clinical evidence from RCTs, clinicians should use the best available data to advise this unique patient population. Moderate-intensity exercise has established its role in multiple favorable cardiovascular outcomes. However, clinical evidence demonstrates a paradoxic J-shaped curve in which chronic high-intensity endurance training predisposes male and middle-aged athletes to an increased risk of AF, a risk that is not observed across both genders. Increased mortality associated with AF in the general population does not seem to be shared by athletes. However, clinically significant morbidities among athletes (eg, reduced exercise capacity, athletic performance, and quality of life) need to be appropriately addressed by application of current available therapies with an individualized approach.

CLINICS CARE POINTS

- Suspicion of AF among an athlete is driven by symptoms, including palpitations and impaired physical performance, with subsequent diagnostic approach including electrocardiographic confirmation and assessment of predisposing risk factors.
- Screening asymptomatic athletes for AF is not recommended.
- Deconditioning, pharmacologic rate-control or rhythm-control, and catheter ablation are reasonable treatment options for managing AF in symptomatic athletes, though these require further clinical research and the noninvasive strategies may be impractical.

DISCLOSURE

No conflicts of interest.

REFERENCES

1. Schwellnus M, Soligard T, Alonso JM, et al. How much is too much? (Part 2) International Olympic Committee consensus statement on load in sport and risk of illness. Br J Sports Med 2016;50(17): 1043–52.
2. Maron BJ, Zipes DP, Kovacs RJ. Eligibility and disqualification recommendations for competitive athletes with cardiovascular abnormalities: preamble, principles, and general considerations: a scientific statement from the American Heart Association and American College of Cardiology. Circulation 2015;132(22):e256–61.
3. Abdulla J, Nielsen JR. Is the risk of atrial fibrillation higher in athletes than in the general population? A systematic review and meta-analysis. Europace 2009;11(9):1156–9.

4. Mont L, Elosua R, Brugada J. Endurance sport practice as a risk factor for atrial fibrillation and atrial flutter. Europace 2009;11(1):11–7.

5. Sanchis-Gomar F, Perez-Quilis C, Lippi G, et al. Atrial fibrillation in highly trained endurance athletes - Description of a syndrome. Int J Cardiol 2017;226:11–20.

6. Warburton DER, Bredin SSD. Health benefits of physical activity: a systematic review of current systematic reviews. Curr Opin Cardiol 2017;32(5):541–56.

7. Franklin BA, Thompson PD, Al-Zaiti SS, et al. Exercise-related acute cardiovascular events and potential deleterious adaptations following long-term exercise training: placing the risks into perspective-an update: a scientific statement from the American Heart Association. Circulation 2020;141(13):e705–36.

8. Wasfy MM, Baggish AL. Exercise dose in clinical practice. Circulation 2016;133(23):2297–313.

9. Myrstad M, Aaronaes M, Graff-Iversen S, et al. Physical activity, symptoms, medication and subjective health among veteran endurance athletes with atrial fibrillation. Clin Res Cardiol 2016;105(2):154–61.

10. Proietti M, Boriani G, Laroche C, et al. Self-reported physical activity and major adverse events in patients with atrial fibrillation: a report from the EURObservational Research Programme Pilot Survey on Atrial Fibrillation (EORP-AF) General Registry. Europace 2017;19(4):535–43.

11. Mohanty S, Mohanty P, Tamaki M, et al. Differential association of exercise intensity with risk of atrial fibrillation in men and women: evidence from a meta-analysis. J Cardiovasc Electrophysiol 2016;27(9):1021–9.

12. Karjalainen J, Kujala UM, Kaprio J, et al. Lone atrial fibrillation in vigorously exercising middle aged men: case-control study. BMJ 1998;316(7147):1784–5.

13. Nielsen JR, Wachtell K, Abdulla J. The relationship between physical activity and risk of atrial fibrillation-A systematic review and meta-analysis. J Atr Fibrillation 2013;5(5):789.

14. Elosua R, Arquer A, Mont L, et al. Sport practice and the risk of lone atrial fibrillation: a case-control study. Int J Cardiol 2006;108(3):332–7.

15. Calvo N, Ramos P, Montserrat S, et al. Emerging risk factors and the dose-response relationship between physical activity and lone atrial fibrillation: a prospective case-control study. Europace 2016;18(1):57–63.

16. Aizer A, Gaziano JM, Cook NR, et al. Relation of vigorous exercise to risk of atrial fibrillation. Am J Cardiol 2009;103(11):1572–7.

17. Thelle DS, Selmer R, Gjesdal K, et al. Resting heart rate and physical activity as risk factors for lone atrial fibrillation: a prospective study of 309,540 men and women. Heart 2013;99(23):1755–60.

18. Svedberg N, Sundstrom J, James S, et al. Long-term incidence of atrial fibrillation and stroke among cross-country skiers. Circulation 2019;140(11):910–20.

19. Ayinde H, Schweizer ML, Crabb V, et al. Age modifies the risk of atrial fibrillation among athletes: a systematic literature review and meta-analysis. Int J Cardiol Heart Vasc 2018;18:25–9.

20. Lachman ME, Teshale S, Agrigoroaei S. Midlife as a pivotal period in the life course: balancing growth and Decline at the crossroads of youth and old age. Int J Behav Dev 2015;39(1):20–31.

21. Boraita A, Santos-Lozano A, Heras ME, et al. Incidence of atrial fibrillation in elite athletes. JAMA Cardiol 2018;3(12):1200–5.

22. Baldesberger S, Bauersfeld U, Candinas R, et al. Sinus node disease and arrhythmias in the long-term follow-up of former professional cyclists. Eur Heart J 2008;29(1):71–8.

23. Heidbuchel H, Panhuyzen-Goedkoop N, Corrado D, et al. Recommendations for participation in leisure-time physical activity and competitive sports in patients with arrhythmias and potentially arrhythmogenic conditions Part I: Supraventricular arrhythmias and pacemakers. Eur J Cardiovasc Prev Rehabil 2006;13(4):475–84.

24. Furlanello F, Lupo P, Pittalis M, et al. Radiofrequency catheter ablation of atrial fibrillation in athletes referred for disabling symptoms preventing usual training schedule and sport competition. J Cardiovasc Electrophysiol 2008;19(5):457–62.

25. Christophersen IE, Ellinor PT. Genetics of atrial fibrillation: from families to genomes. J Hum Genet 2016;61(1):61–70.

26. Mont L, Tamborero D, Elosua R, et al. Physical activity, height, and left atrial size are independent risk factors for lone atrial fibrillation in middle-aged healthy individuals. Europace 2008;10(1):15–20.

27. Carpenter A, Frontera A, Bond R, et al. Vagal atrial fibrillation: what is it and should we treat it? Int J Cardiol 2015;201:415–21.

28. Wernhart S, Halle M. Atrial fibrillation and long-term sports practice: epidemiology and mechanisms. Clin Res Cardiol 2015;104(5):369–79.

29. McClaskey D, Lee D, Buch E. Outcomes among athletes with arrhythmias and electrocardiographic abnormalities: implications for ECG interpretation. Sports Med 2013;43(10):979–91.

30. Liu X, Guo N, Zhu W, et al. Resting heart rate and the risk of atrial fibrillation. Int Heart J 2019;60(4):805–11.

31. Grimsmo J, Grundvold I, Maehlum S, et al. High prevalence of atrial fibrillation in long-term endurance cross-country skiers: echocardiographic findings and possible predictors–a 28-30 years follow-up study. Eur J Cardiovasc Prev Rehabil 2010;17(1):100–5.

32. Kovoor P, Wickman K, Maguire CT, et al. Evaluation of the role of I(KACh) in atrial fibrillation using a mouse knockout model. J Am Coll Cardiol 2001; 37(8):2136–43.

33. Elliott AD, Mahajan R, Lau DH, et al. Atrial fibrillation in endurance athletes: from mechanism to management. Cardiol Clin 2016;34(4):567–78.

34. Nattel S, Harada M. Atrial remodeling and atrial fibrillation: recent advances and translational perspectives. J Am Coll Cardiol 2014;63(22): 2335–45.

35. Stumpf C, Simon M, Wilhelm M, et al. Left atrial remodeling, early repolarization pattern, and inflammatory cytokines in professional soccer players. J Cardiol 2016;68(1):64–70.

36. Calvo N, Brugada J, Sitges M, et al. Atrial fibrillation and atrial flutter in athletes. Br J Sports Med 2012; 46(Suppl 1):i37–43.

37. Gabrieli L, Bijnens BH, Butakoff C, et al. Atrial functional and geometrical remodeling in highly trained male athletes: for better or worse? Eur J Appl Physiol 2014;114(6):1143–52.

38. Tsang TS, Barnes ME, Bailey KR, et al. Left atrial volume: important risk marker of incident atrial fibrillation in 1655 older men and women. Mayo Clin Proc 2001;76(5):467–75.

39. Baggish AL, Wood MJ. Athlete's heart and cardiovascular care of the athlete: scientific and clinical update. Circulation 2011;123(23):2723–35.

40. Pelliccia A, Maron BJ, Di Paolo FM, et al. Prevalence and clinical significance of left atrial remodeling in competitive athletes. J Am Coll Cardiol 2005;46(4): 690–6.

41. Gabrielli L, Herrera S, Contreras-Briceno F, et al. Increased active phase atrial contraction is related to marathon runner performance. Eur J Appl Physiol 2018;118(9):1931–9.

42. Opondo MA, Aiad N, Cain MA, et al. Does high-intensity endurance training increase the risk of atrial fibrillation? a longitudinal study of left atrial structure and function. Circ Arrhythm Electrophysiol 2018; 11(5):e005598.

43. McNamara DA, Aiad N, Howden E, et al. Left atrial electromechanical remodeling following 2 years of high-intensity exercise training in sedentary middle-aged adults. Circulation 2019;139(12): 1507–16.

44. Wilhelm M, Roten L, Tanner H, et al. Atrial remodeling, autonomic tone, and lifetime training hours in nonelite athletes. Am J Cardiol 2011;108(4):580–5.

45. Elliott AD, Mahajan R, Linz D, et al. Atrial remodeling and ectopic burden in recreational athletes: implications for risk of atrial fibrillation. Clin Cardiol 2018; 41(6):843–8.

46. Schotten U, Verheule S, Kirchhof P, et al. Pathophysiological mechanisms of atrial fibrillation: a translational appraisal. Physiol Rev 2011;91(1):265–325.

47. Aschar-Sobbi R, Izaddoustdar F, Korogyi AS, et al. Increased atrial arrhythmia susceptibility induced by intense endurance exercise in mice requires TNFalpha. Nat Commun 2015;6:6018.

48. Calkins H, Hindricks G, Cappato R, et al. 2017 HRS/EHRA/ECAS/APHRS/SOLAECE expert consensus statement on catheter and surgical ablation of atrial fibrillation. Heart Rhythm 2017;14(10):e275–444.

49. Chung MK, Martin DO, Sprecher D, et al. C-reactive protein elevation in patients with atrial arrhythmias: inflammatory mechanisms and persistence of atrial fibrillation. Circulation 2001;104(24): 2886–91.

50. Zipes DP, Link MS, Ackerman MJ, et al. Eligibility and disqualification recommendations for competitive athletes with cardiovascular abnormalities: task force 9: arrhythmias and conduction Defects: a scientific statement from the American heart association and American College of Cardiology. Circulation 2015;132(22):e315–25.

51. Kirchhof P, Benussi S, Kotecha D, et al. 2016 ESC Guidelines for the management of atrial fibrillation developed in collaboration with EACTS. Eur Heart J 2016;37(38):2893–962.

52. Estes NAM 3rd, Madias C. Atrial fibrillation in athletes: a lesson in the virtue of moderation. JACC Clin Electrophysiol 2017;3(9):921–8.

53. January CT, Wann LS, Calkins H, et al. 2019 AHA/ACC/HRS focused update of the 2014 AHA/ACC/HRS guideline for the management of patients with atrial fibrillation: a report of the American College of Cardiology/American heart association task force on clinical practice guidelines and the heart rhythm Society. Heart Rhythm 2019;16(8):e66–93.

54. Guasch E, Mont L. Diagnosis, pathophysiology, and management of exercise-induced arrhythmias. Nat Rev Cardiol 2017;14(2):88–101.

55. January CT, Wann LS, Alpert JS, et al. 2014 AHA/ACC/HRS guideline for the management of patients with atrial fibrillation: a report of the American College of Cardiology/American heart association task force on practice guidelines and the heart rhythm Society. J Am Coll Cardiol 2014;64(21):e1–76.

56. Bunch TJ. The World of wearables – does the data support the Use?. 2020. Available at: www.acc.org/latest-in-cardiology/articles/2020/03/24/14/20/the-world-of-wearables. Accessed May 25, 2020.

57. Myrstad M, Malmo V, Ulimoen SR, et al. Exercise in individuals with atrial fibrillation. Clin Res Cardiol 2019;108(4):347–54.

58. Furlanello F, Bertoldi A, Dallago M, et al. Atrial fibrillation in top-level athletes. Atrial fibrillation: mechanisms therapeutic strategies. Armonk (NY): Futura; 1994. p. 203–4.

59. Hoogsteen J, Schep G, Van Hemel NM, et al. Paroxysmal atrial fibrillation in male endurance athletes. A 9-year follow up. Europace 2004;6(3):222–8.

60. Deligiannis AP, Kouidi EI. Cardiovascular adverse effects of doping in sports. Hellenic J Cardiol 2012;53(6):447–57.

61. Maury P, Rollin A, Galinier M, et al. Role of digoxin in controlling the ventricular rate during atrial fibrillation: a systematic review and a rethinking. Res Rep Clin Cardiol 2014;(5):93–101.

62. Sugiura H, Chinushi M, Komura S, et al. Heart rate variability is a useful parameter for evaluation of anticholinergic effect associated with inducibility of atrial fibrillation. Pacing Clin Electrophysiol 2005; 28(11):1208–14.

63. Calkins H, Kuck KH, Cappato R, et al. 2012 HRS/ EHRA/ECAS Expert Consensus Statement on Catheter and Surgical Ablation of Atrial Fibrillation: recommendations for patient selection, procedural techniques, patient management and follow-up, definitions, endpoints, and research trial design. Europace 2012;14(4):528–606.

64. Calvo N, Mont L, Tamborero D, et al. Efficacy of circumferential pulmonary vein ablation of atrial fibrillation in endurance athletes. Europace 2010; 12(1):30–6.

65. Koopman P, Nuyens D, Garweg C, et al. Efficacy of radiofrequency catheter ablation in athletes with atrial fibrillation. Europace 2011;13(10):1386–93.

66. Zipes DP, Ackerman MJ, Estes NA 3rd, et al. Task force 7: arrhythmias. J Am Coll Cardiol 2005;45(8): 1354–63.

67. Levine BD, Baggish AL, Kovacs RJ, et al. Eligibility and disqualification recommendations for competitive athletes with cardiovascular abnormalities: task force 1: classification of sports: dynamic, static, and impact: a scientific statement from the American Heart Association and American College of Cardiology. Circulation 2015; 132(22):e262–6.

Autonomic Dysfunction and Neurohormonal Disorders in Atrial Fibrillation

Anna Pfenniger, MD, PhD, Gail Elizabeth Geist, DVM, Rishi Arora, MD*

KEYWORDS

• Atrial fibrillation • Autonomic nervous system • Neurohormonal • Autonomic modulation

KEY POINTS

• The autonomic nervous system plays a significant role in the initiation and maintenance of atrial fibrillation.
• Both functional and structural remodeling of the autonomic nervous system occur in atrial fibrillation.
• Both sympathetic and parasympathetic hyperinnervation contribute to atrial fibrillation, with parasympathetic hyperinnervation playing a key role.

INTRODUCTION

Atrial fibrillation (AF) is the most commonly diagnosed arrhythmia and eludes an efficacious cure despite an increasing prevalence and a significant association with morbidity and mortality.[1] In addition to an array of clinical sequelae, the origins and propagation of AF are multifactorial. In recent years, the bidirectional interface between AF and the autonomic nervous system (ANS) has been an area of particular interest.[2–4] This review highlights the relevant physiology of autonomic and neurohormonal contributions to AF origin and maintenance, the current state of the literature on targeted therapies, and the path forward for clinical interventions, summarized in **Fig. 1**.

CARDIAC AUTONOMIC INNERVATION

Briefly, the autonomic innervation of the atria is described as follows. The heart receives direct parasympathetic input from preganglionic fibers extending from the medulla through the vagus nerve and synapsing within the heart.[5] Similarly, sympathetic nerves originate at the level of the medulla, but travel through the spinal cord to exit and synapse at paravertebral ganglia before reaching the heart. From these ganglia, sympathetic fibers distribute to target sites within the heart and the vasculature. At the level of the heart, the intrinsic cardiac nervous system (ICNS) integrates a complex network of extrinsic (central) and intracardiac signaling.[6] The ICNS is dispersed as ganglionated plexi (GPs) throughout the atria and ventricles, composed of parasympathetic and sympathetic efferents and afferents and an array of neuropeptides.[2,7] In relevance to AF, GPs are especially densely distributed within the atria in the regions of the posterior left atrium (PLA) and pulmonary veins (PVs). At the junction of the PVs and left atrium, a circuitry of cardiac afferents arise to generate the atrial stretch-driven autonomic reflexes and maintain cardiac homeostasis.[8,9] These regions, as discussed later, are heavily implicated in the genesis of atrial arrhythmias.

Feinberg Cardiovascular and Renal Research Institute, Northwestern University Feinberg School of Medicine, 251 East Huron, Feinberg 8-503, Chicago, IL 60611, USA
* Corresponding author. Northwestern University-Feinberg School of Medicine, 251 East Huron, Feinberg 8-503, Chicago, IL 60611.
E-mail address: r-arora@northwestern.edu

Card Electrophysiol Clin 13 (2021) 183–190
https://doi.org/10.1016/j.ccep.2020.11.012
1877-9182/21/© 2020 Elsevier Inc. All rights reserved.

AUTONOMIC DYSFUNCTION IN ATRIAL FIBRILLATION

Sympathetic and Parasympathetic Contributions to Dysrhythmia

Within the atria, increases in either sympathetic or parasympathetic signaling have been demonstrated to be proarrhythmogenic.[10,11] High vagal input has been classically associated as a driver of paroxysmal or lone AF,[12] whereas increased adrenergic discharge is implicated in exercise-induced AF and heart failure (HF)-associated arrhythmic disturbances. However, close examination of patients with AF and animal models gives evidence that a spectrum of sympathovagal discharge patterns can precede the onset of AF. Recent research indicates that in the setting of heart disease a mixed model of autonomic dysfunction is likely present, with co-upregulation of both parasympathetic and sympathetic signaling within the atria.[13,14] Both limbs of the ANS seem to exhibit a neural remodeling at the structural and functional level that synergistically promotes a dynamic AF substrate. Investigation into atrial neuroplasticity has demonstrated that once AF is present—whether the result of electrical remodeling in the absence of structural heart disease, or in the presence of congestive HF—autonomic remodeling presents as a spatially heterogeneous increase in neural innervation within the atria.[11,15,16] When combined with a background of fibrosis, stretch, and oxidative stress, these alterations in innervation set a fixed substrate, whereupon fluctuations in adrenergic or vagal tone may exert a profound, dynamic influence on electrophysiology.

Autonomic Effects on Electrophysiology

Shortened effective refractory periods (ERPs) are the hallmark of electrophysiological remodeling in AF. Although high parasympathetic tone prolongs ventricular ERPs, atrial ERPs are shortened. Importantly, this parasympathetic shortening is not uniform through the atria, rather, it is heterogeneously distributed even in healthy hearts.[5] This variegation is due to the rapid effects of local acetylcholinesterase, which swiftly breaks down the acetylcholine near its release from the cholinergic nerve terminal.[17] Acetylcholine, when present, interacts with atrial muscarinic receptors (M_2, G-coupled) and initiates G-protein signaled activation of the inwardly rectifying potassium channel I_{KAch}.[18] As a result, action potential duration (APD) and ERP are shortened in a regionally dependent manner.

Adrenergic stimulation exerts the bulk of its arrhythmogenic influence through alterations in Ca^{2+} handling. Norepinephrine stimulation of β-adrenergic G-coupled receptors initiates a cascade of membrane protein phosphorylation. Among these are membrane channels that regulate calcium entry at the level of the sarcolemma (L-type Ca^{2+} channel, I_{CaL}) and calcium release and reuptake at the sarcoplasmic reticulum (Ca^{2+} release ryanodine channel RyR2, Ca^{2+} reuptake transporter SERC2a).[19] Under these conditions, the availability of intracellular calcium is greatly increased and provides for an enhanced systolic function under sympathetically active conditions. However, this Ca^{2+} loading (increased I_{CaL} and RyR2) with an impaired reuptake mechanism (SERC2a) also permits ideal conditions for Ca^{2+}-triggered arrhythmic activity. When sympathetic stimulation is joined with parasympathetic tone, the influx of Ca^{2+} availability in the presence of a heterogeneously shortened APD produces a condition where ectopic foci for reentry can be established.[20]

Autonomic Implications at the Pulmonary Veins and Posterior Left Atrium

Through recent research, the anatomic region around the PVs and PLA seems to possess a unique autonomic profile[21–24] and is readily coaxed to disarray. When combined with the influences of disease remodeling, the PVs and PLA present a distinctive electrophysiologic climate from which neurally mediated arrhythmic disturbances can arise. In comparison to the rest of the atria, this region is characterized by naturally shortened APDs[5] and an increased responsiveness to autonomic manipulations.[22] The PVs and PLA seem to be particularly replete in both sympathetic and parasympathetic fibers,[24,25] and this rich innervation increases further in the setting of disease. During chronic AF, human and animal studies have demonstrated alterations in the density and ratio of parasympathetic and sympathetic fibers.[11,26] In a recent study, we demonstrated a significant increase in the size and number of autonomic nerve trunks in the PLA in a rapid atrial pacing model of AF; this increase in "parent" nerve trunks in the PLA resulted in a diffuse increase in both parasympathetic and sympathetic innervation in both atria.[27]

Although tonic parasympathetic activity within the ventricle is diminished during HF,[28] the opposite effect is noted in the atria: here, an excessive sprouting of new parasympathetic nerves in the PLA, as has been shown by our group and by others,[11,13] may provide sufficient vagal input to incite a proarrhythmic state.[2] Similarly, with increased adrenergic innervation, small fluctuations in sympathetic discharge may be magnified, exerting a potent arrhythmic stimulus to a diseased tissue bed. This hyperinnervation is accompanied by increased sympathovagal discharge that precedes the onset of atrial arrhythmias in the setting of HF.[13]

THERAPEUTIC STRATEGIES FOR ATRIAL FIBRILLATION TARGETING THE AUTONOMIC NERVOUS SYSTEM
Risk Factor Modification

The development of AF is complex, and the precise contribution of parasympathetic and sympathetic hyperactivation is likely variable between patients. Multiple risk factors for AF have been shown to activate one or more limbs of the ANS. Consequently, risk factor modification can also be used to target the ANS.[29] For example, weight loss was shown to reduce sympathetic activation. Obstructive sleep apnea leads to enhanced parasympathetic activation during periods of apnea, followed by a sympathetic surge.[30] Treatment of sleep apnea was shown to reduce sympathetic activation and likely also reduces parasympathetic activation.[31,32] When evaluated in the setting of AF, treatment of sleep apnea led to improved outcomes after catheter ablation.[33] More general lifestyle modifications such as exercise have also shown to be beneficial for the modulation of the ANS.[29]

Pharmacologic Therapies Targeting the Neurohormonal System

Autonomic blockade
Beta-blockers currently represent the pharmacologic gold standard to achieve sympathetic modulation and have been used for decades for the treatment of arrhythmias, HF, and coronary heart disease. Despite a clear role for beta-blockers in postoperative AF,[34] and a mild effect in the setting of HF,[35] this class of agents does not clearly prevent development of AF in other clinical scenarios and is predominantly reserved for rate control management.

Because of its pharmacologic property of preferentially blocking the N-type calcium channel, the dual (L-/N-) calcium channel blocker cilnidipine primarily blocks release of norepinephrine from sympathetic nerves, with a 20-fold smaller effect on L-type calcium channels. Evaluation in the canine atrial tachypacing model of AF showed that this compound could attenuate norepinephrine release and reduce electrical remodeling (both ERP and conduction velocity) as well as structural remodeling.[36] These promising results in a relevant animal model pave the way for clinical trials with patients with AF.

The main limitation of pharmacologic autonomic blockade is the absence of an effective strategy to target the parasympathetic nervous system, as high sequence homology between all isoforms of muscarinic receptors (M1–M5) makes difficult the development of highly selective M2 inhibitors.[37,38] In the absence of effective small molecule inhibitors of parasympathetic signaling, more "indirect" strategies of autonomic modulation have been investigated, which are reviewed in the following section.

Renin-angiotensin-aldosterone system blockade
Angiotensin-converting enzyme inhibitors (ACEIs) and angiotensin-II receptor blockers (ARBs) are effective antihypertensive drugs and reduce morbidity and mortality in patients with HF (HF) or systolic dysfunction after myocardial infarction.[39] Although both hypertension and HF predispose to AF, animal models suggest a more direct role of the renin-angiotensin-aldosterone system on atrial remodeling. Nakashima and colleagues[40] showed that acute application of captopril or candesartan prevented ERP shortening secondary to rapid atrial pacing in a large animal model. In addition to acute effects on ERP, a long-term effect on structural remodeling was also shown in a canine model of HF, with a reduction in atrial fibrosis, and development of AF after treatment with enalapril.[41] A large meta-analysis including patients with HF, hypertension, or patients who had undergone a cardioversion for AF showed a 28% reduction in relative risk of AF in patients treated with ACEIs or ARBs.[42] This effect was most relevant for patients with HF. Importantly, a study examining patients receiving ACEIs or ARBs after a myocardial infarction in the Swedish registry found no difference in new-onset of AF.[43] And a prospective, randomized, placebo-controlled, multicenter trial in patients with paroxysmal AF but no structural heart disease found no effect of olmesartan on AF burden.[44] Therefore, although animal studies suggest an effect of ACEIs or ARBs on acute electrical remodeling, it seems that the beneficial effect of ACEIs or ARBs is more likely to involve prevention of structural remodeling, which is more relevant in the context of HF, or possibly persistent or long-standing persistent AF. Further randomized trials will be necessary to elucidate this point.

Invasive Strategies for Autonomic Modulation

Ganglionated plexi ablation
Because the parasympathetic limb seems to play a key role in autonomic-induced AF, direct targeting of parasympathetic innervation was

investigated. Ablation of the GPs in the canine atrial tachypacing model reversed acute autonomic remodeling.[45] Human studies have also shown promising results: in 2 randomized clinical trials, Katritsis and colleagues[46,47] showed superior freedom from AF recurrence in patients who received GP ablation in addition to PVI when compared with PVI alone or GP ablation alone. A recent meta-analysis by Kampatsis and colleagues[48] also confirmed better clinical outcomes with a combination of catheter-based PVI and GP ablation for patients with paroxysmal AF, with a less clear effect in patients with persistent AF. Because both radiofrequency wide antrum circumferential PVI and cryoballoon PVI result in partial GP ablation,[49,50] it is hypothesized that inadvertent autonomic denervation contributes to the therapeutic effect of catheter-based PVI in patients with AF. In addition, the STAR AF study showed a superior freedom from after both PVI and complex fractionated atrial electrograms (CFAE) ablation when compared with PVI or CFAE ablation alone.[51] As high local parasympathetic tone colocalizes with CFAE,[11,52] the superiority of PVI and CFAE ablation may represent a more complete autonomic denervation.

Nonablative autonomic modulation

In addition to complete sympathetic or parasympathetic denervation, there is a growing interest for autonomic modulation approaches. This concept has been used for decades for treatment of epilepsy and depression and is based on synaptic plasticity: short-term therapy can have long-lasting effects on the ANS.[53] The strategies with clinical or preclinical results are detailed in the following section.

Modulation of the parasympathetic nervous system: direct vagus nerve stimulation and tragus stimulation

Although direct, high-level vagal stimulation was shown to promote AF, low-level vagus nerve stimulation below the bradycardia threshold seems to produce an antiarrhythmic effect in animal models of AF.[54–56] This effect is mediated at least in part by inhibition of GP activity.[55] In addition, low-level vagus nerve stimulation was also shown to suppress left stellate ganglion activity, thereby affecting both limbs of the ANS.[56] In humans, this modality of autonomic modulation has only been investigated in the postoperative setting, as it requires access to preganglionic fibers in the chest cavity. This randomized study showed a significant reduction in postoperative AF when compared with controls.[57] Further

investigation is limited by the need for access to the vagus nerve.

Stimulation of the tragus of the ear affects the parasympathetic nervous system through the afferent auricular branch of the vagus nerve. This has been used as a noninvasive method of vagal stimulation. Similar to direct vagal stimulation, low-level tragus stimulation was shown to inhibit GP firing in a canine model of AF and was able to reduce electrical remodeling and AF inducibility.[58] The noninvasive nature of tragus stimulation has made it attractive for potential application in humans, with 2 clinical trials showing promising results. First, Stavrakis and colleagues[59] used 1 hour of low-level tragus stimulation at 20 Hz through a metal clip placed on the tragus. When compared with sham, low-level tragus stimulation reduced pacing-induced AF duration and prolonged ERP. After these promising results, a long-term, randomized control trial evaluated low-level tragus stimulation in 53 patients with paroxysmal AF (the TREAT-AF trial).[60] The investigators showed a reduction in AF burden at 6 months in patients who had received 1 hour of low-level tragus stimulation daily.

Modulation of the sympathetic nervous system: renal denervation

Sympathetic ganglia and fibers form a neural network around the proximal renal arteries, with both afferent and efferent connections between the kidneys and the central nervous system. Denervation of this region is thought to modulate the heart and blood vessels through its effect on the afferent sympathetic branches. Although the trials of renal denervation for the treatment of hypertension have led to disappointing results, some studies suggest a potential role for renal denervation in the treatment of AF. Animal studies show reduced sympathetic hyperinnervation in the atria after renal denervation, and reduced AF inducibility, consistent with a central effect of this strategy.[61,62] Two small and one large randomized trials evaluating renal denervation in addition to PVI versus PVI alone showed promising results.[63–65] The ERADICATE-AF trial, in which 302 patients with paroxysmal AF were randomized to PVI with or without renal denervation, showed greater freedom from AF off antiarrhythmic drugs at 12 months in patients with renal denervation (72.1% vs 56.5%).[65] Importantly, it is difficult to separate direct effects of renal denervation from indirect effects on optimized control of blood pressure. In addition, although patients were blinded, operators were not.

Gene Therapy Targeting Parasympathetic and Sympathetic Signaling Pathways

Although the afferent and efferent limbs of the ANS can be modulated via the strategies described earlier, this is likely to cause widespread effects beyond the atria and may therefore lead to deleterious effects in other target tissues (such as the ventricular myocardium). Indeed, animal studies have shown an increased risk of ventricular arrhythmias after GP ablation in the postmyocardial infarction setting.[66] Anatomically defined modulation of the ANS, such as by gene therapy targeting the intracellular signaling pathways for parasympathetic or sympathetic innervation, would circumvent this limitation. Modulation of the ANS by gene therapy was first investigated in the setting of AF rate control, by directly targeting the effect of autonomic innervation on the atrioventricular (AV) node. Donahue and colleagues first explored this strategy in a porcine model of AF by injecting an adenovirus leading to overexpression of $G\alpha_{i2}$ in the AV nodal artery. This is expected to mimic the effect of heightened vagal tone. The investigators described a longer AV nodal ERP and slower ventricular rates during AF

in an acute model of AF[67] and in a model with persistent AF.[68] Inhibition of stimulatory G protein $G\alpha_s$ (responsible for signal transduction of beta-adrenoreceptors) via a similar approach was also effective in rate control, with even better control in the presence of sympathetic agonists.[69] In addition to its effect on the AV node, the ANS (both parasympathetic and sympathetic) also has a direct influence on the electrophysiology of atrial cardiomyocytes, as detailed earlier. Therefore, similar targets used in the AV node could potentially be exploited in a broader biatrial application. It is worth noting that increased parasympathetic signaling leads to slower AV nodal conduction, but shorter refractory period elsewhere in the atria, and thus an opposite strategy should be used when targeting the parasympathetic system in the atria or the AV node. For example, Aistrup and colleagues[37] showed that acute application of inhibitory peptides of $G\alpha_i$ (C-terminal $G\alpha_{i/o}$ peptides), that is, a reduction in parasympathetic signaling, can attenuate vagal-induced ERP shortening and reduce AF inducibility during vagal stimulation in canine hearts. The same group also showed that in vivo subepicardial injection of minigenes expressing these inhibitory peptides

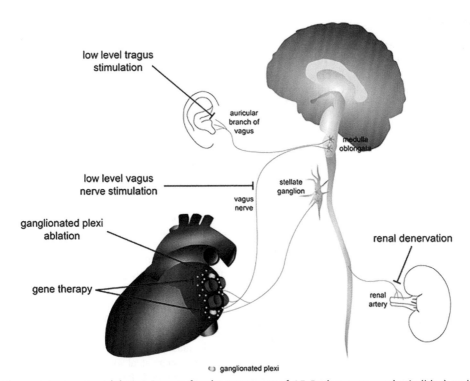

Fig. 1. Therapeutic neuromodulation targets for the treatment of AF. Both parasympathetic (*blue*) and sympathetic (*green*) fibers can be targeted, either by denervation or by low-level stimulation. In addition, ablation of GP, which predominantly contain parasympathetic neurons, shows promising results for the treatment of AF. Finally, gene therapy may lead to promising tissue-specific neuromodulation.

followed by electroporation led to reduced vagal-induced AF in a canine model.[70]

All gene therapy studies targeting the ANS in AF have been of relatively short duration, spanning from 3 to 18 days. Longer term studies will be required before translation to human AF. Finally, as the mechanisms leading to autonomic hyperinnervation become better understood in the near future, therapies promoting regression of the hyperinnervation will likely emerge.

SUMMARY

Taken together, the parasympathetic and sympathetic components of the ANS are positioned as viable therapeutic targets in the modulation of AF (**Fig. 1**). Autonomic dysfunction seems to play an essential role in the development and persistence of AF; however, the pathophysiology and relevance of sympathovagal interactions are intricate and have yet to be fully elucidated. Although clinically applicable strategies for AF have been challenging to establish, novel preclinical developments and an increasing understanding in the underlying mechanisms of autonomic dysfunction yield encouraging prospects for future therapies.

FUNDING SOURCES

Dr. Arora is supported by NIH grants R01 HL093490 and R01 HL140061; the American Heart Association (AHA) Strategically Focused Research Networks AF Center grant; NIH Center for Accelerated Innovations at Cleveland Clinic (NCAI-CC).

DISCLOSURE

R. Arora: Ownership interest, Rhythm Therapeutics, Inc. Other authors have no conflicts related to this study.

CLINICS CARE POINTS

- The beneficial effects of risk factor modification for atrial fibrillation, such as weight loss and treatment of sleep apnea, are partly mediated by their effect on the autonomic nervous system.
- Pulmonary vein isolation by catheter ablation causes partial autonomic denervation by ablation of the ganglionated plexi, likely contributing to the efficacy of ablation.
- Strategies directly targeting the autonomic nervous system, either by denervation or by neuromodulation, are promising avenues for the treatment of atrial fibrillation.

REFERENCES

1. Chugh SS, Havmoeller R, Narayanan K, et al. Worldwide epidemiology of atrial fibrillation. Circulation 2014;129(8):837–47.
2. Shen MJ, Choi E-K, Tan AY, et al. Neural mechanisms of atrial arrhythmias. Nat Rev Cardiol 2012; 9(1):30–9.
3. Malik V, Gallagher C, Linz D, et al. Atrial fibrillation is associated with syncope and falls in older adults. Mayo Clin Proc 2020;95(4):676–87.
4. Malik V, Mishima R, Elliott D, H Lau D, Sanders P. The "road" to atrial fibrillation: the role of the cardiac autonomic nervous system. J Atr Fibrillation 2020;13(1):2400.
5. Chen P-S, Chen LS, Fishbein MC, et al. Role of the autonomic nervous system in atrial fibrillation. Circ Res 2014;114(9):1500–15.
6. Armour JA, Murphy DA, Yuan BX, et al. Gross and microscopic anatomy of the human intrinsic cardiac nervous system. Anat Rec 1997;247(2):289.
7. Stavrakis S, Po S. Ganglionated plexi ablation: physiology and clinical applications. Arrhythm Electrophysiol Rev 2017;6(4):186.
8. Coleridge JCG, Hemingway A, Holmes RL, et al. The location of atrial receptors in the dog: a physiological and histological study. J Physiol 1957;136(1):174–97.
9. Malik V, McKitrick DJ, Lau DH, et al. Clinical evidence of autonomic dysfunction due to atrial fibrillation: implications for rhythm control strategy. J Interv Card Electrophysiol 2019;54(3):299–307.
10. Chen P-S, Tan AY. Autonomic nerve activity and atrial fibrillation. Heart Rhythm 2007;4(3):S61–4.
11. Ng J, Villuendas R, Cokic I, et al. Autonomic remodeling in the left atrium and pulmonary veins in heart failure: creation of a dynamic substrate for atrial fibrillation. Circ Arrhythm Electrophysiol 2011;4(3):388–96.
12. Coumel P. Paroxysmal atrial fibrillation: a disorder of autonomic tone? Eur Heart J 1994;15(suppl A):9–16.
13. Ogawa M, Zhou S, Tan AY, et al. Left stellate ganglion and vagal nerve activity and cardiac arrhythmias in ambulatory dogs with pacing-induced congestive heart failure. J Am Coll Cardiol 2007;50(4):335–43.
14. Amar D, Zhang H, Miodownik S, et al. Competing autonomic mechanisms precedethe onset of postoperative atrial fibrillation. J Am Coll Cardiol 2003; 42(7):1262–8.
15. Jayachandran JV, Sih HJ, Winkle W, et al. Atrial fibrillation produced by prolonged rapid atrial pacing is associated with heterogeneous changes in atrial sympathetic innervation. Circulation 2000;101(10):1185–91.
16. Gould PA, Yii M, McLean C, et al. Evidence for increased atrial sympathetic innervation in persistent human atrial fibrillation. Pacing Clin Electrophysiol 2006;29(8):821–9.
17. Oberhauser V, Schwertfeger E, Rutz T, et al. Acetylcholine release in human heart atrium. Circulation 2001;103(12):1638–43.

18. Grant AO. Cardiac ion channels. Circ Arrhythm Electrophysiol 2009;2(2):185–94.

19. Nattel S, Dobrev D. The multidimensional role of calcium in atrial fibrillation pathophysiology: mechanistic insights and therapeutic opportunities. Eur Heart J 2012;33(15):1870–7.

20. Patterson E, Po SS, Scherlag BJ, et al. Triggered firing in pulmonary veins initiated by in vitro autonomic nerve stimulation. Heart Rhythm 2005;2(6):624–31.

21. Ogawa M, Tan AY, Song J, et al. Cryoablation of stellate ganglia and atrial arrhythmia in ambulatory dogs with pacing-induced heart failure. Heart Rhythm 2009;6(12):1772–9.

22. Arora R, Ng J, Ulphani J, et al. Unique autonomic profile of the pulmonary veins and posterior left atrium. J Am Coll Cardiol 2007;49(12):1340–8.

23. Arora R. Recent insights into the role of the autonomic nervous system in the creation of substrate for atrial fibrillation. Circ Arrhythm Electrophysiol 2012;5(4):850–9.

24. Arora R, Ulphani JS, Villuendas R, et al. Neural substrate for atrial fibrillation: implications for targeted parasympathetic blockade in the posterior left atrium. Am J Physiol Heart Circ Physiol 2008;294(1):H134–44.

25. Tan AY, Li H, Wachsmann-Hogiu S, et al. Autonomic innervation and segmental muscular disconnections at the human pulmonary vein-atrial junction. J Am Coll Cardiol 2006;48(1):132–43.

26. Deneke T, Chaar H, De Groot JR, et al. Shift in the pattern of autonomic atrial innervation in subjects with persistent atrial fibrillation. Heart Rhythm 2011;8(9):1357–63.

27. Gussak G, Pfenniger A, Wren L, et al. Region-specific parasympathetic nerve remodeling in the left atrium contributes to creation of a vulnerable substrate for atrial fibrillation. JCI Insight 2019;4(20):e130532.

28. Olshansky B, Sabbah HN, Hauptman PJ, et al. Parasympathetic nervous system and heart failure. Circulation 2008;118(8):863–71.

29. Linz D, Elliott AD, Hohl M, et al. Role of autonomic nervous system in atrial fibrillation. Int J Cardiol 2019;287:181–8.

30. May AM, Van Wagoner DR, Mehra R. OSA and cardiac arrhythmogenesis: mechanistic insights. Chest 2017;151(1):225–41.

31. Usui K, Bradley TD, Spaak J, et al. Inhibition of awake sympathetic nerve activity of heart failure patients with obstructive sleep apnea by nocturnal continuous positive airway pressure. J Am Coll Cardiol 2005;45(12):2008–11.

32. Narkiewicz K, Kato M, Phillips BG, et al. Nocturnal continuous positive airway pressure decreases daytime sympathetic traffic in obstructive sleep apnea. Circulation 1999;100(23):2332–5.

33. Fein AS, Shvilkin A, Shah D, et al. Treatment of obstructive sleep apnea reduces the risk of atrial fibrillation recurrence after catheter ablation. J Am Coll Cardiol 2013;62(4):300–5.

34. Bessissow A, Khan J, Devereaux PJ, et al. Postoperative atrial fibrillation in non-cardiac and cardiac surgery: an overview. J Thromb Haemost 2015;13(Suppl 1):S304–12.

35. Nasr IA, Bouzamondo A, Hulot JS, et al. Prevention of atrial fibrillation onset by beta-blocker treatment in heart failure: a meta-analysis. Eur Heart J 2007;28(4):457–62.

36. Tajiri K, Guichard JB, Qi X, et al. An N-/L-type calcium channel blocker, cilnidipine, suppresses autonomic, electrical, and structural remodelling associated with atrial fibrillation. Cardiovasc Res 2019;115(14):1975–85.

37. Aistrup GL, Villuendas R, Ng J, et al. Targeted G-protein inhibition as a novel approach to decrease vagal atrial fibrillation by selective parasympathetic attenuation. Cardiovasc Res 2009;83(3):481–92.

38. Watson N, Eglen RM. Muscarinic receptor antagonists. Pulm Pharmacol Ther 1999;12(2):115–8.

39. Burnett H, Earley A, Voors AA, et al. Thirty years of evidence on the efficacy of drug treatments for chronic heart failure with reduced ejection fraction: a network meta-analysis. Circ Heart Fail 2017;10(1):e003529.

40. Nakashima H, Kumagai K, Urata H, et al. Angiotensin II antagonist prevents electrical remodeling in atrial fibrillation. Circulation 2000;101(22):2612–7.

41. Shi Y, Li D, Tardif JC, et al. Enalapril effects on atrial remodeling and atrial fibrillation in experimental congestive heart failure. Cardiovasc Res 2002;54(2):456–61.

42. Healey JS, Baranchuk A, Crystal E, et al. Prevention of atrial fibrillation with angiotensin-converting enzyme inhibitors and angiotensin receptor blockers: a meta-analysis. J Am Coll Cardiol 2005;45(11):1832–9.

43. Batra G, Lindhagen L, Andell P, et al. Angiotensin-converting enzyme inhibitors and angiotensin II receptor blockers are associated with improved outcome but do not prevent new-onset atrial fibrillation after acute myocardial infarction. J Am Heart Assoc 2017;6(3):e005165.

44. Goette A, Schon N, Kirchhof P, et al. Angiotensin II-antagonist in paroxysmal atrial fibrillation (ANTIPAF) trial. Circ Arrhythm Electrophysiol 2012;5(1):43–51.

45. Lu Z, Scherlag BJ, Lin J, et al. Atrial fibrillation begets atrial fibrillation: autonomic mechanism for atrial electrical remodeling induced by short-term rapid atrial pacing. Circ Arrhythm Electrophysiol 2008;1(3):184–92.

46. Katritsis DG, Giazitzoglou E, Zografos T, et al. Rapid pulmonary vein isolation combined with autonomic

ganglia modification: a randomized study. Heart Rhythm 2011;8(5):672–8.

47. Katritsis DG, Pokushalov E, Romanov A, et al. Autonomic denervation added to pulmonary vein isolation for paroxysmal atrial fibrillation a randomized clinical trial. J Am Coll Cardiol 2013;62(24):2318–25.

48. Kampaktsis PN, Oikonomou EK, Choi DY, et al. Efficacy of ganglionated plexi ablation in addition to pulmonary vein isolation for paroxysmal versus persistent atrial fibrillation: a meta-analysis of randomized controlled clinical trials. J Interv Card Electrophysiol 2017;50(3):253–60.

49. Stavrakis S, Nakagawa H, Po SS, et al. The role of the autonomic ganglia in atrial fibrillation. JACC Clin Electrophysiol 2015;1(1–2):1–13.

50. Garabelli P, Stavrakis S, Kenney JFA, et al. Effect of 28-mm cryoballoon ablation on major atrial ganglionated plexi. JACC Clin Electrophysiol 2018;4(6):831–8.

51. Verma A, Mantovan R, Macle L, et al. Substrate and trigger ablation for reduction of atrial fibrillation (STAR AF): a randomized, multicentre, international trial. Eur Heart J 2010;31(11):1344–56.

52. Pokushalov E, Romanov A, Artyomenko S, et al. Ganglionated plexi ablation directed by high-frequency stimulation and complex fractionated atrial electrograms for paroxysmal atrial fibrillation. Pacing Clin Electrophysiol 2012;35(7):776–84.

53. Stavrakis S, Kulkarni K, Singh JP, et al. Autonomic modulation of cardiac arrhythmias: methods to assess treatment and outcomes. JACC Clin Electrophysiol 2020;6(5):467–83.

54. Sheng X, Scherlag BJ, Yu L, et al. Prevention and reversal of atrial fibrillation inducibility and autonomic remodeling by low-level vagosympathetic nerve stimulation. J Am Coll Cardiol 2011;57(5):563–71.

55. Yu L, Scherlag BJ, Li S, et al. Low-level vagosympathetic nerve stimulation inhibits atrial fibrillation inducibility: direct evidence by neural recordings from intrinsic cardiac ganglia. J Cardiovasc Electrophysiol 2011;22(4):455–63.

56. Shen MJ, Shinohara T, Park HW, et al. Continuous low-level vagus nerve stimulation reduces stellate ganglion nerve activity and paroxysmal atrial tachyarrhythmias in ambulatory canines. Circulation 2011;123(20):2204–12.

57. Stavrakis S, Humphrey MB, Scherlag B, et al. Low-level vagus nerve stimulation suppresses postoperative atrial fibrillation and inflammation: a randomized study. JACC Clin Electrophysiol 2017;3(9):929–38.

58. Yu L, Scherlag BJ, Li S, et al. Low-level transcutaneous electrical stimulation of the auricular branch of the vagus nerve: a noninvasive approach to treat the initial phase of atrial fibrillation. Heart Rhythm 2013;10(3):428–35.

59. Stavrakis S, Humphrey MB, Scherlag BJ, et al. Low-level transcutaneous electrical vagus nerve stimulation suppresses atrial fibrillation. J Am Coll Cardiol 2015;65(9):867–75.

60. Stavrakis S, Stoner JA, Humphrey MB, et al. TREAT AF (transcutaneous electrical vagus nerve stimulation to suppress atrial fibrillation): a randomized clinical trial. JACC Clin Electrophysiol 2020;6(3):282–91.

61. Linz D, Mahfoud F, Schotten U, et al. Renal sympathetic denervation suppresses postapneic blood pressure rises and atrial fibrillation in a model for sleep apnea. Hypertension 2012;60(1):172–8.

62. Linz D, van Hunnik A, Hohl M, et al. Catheter-based renal denervation reduces atrial nerve sprouting and complexity of atrial fibrillation in goats. Circ Arrhythm Electrophysiol 2015;8(2):466–74.

63. Pokushalov E, Romanov A, Corbucci G, et al. A randomized comparison of pulmonary vein isolation with versus without concomitant renal artery denervation in patients with refractory symptomatic atrial fibrillation and resistant hypertension. J Am Coll Cardiol 2012;60(13):1163–70.

64. Feyz L, Theuns DA, Bhagwandien R, et al. Atrial fibrillation reduction by renal sympathetic denervation: 12 months' results of the AFFORD study. Clin Res Cardiol 2019;108(6):634–42.

65. Steinberg JS, Shabanov V, Ponomarev D, et al. Effect of renal denervation and catheter ablation vs catheter ablation alone on atrial fibrillation recurrence among patients with paroxysmal atrial fibrillation and hypertension: the ERADICATE-AF randomized clinical trial. JAMA 2020;323(3):248–55.

66. Wu B, Xu S, Dai R, et al. Epicardial ganglionated plexi ablation increases the inducibility of ventricular tachyarrhythmias in a canine postmyocardial infarction model. J Cardiovasc Electrophysiol 2019;30(5):741–6.

67. Donahue JK, Heldman AW, Fraser H, et al. Focal modification of electrical conduction in the heart by viral gene transfer. Nat Med 2000;6(12):1395–8.

68. Bauer A, McDonald AD, Nasir K, et al. Inhibitory G protein overexpression provides physiologically relevant heart rate control in persistent atrial fibrillation. Circulation 2004;110(19):3115–20.

69. Lugenbiel P, Thomas D, Kelemen K, et al. Genetic suppression of Galphas protein provides rate control in atrial fibrillation. Basic Res Cardiol 2012;107(3):265.

70. Aistrup GL, Cokic I, Ng J, et al. Targeted nonviral gene-based inhibition of Galpha(i/o)-mediated vagal signaling in the posterior left atrium decreases vagal-induced atrial fibrillation. Heart Rhythm 2011;8(11):1722–9.

Pathophysiology, Risk Factors, and Management of Atrial Fibrillation in Adult Congenital Heart Disease

Victor Waldmann, MD, PhD[a], Paul Khairy, MD, PhD[b],*

KEYWORDS

• Atrial fibrillation • Adult congenital heart disease • Atrial arrhythmias • Catheter ablation

KEY POINTS

• Atrial fibrillation is increasing in prevalence in adults with congenital heart disease and is the most common presenting arrhythmia over the age of 50 years.
• Atrial fibrillation has been associated with several predisposing features, including older age, number of cardiac surgeries, complexity of congenital heart disease, left atrial dilatation, and standard cardiovascular risk factors.
• Anticoagulation is recommended in patients with atrial fibrillation and moderate or complex congenital heart disease and in those with simple defects with established risk factors for stroke.
• Catheter ablation is increasingly performed for atrial fibrillation in adults with congenital heart disease, with modest success rates.
• Catheter ablation outcomes stand to improve with a greater understanding of underlying mechanisms and substrates, particularly with regards to extra pulmonary vein triggers.

INTRODUCTION

Advances in pediatric cardiac care have resulted in an increasing number of patients with congenital heart disease (CHD) surviving to adulthood, with adults now outnumbering children with CHD.[1] Major successes in long-term outcomes have generated new challenges, including the management of atrial arrhythmias, which are among the most common late complications encountered. As life expectancy in adults with CHD increases, a convergence of factors is driving an upsurge in the prevalence of atrial fibrillation (AF), which has been regarded as the next arrhythmic epidemic to afflict this population.[2,3] This review synthesizes current knowledge on AF in adults with CHD, addresses management issues, and highlights knowledge gaps and areas for future research.

EPIDEMIOLOGY

It has been estimated that, in the United States alone, approximatively 1.4 million adults lived with CHD in 2010, with a prevalence that has continued to increase since.[4] Atrial arrhythmias are associated with considerable morbidity in this population, with increased risks of heart failure, sudden death, stroke, and hospitalizations.[5] Atrial arrhythmias have been documented in 15% of patients with CHD, with higher reported rates in those with complex phenotypes. Indeed, projections indicate that 50% of 20-year-old

[a] Electrophysiology and Adult Congenital Heart Disease Unit, Hôpital Européen Georges Pompidou, Université de Paris, 20 Rue Leblanc, 75015 Paris, France; [b] Electrophysiology Service and Adult Congenital Heart Center, Montreal Heart Institute, Université de Montréal, Montreal, Quebec, Canada
* Corresponding author. Adult Congenital Heart Center, Montreal Heart Institute, 5000 Belanger Street East, Montreal, Quebec H1T 1C8, Canada.
E-mail address: paul.khairy@umontreal.ca

Card Electrophysiol Clin 13 (2021) 191–199
https://doi.org/10.1016/j.ccep.2020.10.007

patients with severe CHD will have an atrial tachyarrhythmia during their lifespan. The risk of developing intra-atrial reentrant tachycardia (IART) or AF has been estimated to be 22-fold higher in patients with CHD than matched controls.[6]

In a multicenter study conducted across 12 North American centers, AF accounted for 29% of presenting arrhythmias in patients with CHD, whereas IART and focal atrial tachycardia were responsible for 62% and 9.5%, respectively.[2] However, AF surpassed IART as the most common presenting arrhythmia in patients 50 years of age or older (**Fig. 1**). Coexistence of AF and organized atrial arrhythmias are frequent. Typically, patients initially present with episodes of atrial tachycardia or IART that then progress toward AF.[7] The arrhythmia pattern also tends to evolve progressively from paroxysmal to persistent or permanent forms.[2]

PATHOPHYSIOLOGY

The pathophysiologic mechanisms underlying AF involve triggers and a substrate that sustains the arrhythmia. In structurally normal hearts, most triggers arise from pulmonary veins, particularly in those with paroxysmal AF, whereas mechanisms perpetuating persistent and long-standing AF remain controversial. Considering the unique anatomic and physiologic features of patients with CHD, it should not be assumed that pathophysiologic mechanisms for AF are identical. Surgical scars, altered hemodynamics, chronic cyanosis, abnormal pulmonary or systemic venous connections, common atrial chambers, juxtaposed appendages, atrialized ventricular tissue, and a myriad of other influential factors may produce different arrhythmogenic substrates.

Few studies have described specific electrophysiologic features of AF in adults with CHD. Focal drivers were reported in 2 patients with

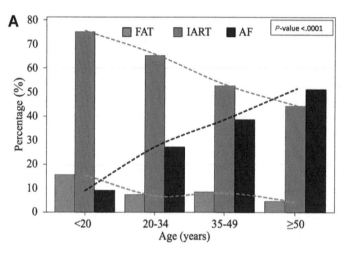

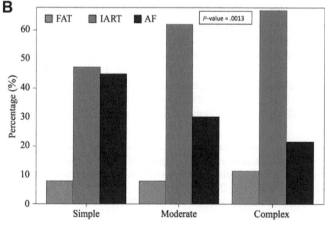

Fig. 1. Distribution of the type of atrial arrhythmia according to age (*A*) and to congenital heart disease complexity (*B*). FAT, focal atrial tachycardia. (*From* Labombarda F, Hamilton R, Shohoudi A et al. Increasing prevalence of atrial fibrillation and permanent atrial arrhythmias in congenital heart disease. J Am Coll Cardiol 2017;70:857-865; with permission.)

CHD and AF where circumscribed areas of continuous electrical activity coexisted with parts of the atrium activated in a standard fashion. Radiofrequency ablation within the abnormal circumscribed areas terminated AF[8] (**Fig. 2**). Detailed intracardiac electroanatomic maps in patients with electrocardiographic patterns consistent with AF sometimes reveal stable single- or multiple-loop circuits, which may produce seemingly irregularly irregular atrial activity especially when atrial scarring results in electrical dissociation of portions of the atrial chambers. Other studies using intraoperative epicardial mapping demonstrated that activation patterns differed in paroxysmal versus persistent AF. For example, in patients with atrial septal defects (ASD), atrial reentry or focal drivers confined to the right atrium often triggered AF, whereas multiple sources arising from pulmonary veins or the posterior left atrium were identified in patients with persistent AF.[9] In our experience, extrapulmonary triggers are more common than in patients with normal hearts. Identifying and eliminating these triggers can result in arrhythmia-free survival. This observation is consistent with reports demonstrating that patients with AF triggered by nonpulmonary vein foci tend to be younger and have right atrial enlargement and biatrial remodeling.[10]

RISK FACTORS FOR ATRIAL FIBRILLATION IN CONGENITAL HEART DISEASE

Most studies exploring factors associated with atrial arrhythmias in adults with CHD have either focused on IART or lacked the granularity to distinguish between different types of atrial arrhythmias. Factors specifically associated with AF were reported in a multicenter study of adults with

tetralogy of Fallot. In contrast with IART, which was associated with right atrial enlargement, factors that independently predicted AF were older age, number of cardiac surgeries, lower left ventricular ejection fraction, and left atrial dilatation.[11] The link between AF and age seems to be universal, regardless of the underlying cardiac anatomy, with younger age conferring a protective effect.[12] Older age is associated with alterations in ion channel function, action potential properties, and calcium homeostasis, which enable afterdepolarizations and ectopic atrial activity that promote AF.[13] Atrial fibrosis increases with age and contributes to structural remodeling that promotes and maintains AF. In addition, as patients with CHD age, they may acquire comorbidities such as hypertension, diabetes, and obesity that further contribute to arrhythmogenesis by virtue of atrial dilation, fibrosis, and electrical remodeling[2] (**Fig. 3**).

Consistently, a retrospective review of patients with CHD who underwent cardioversion for AF or IART found that those with AF tended to be older and had a higher prevalence of residual left-sided obstructive lesions.[14] Adults with CHD are also subject to developing heart failure that leads to structural, electrophysiologic, and neurohormonal modifications that can provoke and perpetuate AF. Last, the complexity of CHD has been associated with an increased risk for developing AF in different studies.[6,15]

ATRIAL FIBRILLATION IN PATIENTS WITH ATRIAL SEPTAL DEFECTS

ASDs account for approximately 30% of congenital heart defects in adults. Whereas large defects can provoke heart failure in children, many patients

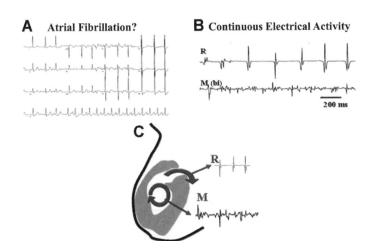

A Atrial Fibrillation?

B Continuous Electrical Activity

C

Fig. 2. Focal continuous electrical activity giving rise to fibrillatory conduction. Mapping during AF (*A*) revealed an area of continuous electrical activity at the right atrial free wall (*B* and *C*), whereas other parts of the atrium were activated in a regular manner. (*From* de Groot NM, Zeppenfeld K, Wijffels MC et al. Ablation of focal atrial arrhythmia in patients with congenital heart defects after surgery: role of circumscribed areas with heterogeneous conduction. Heart Rhythm 2006;3:526-35; with permission.)

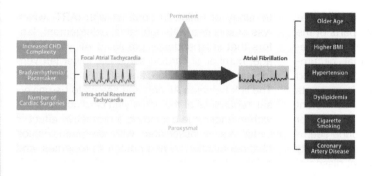

Fig. 3. Atrial arrhythmias in the aging population with CHD: changing types and patterns. Factors associated with focal atrial tachycardia and IART in patients with CHD include younger age, more complex disease, a greater number of cardiac surgeries, and bradyarrhythmias/pacemakers. By contrast, factors associated with AF include older age, higher body mass index, cardiovascular risk factors, and coronary artery disease. As age advances, AF surpasses IART to become the most prevalent atrial arrhythmia, and the pattern transitions from predominantly paroxysmal to permanent forms. (*From* Labombarda F, Hamilton R, Shohoudi A et al. Increasing prevalence of atrial fibrillation and permanent atrial arrhythmias in congenital heart disease. J Am Coll Cardiol 2017;70:857-865; with permission.)

with smaller ASDs remain asymptomatic or with subclinical manifestations well into adulthood. AF is one of the main causes of morbidity in adults with ASDs and is an outcome that reflects age-related increases in atrial dilation and stretch. Approximately 10% of nontreated patients with ASDs develop atrial arrhythmias, predominantly AF, by 40 years of age.[16] More than one-half the patient population with ASDs develops AF after 60 years of age.[17] The burden of AF can be decreased by ASD closure, if performed early enough. Older age at the time of shunt closure is the main factor associated with persistent or new-onset AF.[18] Atrial arrhythmias rarely occur when the ASD is closed during childhood or early adulthood.[19] A 4.1% annual incidence of new-onset AF was reported in a cohort of 1062 patients aged 50 ± 15 years with transcatheter ASD closure.[20]

MANAGEMENT OF ATRIAL FIBRILLATION IN ADULTS WITH CONGENITAL HEART DISEASE

In patients with CHD with new-onset, or increased cadence of, atrial arrhythmias, potential contributing causes should be ruled out, including regurgitant or obstructive lesions, shunts, and ventricular dysfunction. Arrhythmias are intricately linked to hemodynamic conditions such that consideration should be given to addressing the latter before or in conjunction with rhythm disorders. For example, in adults with CHD who require open heart surgery to address a hemodynamic condition, a left atrial Cox–Maze III procedure with right atrial cavotricuspid isthmus ablation can be considered in the setting of documented AF.[21]

Prevention of Thromboembolism

Thromboembolic complications are a central issue in adults with CHD. The prevalence of cerebrovascular accidents has been estimated to be 10- to 100-fold higher than in age-matched controls.[22] Thromboembolic events are thought to account for approximately 4% of all-cause mortality in CHD.[23] In patients with CHD, atrial arrhythmias are associated with a 60% to 190% increased risk of thromboembolic complications compared with those without atrial arrhythmias. There are currently no randomized trials of anticoagulation for AF in patients with CHD. In the multicenter observational *The AntiCoagulation Therapy In Congenital Heart Disease* (TACTIC) study, increased complexity of CHD was identified as the factor most strongly associated with thromboembolic events.[24] In patients with atrial arrhythmias, thromboembolic complication rates were 0.00%, 0.93%, and 1.95% per year in those with simple, moderate, and severe forms of CHD, respectively. The mean annual rate of thromboembolic events was 1.14%, which was comparable with rates observed in studies of patients without CHD with nonvalvular AF, despite the CHD population being younger and having fewer traditional risk factors.

In the absence of randomized trials specific to the CHD population with AF, in 2014 the Pediatric and Congenital Electrophysiology Society in conjunction with the Heart Rhythm Society issued an expert consensus statement on the management of arrhythmias in adults with CHD, which included recommendations on anticoagulation.[21] Updated modifications, albeit unvetted, to the consensus-based algorithm for pericardioversion and long-term anticoagulation were proposed in 2019 and are summarized in **Fig. 4**.[25]

Non–vitamin K Antagonist Oral Anticoagulants

Non–vitamin K antagonist oral anticoagulants (NOACs) have emerged as alternatives to vitamin K antagonists. In patients without CHD with

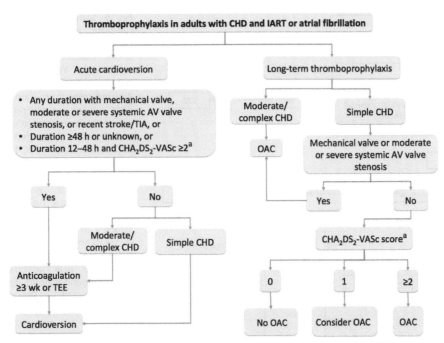

Fig. 4. Pericardioversion and long-term anticoagulation for IART or AF in adults with CHD. AV, atrioventricular; CHA_2DS_2-VASc, Congestive heart failure; Hypertension; Age ($\geq$75 years, 2 points; 65–74 years, 1 point); Diabetes; Stroke, transient ischemic attack, or thromboembolism (2 points); VAscular disease; Sex category (female); OAC, oral anticoagulation; TEE, transesophageal echocardiography; TIA, transient ischemic attack. [a] Excluding female sex from the CHA_2DS_2-VASc score. (*From* Khairy P. Arrhythmias in adults with congenital heart disease: what the practicing cardiologist needs to know. Can J Cardiol 2019;35:1698-1707; with permission.)

nonvalvular AF, the noninferior to superior efficacy of NOACs combined with a more favorable safety profile have prompted guidelines to recommend NOACs as a first-line therapy in eligible patients. The convenience of NOACs, with no need for monitoring or frequent dose adjustments, may be particularly attractive to a young and active population, such as patients with CHD. Indeed, observational data are emerging in support of a favorable safety and efficacy profile among most patients with CHD who have an indication for anticoagulation.[26,27] Nevertheless, a recent assessment of the literature suggested that the evidence is currently insufficient to recommend NOACs in patients with a Fontan circulation or in those with cyanotic CHD.[26] Moreover, NOACs are considered contraindicated in patients with a mechanical valve or mitral or tricuspid valve stenosis with enlarged and diseased atria, and after recent cardiac surgery (<3 months). **Fig. 5** summarizes scenarios where NOACs are thought to be reasonable, nondesirable, or should be used with caution.[26]

Antiarrhythmics

There is a paucity of safety and efficacy data on antiarrhythmic drugs in adults with CHD.[28]

Conversion rates for acute termination of AF with ibutilide and sotalol have ranged from 50% to 80%, with bradycardia, hypotension, and torsades de pointes described as complications.[29,30] Data on class IA, IC, or other class III agents in this context are lacking.

As an initial approach to management, rhythm control is generally preferred to rate control in patients with moderate or complex CHD who may poorly tolerate supraventricular arrhythmias. The choice of pharmacologic therapies should take into consideration various factors such as coexisting bradyarrhythmias, systemic or subpulmonary ventricular dysfunction, polypharmacy, and childbearing potential in women.[21] Class I antiarrhythmic drugs should be discouraged in patients with CHD and concomitant coronary artery disease or systolic dysfunction of a systemic or subpulmonary ventricle.[21] Amiodarone is the most effective agent to prevent AF recurrence, and is considered a drug of choice in the setting of heart failure. Nevertheless, long-term administration is limited by time- and dose-dependent side effects especially in this relatively young population. Particular to patients with CHD, the risk of amiodarone-induced thyrotoxicosis is 4- to 7-fold higher in those with cyanotic CHD and Fontan

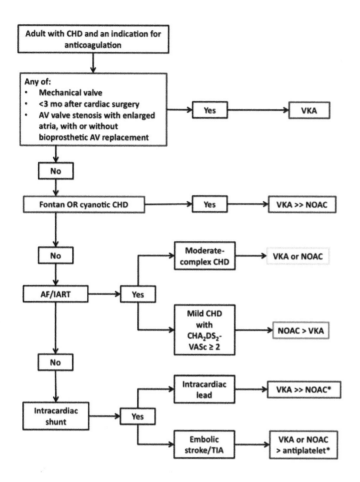

Fig. 5. Suggested choices of antithrombotic medications for selected clinical situations in adults with CHD. Green indicates that NOAC use is reasonable. Yellow indicates that NOACs should be used with caution. Red indicates that vitamin K antagonists (VKAs) are strongly preferred over NOACs or that NOACs are contraindicated. >, preferred to; AV, atrioventricular; CHA2DS2-VASc, Congestive Heart Failure, Hypertension, Age (≥75 years), Diabetes, Stroke/Transient Ischemic Attack, Vascular Disease, Age (65–74 years), Sex (Female); TIA, transient ischemic attack. [a] In absence of shunt closure. (*From* Mongeon FP, Macle L, Beauchesne LM et al. Non-vitamin K antagonist oral anticoagulants in adult congenital heart disease. Can J Cardiol 2019;35:1686-1697; with permission.)

palliation.[31] The use of sotalol has been relegated to a class IIb indication as a first-line agent given concerns over proarrhythmia and meta-analyses that reported increased all-cause mortality in the general population.[32] Dofetilide (a class III agent) is another reasonable alternative to amiodarone as a first-line antiarrhythmic drug in adults with CHD and ventricular dysfunction. Limitations include the required strict protocol of initiation and hospitalization owing to the risk of life-threatening torsades de pointes associated with excessive QT prolongation, and lack of availability in many countries worldwide.

Catheter Ablation

Limited success of pharmacologic therapy for AF in adults with CHD combined with considerable advances in ablative technologies have resulted in a growing preference for interventional approaches. Although numerous studies have reported outcomes for catheter ablation of IART or focal atrial tachycardia, the literature regarding AF ablation in CHD is just emerging.

In patients with ASDs, transseptal access across a portion of the native septum is often possible. In those with larger devices that cover most of the atrial septum, direct puncture through the prosthesis has been described.[33] Successful transseptal access has ranged from 90% to 98%, with 75% freedom from recurrence at 1 year.[33,34] Importantly, for adults with AF and newly diagnosed ASDs, it is preferable to proceed with catheter ablation before ASD closure whenever possible.

The first AF ablation study that included a mixed cohort of patients with CHD (n = 36) was published in 2012.[35] Most had paroxysmal AF (72%) and ASDs (61%) or ventricular septal defects (17%). Antral pulmonary vein isolation was performed in all patients, with individualized additional target sites that included the superior vena cava junction, left atrial septum and posterior wall, coronary sinus, and crista terminalis. After a single procedure, survival rates free from AF recurrence off antiarrhythmic drugs were 42% at 300 days and 27% at 4 years. Corresponding rates with or without antiarrhythmic drugs were 84%

and 61%, respectively. Another series of pulmonary vein isolation-based AF ablation reported outcomes in 57 patients with CHD, average age 51 years, 61% of whom had simple, 18% moderate, and 21% complex CHD.[36] The AF pattern was paroxysmal in 37% and persistent in 63%. Arrhythmia-free survival (on or off antiarrhythmic drugs) was 63% at 1 year and 22% at 5 years. During follow-up, 56% of patients had repeat interventions. At the second procedure, 65% had recovered pulmonary vein conduction. Cryoballoon ablation for AF has also been shown to be feasible in adults with CHD, with a similarly modest freedom from recurrent arrhythmias at 1 year.[37] Greater complexity of CHD seems to be associated with poorer outcomes. In a series of 58 patients, 57% of whom had moderate or complex CHD, only 33% remained free of recurrence at 1 year.[38] It remains possible that reluctance to proceed with AF ablation in adults with CHD contributes to poorer outcomes owing to an indication bias, with procedures often performed late in the disease course in patients with recalcitrant and persistent AF.

SUMMARY

AF is the next arrhythmic tsunami to strike adults with CHD and is already the most common presenting arrhythmia in patients over the age of 50 years. It has a compounding affect on morbidity in a patient population with an already high risk before AF of developing heart failure and thromboembolic complications. The limited efficacy of antiarrhythmic drugs and advances in catheter ablation technologies are resulting in an increased uptake of ablative techniques. The budding literature on catheter ablation supports feasibility and safety, yet suggests modest efficacy. Much remains to be learned about the impact of congenital heart defects and associated abnormalities on the pathophysiology and determinants of AF. It seems to be likely than non–pulmonary vein triggers, be they focal or reentrant, play a relatively more important role in the CHD population. A deeper understanding of these mechanisms and substrates may contribute to further improving outcomes in adults with CHD and AF.

CLINICS CARE POINTS

- In patients with CHD and new-onset or worsening atrial arrhythmias, potential contributing factors should be sought including regurgitant and obstructive lesions, shunts, and ventricular dysfunction.

- An initial strategy of rhythm control is generally favored in patients with moderate or complex CHD who may poorly tolerate supraventricular arrhythmias.
- Anticoagulation is recommended in patients with atrial fibrillation and moderate or complex CHD and in those with simple defects and risk factors for stroke.
- Non-vitamin K oral anticoagulants are not currently recommended in patients with a Fontan circulation or cyanotic CHD, and are contraindicated in the setting of a mechanical valve or mitral or tricuspid valve stenosis with enlarged and diseased atria.
- Non-pulmonary vein triggers should be identified and treated during catheter ablation procedures for atrial fibrillation in adults with CHD.

DISCLOSURE

Dr. Khairy is supported by the André Chagnon Research Chair in Electrophysiology and Congenital heart disease.

REFERENCES

1. Khairy P, Ionescu-Ittu R, Mackie AS, et al. Changing mortality in congenital heart disease. J Am Coll Cardiol 2010;56:1149–57.
2. Labombarda F, Hamilton R, Shohoudi A, et al. Increasing prevalence of atrial fibrillation and permanent atrial arrhythmias in congenital heart disease. J Am Coll Cardiol 2017;70:857–65.
3. Waldmann V, Laredo M, Abadir S, et al. Atrial fibrillation in adults with congenital heart disease. Int J Cardiol 2019;287:148–54.
4. Gilboa SM, Devine OJ, Kucik JE, et al. Congenital heart defects in the United States: estimating the magnitude of the affected population in 2010. Circulation 2016;134:101–9.
5. Bouchardy J, Therrien J, Pilote L, et al. Atrial arrhythmias in adults with congenital heart disease. Circulation 2009;120:1679–86.
6. Mandalenakis Z, Rosengren A, Lappas G, et al. Atrial fibrillation burden in young patients with congenital heart disease. Circulation 2018;137:928–37.
7. Teuwen CP, Ramdjan TT, Gotte M, et al. Time course of atrial fibrillation in patients with congenital heart defects. Circ Arrhythm Electrophysiol 2015;8:1065–72.
8. de Groot NM, Zeppenfeld K, Wijffels MC, et al. Ablation of focal atrial arrhythmia in patients with congenital heart defects after surgery: role of circumscribed areas with heterogeneous conduction. Heart Rhythm 2006;3:526–35.

9. Nitta T, Sakamoto S, Miyagi Y, et al. Reentrant and focal activations during atrial fibrillation in patients with atrial septal defect. Ann Thorac Surg 2013;96:1266–72.

10. Chang HY, Lo LW, Lin YJ, et al. Long-term outcome of catheter ablation in patients with atrial fibrillation originating from nonpulmonary vein ectopy. J Cardiovasc Electrophysiol 2013;24:250–8.

11. Khairy P, Aboulhosn J, Gurvitz MZ, et al. Arrhythmia burden in adults with surgically repaired tetralogy of Fallot: a multi-institutional study. Circulation 2010;122:868–75.

12. Laredo M, Waldmann V, Khairy P, et al. Age as a critical determinant of atrial fibrillation: a two-sided relationship. Can J Cardiol 2018;34:1396–406.

13. Andrade J, Khairy P, Dobrev D, et al. The clinical profile and pathophysiology of atrial fibrillation: relationships among clinical features, epidemiology, and mechanisms. Circ Res 2014;114:1453–68.

14. Kirsh JA, Walsh EP, Triedman JK. Prevalence of and risk factors for atrial fibrillation and intra-atrial reentrant tachycardia among patients with congenital heart disease. Am J Cardiol 2002;90:338–40.

15. Teuwen CP, Korevaar TI, Coolen RL, et al. Frequent atrial extrasystolic beats predict atrial fibrillation in patients with congenital heart defects. Europace 2018;20:25–32.

16. Craig RJ, Selzer A. Natural history and prognosis of atrial septal defect. Circulation 1968;37:805–15.

17. Sutton JMG, Tajik AJ, McGoon DC. Atrial septal defect in patients ages 60 years or older: operative results and long-term postoperative follow-up. Circulation 1981;64:402–9.

18. Vecht JA, Saso S, Rao C, et al. Atrial septal defect closure is associated with a reduced prevalence of atrial tachyarrhythmia in the short to medium term: a systematic review and meta-analysis. Heart 2010;96:1789–97.

19. Roos-Hesselink JW, Meijboom FJ, Spitaels SE, et al. Excellent survival and low incidence of arrhythmias, stroke and heart failure long-term after surgical ASD closure at young age. A prospective follow-up study of 21-33 years. Eur Heart J 2003;24:190–7.

20. Spies C, Khandelwal A, Timmermanns I, et al. Incidence of atrial fibrillation following transcatheter closure of atrial septal defects in adults. Am J Cardiol 2008;102:902–6.

21. Khairy P, Van Hare GF, Balaji S, et al. PACES/HRS Expert consensus statement on the recognition and management of arrhythmias in adult congenital heart disease: developed in partnership between the Pediatric and Congenital Electrophysiology Society (PACES) and the Heart Rhythm Society (HRS). Endorsed by the governing bodies of PACES, HRS, the American College of Cardiology (ACC), the American Heart Association (AHA), the European Heart Rhythm Association (EHRA), the Canadian Heart Rhythm Society (CHRS), and the International Society for Adult Congenital Heart Disease (ISACHD). Heart Rhythm 2014;11:e102–65.

22. Hoffmann A, Chockalingam P, Balint OH, et al. Cerebrovascular accidents in adult patients with congenital heart disease. Heart 2010;96:1223–6.

23. Karsenty C, Zhao A, Marijon E, et al. Risk of thromboembolic complications in adult congenital heart disease: a literature review. Arch Cardiovasc Dis 2018;111:613–20.

24. Khairy P, Aboulhosn J, Broberg CS, et al. Thromboprophylaxis for atrial arrhythmias in congenital heart disease: a multicenter study. Int J Cardiol 2016;223:729–35.

25. Khairy P. Arrhythmias in adults with congenital heart disease: what the practicing cardiologist needs to know. Can J Cardiol 2019;35:1698–707.

26. Mongeon FP, Macle L, Beauchesne LM, et al. Nonvitamin K antagonist oral anticoagulants in adult congenital heart disease. Can J Cardiol 2019;35:1686–97.

27. Yang H, Bouma BJ, Dimopoulos K, et al. Non-vitamin K antagonist oral anticoagulants (NOACs) for thromboembolic prevention, are they safe in congenital heart disease? Results of a worldwide study. Int J Cardiol 2020;299:123–30.

28. Brida M, Diller GP, Nashat H, et al. Pharmacological therapy in adult congenital heart disease: growing need, yet limited evidence. Eur Heart J 2019;40:1049–56.

29. Hoyer AW, Balaji S. The safety and efficacy of ibutilide in children and in patients with congenital heart disease. Pacing Clin Electrophysiol 2007;30:1003–8.

30. Rao SO, Boramanand NK, Burton DA, et al. Atrial tachycardias in young adults and adolescents with congenital heart disease: conversion using single dose oral sotalol. Int J Cardiol 2009;136:253–7.

31. Thorne SA, Barnes I, Cullinan P, et al. Amiodarone-associated thyroid dysfunction: risk factors in adults with congenital heart disease. Circulation 1999;100:149–54.

32. Lafuente-Lafuente C, Longas-Tejero MA, Bergmann JF, et al. Antiarrhythmics for maintaining sinus rhythm after cardioversion of atrial fibrillation. Cochrane Database Syst Rev 2012;5:CD005049.

33. Santangeli P, Di Biase L, Burkhardt JD, et al. Transseptal access and atrial fibrillation ablation guided by intracardiac echocardiography in patients with atrial septal closure devices. Heart Rhythm 2011;8:1669–75.

34. Lakkireddy D, Rangisetty U, Prasad S, et al. Intracardiac echo-guided radiofrequency catheter ablation of atrial fibrillation in patients with atrial septal defect or patent foramen ovale repair: a feasibility, safety, and efficacy study. J Cardiovasc Electrophysiol 2008;19:1137–42.

35. Philip F, Muhammad KI, Agarwal S, et al. Pulmonary vein isolation for the treatment of drug-refractory atrial fibrillation in adults with congenital heart disease. Congenit Heart Dis 2012;7:392–9.

36. Sohns C, Nurnberg JH, Hebe J, et al. Catheter ablation for atrial fibrillation in adults with congenital heart disease: lessons learned from more than 10 years following a sequential ablation approach. JACC Clin Electrophysiol 2018;4:733–43.

37. Abadir S, Waldmann V, Dyrda K, et al. Feasibility and safety of cryoballoon ablation for atrial fibrillation in patients with congenital heart disease. World J Cardiol 2019;11:149–58.

38. Guarguagli S, Kempny A, Cazzoli I, et al. Efficacy of catheter ablation for atrial fibrillation in patients with congenital heart disease. Europace 2019;21: 1334–44.

Risk Factors for Atrial Fibrillation Progression

Jordi Heijman, PhD[a], Justin G.L.M. Luermans, MD, PhD[a], Dominik Linz, MD, PhD[a],
Isabelle C. van Gelder, MD, PhD[b], Harry J.G.M. Crijns, MD, PhD[a],*

KEYWORDS

• Atrial fibrillation • Burden • Dynamics • Progression • Risk factors • Vulnerable substrate

KEY POINTS

- Atrial fibrillation (AF) progression is common but variable, occurring in approximately 2% to 20% of patients per year and is more common during the first year of follow-up.
- AF progression is caused by progressive atrial remodeling resulting from AF risk factors and AF itself.
- Advanced age and obesity are independently associated with AF progression in multiple studies.
- Similarly, a more vulnerable substrate (ie, increased left-atrial size and longer AF duration at baseline) is consistently identified as a risk factor for AF progression.
- Advanced forms of AF and AF progression itself are independently associated with worse outcomes, suggesting a role for early aggressive AF and risk factor management to reduce AF progression.

INTRODUCTION

Atrial fibrillation (AF) is a major health burden, negatively affecting morbidity and mortality of millions of individuals.[1] AF is promoted by advancing age and a wide range of cardiovascular risk factors.[2] The prevalence of AF continues to increase as a result of its progressive nature, and the aging of the population and increased prevalence of risk factors. Traditionally, AF is classified as paroxysmal when episodes last less than 7 days, persistent when episodes last greater than or equal to 7 days, or permanent AF when no further attempts to restore normal sinus rhythm are made.[3] The progressive nature of AF has been known for several decades and has classically been defined as a transition from paroxysmal to persistent/permanent forms or from persistent to permanent AF. Dozens of studies with 10,000s of patients have assessed the rate of clinical AF progression (**Table 1**). These studies have demonstrated that AF progression is common but variable, affecting approximately 2% to 20% of patients per year.[4–13] Progression from persistent to permanent AF is more common than progression from paroxysmal to persistent AF (>15%/year vs <10%/year, respectively; see **Table 1**) and yearly progression rates decrease with longer follow-up durations (yearly rates of 20.2%, 8.3%, 5.3%, and 4.2% with <1.5 years, 1.5–4.0 years, 4.0–6.5 years, and >6.5 years follow-up, respectively[4]). Moreover, this definition of AF progression critically depends on the detection of AF and the clinical judgment of patient-reported symptoms, which have limited accuracy with occasional rhythm monitoring.[14] Recently, long-term or continuous rhythm monitoring has enabled a more detailed characterization of AF

a Department of Cardiology, CARIM School for Cardiovascular Diseases, Maastricht University Medical Center+, PO Box 5800, Maastricht 6202 AZ, The Netherlands; b Department of Cardiology, University Medical Center Groningen, University of Groningen, PO Box 30.001, Groningen 9700 RB, The Netherlands
* Corresponding author.
E-mail address: hjgm.crijns@mumc.nl
Twitter: @JordiHeijman (J.H.); @JLuermans (J.G.L.M.L.); @Dominik_Linz (D.L.)

Card Electrophysiol Clin 13 (2021) 201–209
https://doi.org/10.1016/j.ccep.2020.10.011
1877-9182/21/© 2020 Elsevier Inc. All rights reserved.

Table 1
Overview of studies on AF progression and its risk factors

Study	Population	Definition of Progression	Follow-up	Progression	Risk Factors
Studies based on clinical AF types					
Meta-analysis of studies until August 2017, Blum et al,[4] 2019	27,266 patients from 47 studies	Progression from pAF to PersAF/permanent AF or from PersAF to permanent AF	105,912 patient-years	8.1%/y; 7.1%/y from pAF to PersAF, 18.6%/y from PersAF to permanent AF	Advanced age, hypertension
De With et al,[6] 2018; Marcos et al,[54] 2019	468 patients with pAF or PersAF starting <60 y of age	Development of permanent AF	7.2 (2.7–10.0) y	56 (11%) = (2.0%/y)	LA size diastolic blood pressure No sex difference
Dudink et al,[7] 2018	967 patients with pAF or first-detected AF with spontaneous or pharmacologic cardioversion during admission	Progression from pAF to PersAF/permanent	1 y	132 (13.7%) = (13.7%/y)	Advanced age, increased LA diameter, higher CHA_2DS_2VASc-score and HATCH-score
Middeldorp et al,[8] 2018	355 patients in 3 groups: A (<3% weight loss), B (3%–9% weight loss), and C (≥10% weight loss)	Change in AF type determined by clinical review and 7-d Holter yearly	4.0 ± 1.5, 3.8 ± 1.4, and 4.0 ± 1.5 y	A: 41% from pAF to PersAF and 26% from PersAF to pAF or no AF B: 32% from pAF to PersAF and 49% from PersAF to pAF or no AF C: 3% to PersAF and 88% reversed from PersAF to pAF or no AF	Obesity
Ogawa et al,[9] 2018	4045 patients (1974 with pAF; 2071 sustained AF)	Progression from pAF to PersAF	Mean 3.0 y	252 (12.8%) = (4.22%/y)	Longer time since first detection, larger LA diameter, more frequent drinkers, presence of cardiomyopathy

Study	Sample	Outcome	Follow-up	Progression	Risk factors
Schnabel et al,[10] 2018	PREFER in AF prolongation dataset (3223 patients)	Progression from pAF to PersAF/permanent AF or from PersAF to permanent AF	Complete 1-y follow-up	506 (17%) = (17%/y)	Sinus rhythm at baseline, AF duration, cardioversion, hyperthyroidism, valvular heart disease, diabetes mellitus, and heart failure
Blum et al,[5] 2019	2869 patients from the Swiss-AF study	Progression from pAF to PersAF/permanent AF or from PersAF to permanent AF	Median 3 y	5.2%/y	BMI, heart rate, age, systolic blood pressure, hyperthyroidism, stroke, and heart failure
Uetake et al,[11] 2019	306 patients with pAF with structurally normal hearts	Progression to PersAF	2.9 ± 1.6 y	60 of 172 (35%) in medication group; 3 of 134 (2%) in RFCA group	Diastolic wall strain, LA volume index
Jurin et al,[12] 2020	409 patients with nonpermanent AF (pAF or early PersAF)	Progression to permanent AF	Median 1.75 y	109 (26.6%)	Increased LA diameter, increased red cell distribution width
Olivia et al,[13] 2020	Retrospective analysis on clinical records of 136 patients	Progression from pAF to PersAF/permanent AF or from PersAF to permanent AF	Mean 233 d	42 (31%)	Advanced age, obesity, excessive alcohol intake
Studies based (partially) on AF burden					
Boriani et al,[15] 2018	2244 patients with new AF with an AF burden of ≥5 min	CIED-based increase in thresholds of daily AF burden (5 min and 1, 6, 12, and 23 h)	2.4 ± 1.7 y	1091 (49.8%)	Higher duration of daily AF burden manifest at first detection and CHADS$_2$ score ≥2
Wong et al,[17] 2018	415 patients from ASSERT whose longest SCAF episode during the first year after enrollment was >6 min but ≤24 h	CIED-based progression to >24-h episodes or clinical AF	Mean 2 y	65 (15.7%) = (8.8%/y)	Older age, greater BMI, and longer SCAF duration within the first year

(continued on next page)

Table 1
(continued)

Study	Population	Definition of Progression	Follow-up	Progression	Risk Factors
Diederichsen et al,[16] 2019	590 individuals ≥70 y of age with ≥1 of hypertension, diabetes, previous stroke, or heart failure, without history of AF	CIED-based progression to 24-h episodes	Median 3.35 y	33 of 205 with SCAF (16%)	Hypertension, previous stroke, and HF
De With et al,[43] 2020	392 patients with recent-onset pAF or PersAF	(i) doubling in AF burden at 1 y and minimum AF burden of 10% in pAF; or (ii) transition from pAF to PersAF or permanent AF; or (iii) PersAF to permanent AF	1 y	52 (13%); 11% in pAF; 26% in PersAF AF	LA volume NT-proBNP plasminogen activator inhibitor-1
De With et al,[18] 2020	179 patients with pAF	(i) increase in AF burden; or (ii) development of PersAF	Complete 1-y follow-up	Compared with the first 6 mo, 111 patients (62%) remained stable, 39 (22%) progressed, 8 (3%) developed PersAF, 29 (16%) regressed	
Krisai et al,[55] 2020	54 participants with recently documented pAF or PersAF	A relative change ≥10% or an absolute change >0.5% in AF burden between 2 yearly 7-d Holter-ECG	4 y	23.7% of participants had a decrease and 23.7% an increase in AF burden	Prior stroke, BNP

Studies published after the recent meta-analysis by Blum et al[4] (ie, from 2018 onward) were included based on a search for "atrial fibrillation progression" in PubMed.
Abbreviations: BMI, body mass index; BNP, brain natriuretic peptide; CIED, cardiac implantable electronic device; ECG, electrocardiogram; LA, left atrium; NT-proBNP, N-terminal pro– B-type natriuretic peptide; pAF, paroxysmal atrial fibrillation; PersAF, persistent AF; SCAF, subclinical atrial fibrillation.

progression by quantifying changes in AF burden or progression to specific durations of AF episodes.[15–18] These studies have similarly shown that many patients with AF progress toward AF episodes of longer duration (see **Table 1**).

However, a substantial proportion of patients initially present with nonparoxysmal forms,[19] subclinical AF is often a self-limiting or transient entity,[16] and it is increasingly appreciated that patients may also have a decrease in AF burden or show reverse progression (from persistent to paroxysmal forms).[8,18] Thus, although AF progression is common it is not a *sine qua non*.

In the remainder of this review, we describe the mechanisms underlying AF progression, summarize recent studies assessing the risk factors for AF progression, and discuss the clinical implications of the progressive nature of AF.

PATHOPHYSIOLOGY OF ATRIAL FIBRILLATION PROGRESSION

AF pathophysiology has been summarized in detail in recent reviews.[20–22] In brief, AF episodes are initiated by triggers acting on a vulnerable substrate. Ectopic (triggered) activity, often from the pulmonary veins, is an accepted trigger, with ambulatory monitoring revealing premature atrial complexes (PACs) initiating greater than 95% of paroxysmal AF episodes[23] and an increasing frequency of PACs in the 5 days preceding AF onset in pacemaker patients.[24] Ectopic (triggered) activity can produce reentry-initiating unidirectional block in a vulnerable substrate. The vulnerable substrate is characterized by the presence of short effective refractory periods and slow, heterogeneous conduction. The former is referred to as electrical remodeling, whereas the latter is caused by electrical remodeling (alterations in electrical cell-to-cell connections via gap-junctions) and structural remodeling (notably increased fibrosis). Atrial remodeling is promoted by a wide range of AF risk factors.[2] The degree of electrical and structural remodeling largely determines the likelihood of AF maintenance. Indeed, numerous studies have identified molecular, cellular, and tissue-level differences between patients with paroxysmal and persistent AF.[21] However, because these studies require invasive procedures, only cross-sectional data are available in patients, which are not necessarily suitable to determine the contribution of these differences to AF progression. Nonetheless, it is likely that AF progression is primarily caused by advances in atrial remodeling resulting from persistent effects of AF risk factors and AF-induced remodeling.

RISK FACTORS FOR ATRIAL FIBRILLATION PROGRESSION
Atrial Fibrillation Begets Atrial Fibrillation

The progressive increase in duration of individual AF episodes gave rise to the concept of "AF-begets-AF." Animal models with atrial tachypacing-induced remodeling or repeated pacing-induced AF have provided important insights into the underlying pathophysiologic mechanisms.[25–28] Atrial tachycardia produces rapid electrical remodeling that shortens effective refractory period, promoting AF maintenance within hours to days. In a sheep model of atrial tachypacing-induced, self-sustained AF, the rate of dominant frequency increase, reflecting changes in electrical properties, predicts the transition to persistent AF.[28] This model also shows that even in a well-controlled animal model AF progression is variable,[28] suggesting an individual susceptibility to AF progression that may partially explain the wide range of progression rates observed in clinical studies. These results have recently been translated to patients using atrial activation rates during AF detected using implantable devices.[29] This study confirms the existence of variable, patient-specific progression patterns that could not be predicted based on clinical parameters, but could be estimated based on the slope of atrial activation rate changes.[29]

Nonetheless, electrical remodeling is considered largely reversible[27] and absent in isolated right-atrial samples from patients with paroxysmal AF.[30] It is therefore unlikely to fully explain clinical AF progression when AF episodes are infrequent. Over the course of days to weeks, atrial tachycardia also promotes irreversible structural remodeling, contributing to AF progression.[27] In agreement, transgenic CREM-IbΔC-X mice, one of the few animal models with spontaneous AF development and progression, develop progressive structural remodeling.[31] In the sheep AF model, aldosterone inhibition mitigates structural remodeling and prolongs the transition to persistent AF in 26% of animals, but does not prevent AF-induced electrical remodeling or AF persistence.[32] Thus, AF itself is an important mechanistic driver of AF progression by promoting electrical and structural remodeling.

Clinical Risk Factors for Atrial Fibrillation Progression

Because AF progression strongly depends on progression of the atrial vulnerable substrate and many clinical comorbidities and risk factors promote atrial remodeling, it is not surprising that several clinical risk factors are independently associated with AF progression. Among these, several studies have identified advancing age as a risk factor for AF progression that is itself inherently progressive (see **Table 1**). Aging promotes atrial structural remodeling through multiple mechanisms.[33] Heart failure (HF) and biomarkers associated with HF (eg, brain natriuretic peptide) have also been associated with AF progression (see **Table 1**), whereby brain natriuretic peptide improves the prediction of AF progression compared with conventional risk estimates.[34,35] In animal models HF promotes progressive atrial electrical and structural remodeling with a time course of weeks, whereby structural remodeling seems critical for AF promotion.[36] HF is itself also often progressive and AF may promote HF,[37] creating additional positive feedforward loops that may further promote AF progression (HF begets AF and AF begets HF). Finally, obesity and chronic obstructive pulmonary disease are also independent predictors of AF progression (see **Table 1**)[38] and are known to promote atrial remodeling by promoting inflammation and oxidative stress. Other known and emerging AF risk factors have a more transient nature (eg, alcohol, exercise, and sleep disorder breathing), although these transient risk factors do produce atrial remodeling that accumulates over time, suggesting that they may contribute to AF progression.[39–41] However, they have so far not been identified as independent predictors in current studies, possibly because their dynamic nature makes them more difficult to study.

The commonly identified clinical risk factors have previously been summarized in the HATCH score (1x hypertension, 1x age>75 years, 2x previous transient ischemic attack/stroke, 1x chronic obstructive pulmonary disease, 2x HF) to estimate the probability of AF progression in patients with paroxysmal AF.[42] The CHA_2DS_2(-VASc) score for predicting stroke risk in patients with AF similarly incorporates many of these risk factors and has also been shown to predict AF progression risk.[7,15]

In addition to clinical risk factors, left atrial size,[6,7,11,12,43] electrocardiographic P-wave properties,[35] and initial burden or duration of AF episodes[15,17] are consistently associated with AF progression. Because dilation and electrical remodeling typically develop faster than fibrosis,[27,36] these parameters may be early markers of the strength of the atrial remodeling-promoting processes and/or the individual susceptibility to remodeling, thus explaining their association with AF progression. Moreover, the observation that yearly AF progression rates decline with longer follow-up periods[4] suggests that most of the relevant atrial remodeling occurs within the first year.

DISCUSSION AND CLINICAL RELEVANCE

It is widely accepted that more advanced forms of AF are harder to treat. Success rates of catheter ablation are significantly lower in persistent AF than in paroxysmal AF[44,45] and permanent AF represents an advanced, therapy-resistant form of AF. In addition, patients with more advanced forms of AF have a worse outcome.[46–48] AF progression itself is independently associated with worse outcomes in several studies.[6,9,17,42,43] This holds true for the progression in clinical AF types and for progression of AF burden. For example, in patients with young-onset AF (paroxysmal or persistent AF starting <60 years of age), progression to permanent AF was associated with a higher yearly rate of adverse cardiovascular events compared with patients without progression (4.9% [2.3%–9.0%] vs 1.9% [1.4%–2.6%]; $P = .006$).[6] Similarly, progression of subclinical AF (from >6 minutes but ≤24 hours to >24 hours) was independently associated with hospitalization for HF (hazard ratio, 3.68; 95% confidence interval, 1.27–10.70; $P = .016$).[17] Consistent with these unfavorable clinical outcomes, AF progression is also associated with a significantly reduced health-related quality of life.[7] Finally, progression of AF burden was accelerated in the weeks leading to death in 3131 patients age greater than or equal to 55 years implanted with dual-chamber pacemaker from the Merlin.net remote monitoring data,[49] suggesting that progression of AF burden may be used as a risk marker in patients with continuous rhythm monitoring. However, there was no strong correlation between AF progression and outcome in the large PREFER in AF cohort,[10] possibly caused by the limitations associated with assessing the progression of AF based on clinical AF types.

At present, the definition of AF progression and methodologies for determining AF burden are heterogeneous and a direct comparison between studies based on clinical AF types and AF burden may not be reliable. Technological advances, including smaller implantable monitors with larger storage and longer battery life and wearables, will facilitate quantitative assessment of AF progression and its risk factors in much larger cohorts. However, standardization of approaches may be needed to enable comparisons between studies. Moreover, detailed monitoring of AF progression will only become widespread if it has consequences for AF management.

Cardiovascular risk factors and comorbidities, particularly obesity, are key modifiable predictors of clinical AF progression (see **Table 1**).[5,8] Risk factor management, which has already been shown to improve sinus rhythm maintenance,[50,51] may therefore reduce the risk of AF progression and improve outcomes. However, because progression occurs primarily during the first year of follow-up,[4] early detection and early aggressive therapy may be required to successfully prevent AF progression. Such an approach is currently evaluated in several clinical trials.[52,53] Moreover, comparing the results from early rhythm control therapy with integrated risk factor management may help to establish whether AF progression is only a risk marker or a causal contributor to worse outcomes.

SUMMARY

AF progression is common but variable. It results primarily from atrial electrical and structural remodeling promoted by AF risk factors and AF itself. Accordingly, a wide range of clinical risk factors (eg, age, HF, chronic obstructive pulmonary disease, and obesity), and markers of the severity of an underlying atrial cardiomyopathy (left-atrial size, initial duration/burden of subclinical AF) are independent predictors of AF progression. Finally, AF progression is independently associated with worse clinical outcomes in many studies. Together, these data suggest a role for early detection and aggressive AF and risk factor management to reduce AF progression and improve outcomes in patients with AF.

CLINICS CARE POINTS

- Guidelines-based clinical characterisation of the atrial substrate substantiates risk of AF progression.
- Rhythm control and life style measures in early AF improves prognosis with prevention of AF progression.
- Definition of AF progression and methodologies for determining AF burden are heterogeneous precluding a direct comparison between studies.
- Benefits of early detection of AF and of atrial substrate progression in the prevention of AF progression as yet unproven.
- Detailed monitoring of AF progression will only become widespread if it has consequences for AF management.

ACKNOWLEDGMENTS

The authors acknowledge the support from the Netherlands Cardiovascular Research Initiative, an initiative with support of the Dutch Heart Foundation, CVON 2014 to 9: Reappraisal of Atrial Fibrillation: interaction between hypercoagulability, Electrical remodeling, and Vascular destabilization in the progression of AF (RACE V); and grant support from Medtronic to the institution.

DISCLOSURE

The authors have nothing to disclose.

REFERENCES

1. Chugh SS, Havmoeller R, Narayanan K, et al. Worldwide epidemiology of atrial fibrillation: a global burden of disease 2010 Study. Circulation 2014; 129(8):837–47.
2. Andrade J, Khairy P, Dobrev D, et al. The clinical profile and pathophysiology of atrial fibrillation: relationships among clinical features, epidemiology, and mechanisms. Circ Res 2014;114(9):1453–68.
3. Gallagher MM, Camm J. Classification of atrial fibrillation. Am J Cardiol 1998;82(8A):18N–28N.
4. Blum S, Meyre P, Aeschbacher S, et al. Incidence and predictors of atrial fibrillation progression: a systematic review and meta-analysis. Heart Rhythm 2019;16(4):502–10.
5. Blum S, Aeschbacher S, Meyre P, et al. Incidence and predictors of atrial fibrillation progression. J Am Heart Assoc 2019;8(20):e012554.
6. De With RR, Marcos EG, Van Gelder IC, et al. Atrial fibrillation progression and outcome in patients with young-onset atrial fibrillation. Europace 2018;20(11): 1750–7.
7. Dudink E, Erkuner O, Berg J, et al. The influence of progression of atrial fibrillation on quality of life: a report from the Euro Heart Survey. Europace 2018; 20(6):929–34.
8. Middeldorp ME, Pathak RK, Meredith M, et al. PREVEntion and regReSsive effect of weight-loss and risk factor modification on atrial fibrillation: the REVERSE-AF study. Europace 2018;20(12): 1929–35.
9. Ogawa H, An Y, Ikeda S, et al. Progression from paroxysmal to sustained atrial fibrillation is associated with increased adverse events. Stroke 2018; 49(10):2301–8.
10. Schnabel RB, Pecen L, Engler D, et al. Atrial fibrillation patterns are associated with arrhythmia progression and clinical outcomes. Heart 2018; 104(19):1608–14.
11. Uetake S, Maruyama M, Mitsuishi T, et al. Diastolic wall strain predicts progression from paroxysmal to persistent or permanent atrial fibrillation in structurally normal hearts. J Cardiol 2019;74(4):339–46.
12. Jurin I, Hadzibegovic I, Durlen I, et al. Left atrium size and red cell distribution width predict atrial

fibrillation progression from paroxysmal or persistent to permanent. Acta Clin Belg 2020;75(3):205–11.

13. Olivia C, Hastie C, Farshid A. Adherence to guidelines regarding anticoagulation and risk factors for progression of atrial fibrillation in a nurse-led clinic. Intern Med J 2020. https://doi.org/10.1111/imj.14874.

14. Charitos EI, Purerfellner H, Glotzer TV, et al. Clinical classifications of atrial fibrillation poorly reflect its temporal persistence: insights from 1,195 patients continuously monitored with implantable devices. J Am Coll Cardiol 2014;63(25 Pt A):2840–8.

15. Boriani G, Glotzer TV, Ziegler PD, et al. Detection of new atrial fibrillation in patients with cardiac implanted electronic devices and factors associated with transition to higher device-detected atrial fibrillation burden. Heart Rhythm 2018;15(3):376–83.

16. Diederichsen SZ, Haugan KJ, Brandes A, et al. Natural history of subclinical atrial fibrillation detected by implanted loop recorders. J Am Coll Cardiol 2019;74(22):2771–81.

17. Wong JA, Conen D, Van Gelder IC, et al. Progression of device-detected subclinical atrial fibrillation and the risk of heart failure. J Am Coll Cardiol 2018;71(23):2603–11.

18. De With RR, Erkuner O, Rienstra M, et al. Temporal patterns and short-term progression of paroxysmal atrial fibrillation: data from RACE V. Europace 2020;22(8):1162–72.

19. Ruperti Repilado FJ, Doerig L, Blum S, et al. Prevalence and predictors of atrial fibrillation type among individuals with recent onset of atrial fibrillation. Swiss Med Wkly 2018;148:w14652.

20. Schotten U, Verheule S, Kirchhof P, et al. Pathophysiological mechanisms of atrial fibrillation: a translational appraisal. Physiol Rev 2011;91(1):265–325.

21. Heijman J, Voigt N, Nattel S, et al. Cellular and molecular electrophysiology of atrial fibrillation initiation, maintenance, and progression. Circ Res 2014; 114(9):1483–99.

22. Nattel S, Heijman J, Zhou L, et al. Molecular basis of atrial fibrillation pathophysiology and therapy; a translational perspective. Circ Res 2020;127(1): 51–72.

23. Vincenti A, Brambilla R, Fumagalli MG, et al. Onset mechanism of paroxysmal atrial fibrillation detected by ambulatory Holter monitoring. Europace 2006; 8(3):204–10.

24. Boriani G, Botto GL, Pieragnoli P, et al. Temporal patterns of premature atrial complexes predict atrial fibrillation occurrence in bradycardia patients continuously monitored through pacemaker diagnostics. Intern Emerg Med 2020;15(4):599–606.

25. Wijffels MC, Kirchhof CJ, Dorland R, et al. Atrial fibrillation begets atrial fibrillation. A study in awake chronically instrumented goats. Circulation 1995; 92(7):1954–68.

26. Yue L, Feng J, Gaspo R, et al. Ionic remodeling underlying action potential changes in a canine model of atrial fibrillation. Circ Res 1997;81(4):512–25.

27. Allessie M, Ausma J, Schotten U. Electrical, contractile and structural remodeling during atrial fibrillation. Cardiovasc Res 2002;54(2):230–46.

28. Martins RP, Kaur K, Hwang E, et al. Dominant frequency increase rate predicts transition from paroxysmal to long-term persistent atrial fibrillation. Circulation 2014;129(14):1472–82.

29. Lillo-Castellano JM, Gonzalez-Ferrer JJ, Marina-Breysse M, et al. Personalized monitoring of electrical remodelling during atrial fibrillation progression via remote transmissions from implantable devices. Europace 2020;22(5):704–15.

30. Voigt N, Heijman J, Wang Q, et al. Cellular and molecular mechanisms of atrial arrhythmogenesis in patients with paroxysmal atrial fibrillation. Circulation 2014;129(2):145–56.

31. Li N, Chiang DY, Wang S, et al. Ryanodine receptor-mediated calcium leak drives progressive development of an atrial fibrillation substrate in a transgenic mouse model. Circulation 2014;129(12):1276–85.

32. Takemoto Y, Ramirez RJ, Kaur K, et al. Eplerenone reduces atrial fibrillation burden without preventing atrial electrical remodeling. J Am Coll Cardiol 2017;70(23):2893–905.

33. Laredo M, Waldmann V, Khairy P, et al. Age as a critical determinant of atrial fibrillation: a two-sided relationship. Can J Cardiol 2018;34(11):1396–406.

34. Inohara T, Kim S, Pieper K, et al. B-type natriuretic peptide, disease progression and clinical outcomes in atrial fibrillation. Heart 2019;105(5):370–7.

35. Akutsu Y, Kaneko K, Kodama Y, et al. A combination of P wave electrocardiography and plasma brain natriuretic peptide level for predicting the progression to persistent atrial fibrillation: comparisons of sympathetic activity and left atrial size. J Interv Card Electrophysiol 2013;38(2):79–84.

36. Shinagawa K, Shi YF, Tardif JC, et al. Dynamic nature of atrial fibrillation substrate during development and reversal of heart failure in dogs. Circulation 2002;105(22):2672–8.

37. Sugumar H, Nanayakkara S, Prabhu S, et al. Pathophysiology of atrial fibrillation and heart failure: dangerous interactions. Cardiol Clin 2019;37(2): 131–8.

38. Chen X, Lin M, Wang W. The progression in atrial fibrillation patients with COPD: a systematic review and meta-analysis. Oncotarget 2017;8(60): 102420–7.

39. Linz D, Baumert M, Desteghe L, et al. Nightly sleep apnea severity in patients with atrial fibrillation: potential applications of long-term sleep apnea monitoring. Int J Cardiol Heart Vasc 2019;24:100424.

40. Guasch E, Benito B, Qi X, et al. Atrial fibrillation promotion by endurance exercise: demonstration and

mechanistic exploration in an animal model. J Am Coll Cardiol 2013;62(1):68–77.

41. Voskoboinik A, Prabhu S, Ling LH, et al. Alcohol and atrial fibrillation: a sobering review. J Am Coll Cardiol 2016;68(23):2567–76.

42. de Vos CB, Pisters R, Nieuwlaat R, et al. Progression from paroxysmal to persistent atrial fibrillation clinical correlates and prognosis. J Am Coll Cardiol 2010;55(8):725–31.

43. De With RR, Marcos EG, Dudink E, et al. Atrial fibrillation progression risk factors and associated cardiovascular outcome in well-phenotyped patients: data from the AF-RISK study. Europace 2020; 22(3):352–60.

44. Piccini JP, Lopes RD, Kong MH, et al. Pulmonary vein isolation for the maintenance of sinus rhythm in patients with atrial fibrillation: a meta-analysis of randomized, controlled trials. Circ Arrhythm Electrophysiol 2009;2(6):626–33.

45. Clarnette JA, Brooks AG, Mahajan R, et al. Outcomes of persistent and long-standing persistent atrial fibrillation ablation: a systematic review and meta-analysis. Europace 2018;20(FI_3):f366–76.

46. Steinberg BA, Hellkamp AS, Lokhnygina Y, et al. Higher risk of death and stroke in patients with persistent vs. paroxysmal atrial fibrillation: results from the ROCKET-AF Trial. Eur Heart J 2015;36(5): 288–96.

47. Vanassche T, Lauw MN, Eikelboom JW, et al. Risk of ischaemic stroke according to pattern of atrial fibrillation: analysis of 6563 aspirin-treated patients in ACTIVE-A and AVERROES. Eur Heart J 2015;36(5): 281–287a.

48. An Y, Ogawa H, Esato M, et al. Age-dependent prognostic impact of paroxysmal versus sustained atrial fibrillation on the incidence of cardiac death and heart failure hospitalization (the Fushimi AF Registry). Am J Cardiol 2019;124(9):1420–9.

49. Piccini JP, Passman R, Turakhia M, et al. Atrial fibrillation burden, progression, and the risk of death: a case-crossover analysis in patients with cardiac implantable electronic devices. Europace 2019; 21(3):404–13.

50. Rienstra M, Hobbelt AH, Alings M, et al. Targeted therapy of underlying conditions improves sinus rhythm maintenance in patients with persistent atrial fibrillation: results of the RACE 3 trial. Eur Heart J 2018;39(32):2987–96.

51. Lau DH, Nattel S, Kalman JM, et al. Modifiable risk factors and atrial fibrillation. Circulation 2017; 136(6):583–96.

52. Nattel S, Guasch E, Savelieva I, et al. Early management of atrial fibrillation to prevent cardiovascular complications. Eur Heart J 2014;35(22):1448–56.

53. Brandes A, Smit MD, Nguyen BO, et al. Risk factor management in atrial fibrillation. Arrhythm Electrophysiol Rev 2018;7(2):118–27.

54. Marcos EG, De With RR, Mulder BA, et al. Young-onset atrial fibrillation: sex differences in clinical profile, progression rate and cardiovascular outcome. Int J Cardiol Heart Vasc 2019;25:100429.

55. Krisai P, Aeschbacher S, Bossard M, et al. Change in atrial fibrillation burden over time in patients with nonpermanent atrial fibrillation. Cardiol Res Pract 2020;2020:9583409.

Diagnostic Tests

Electrocardiographic and Echocardiographic Abnormalities in Patients with Risk Factors for Atrial Fibrillation

Andrés Ricardo Pérez-Riera, MD, PhD[a], Raimundo Barbosa-Barros, MD[b], Luciano Evaristo Pereira-Rejálaga, MD[c], Kjell Nikus, MD, PhD[d], Mohammad Shenasa, MD[e],*

KEYWORDS

- Atrial fibrillation • 12-lead electrocardiogram • Echocardiogram • Risk factors

KEY POINTS

- The electrocardiogram and various echocardiography modalities are important risk markers for atrial fibrillation (AF).
- Electrocardiographic criteria of left atrial enlargement, advanced interatrial block, and PR-interval prolongation are atrial risk markers for AF.
- Transthoracic echocardiography is elementary for risk stratification of AF.
- Transesophageal echocardiography is a valuable tool to detect cardiac sources of embolism if early cardioversion is necessary.
- Intracardiac echocardiography is a real-time tool for guidance of percutaneous interventions, including radiofrequency ablation and left atrial appendage closure in patients with AF.

INTRODUCTION

Atrial fibrillation (AF) is the most commonly sustained irregular cardiac arrhythmia. The prevalence of AF is 0.12% to 0.16% in less than 49-year-old, 3.7% to 4.2% in those between 60 and 70 years, and 10% to 17% of ≥80-year-old individuals. Male-to-female ratio is 1.2:1. The incidence of AF ranges between 0.21 and 0.41 per 1000 person-years. AF is permanent in ≈50% of patients, whereas the prevalence is 25% in both paroxysmal and persistent AF. AF may present without comorbidities, or it may be associated with hypertension, hyperthyroidism, coronary or valvular heart disease, cardiomyopathies, heart failure, obesity, obstructive sleep apnea, and so forth.[1] AF is associated with a two- to threefold increased risk of cardiovascular mortality and sudden cardiac death,[2] a fivefold increased risk of stroke,[3] and a threefold increased risk of heart failure.[4]

ELECTROCARDIOGRAPHIC MARKERS FOR ATRIAL FIBRILLATION
Prolonged P-Wave Duration

Prolonged P-wave duration (PWD) is an electrocardiogram (ECG) risk factor marker for AF that

[a] Centro Universitário Saúde ABC, Laboratório de Metodologia de Pesquisa e Escrita Científica, Santo André, São Paulo, Brazil; [b] Coronary Center of the Hospital de Messejana Fortaleza, Ceará, Brazil; [c] Sanatorio Medicordis; [d] Heart Center, Tampere University Hospital and Faculty of Medicine and Health Technology, Tampere University, Finland; [e] Department of Cardiovascular Services, Heart and Rhythm Medical Group, 18324 Twin Creeks Road, Monte Sereno, CA 95030, USA
* Corresponding author.
E-mail address: mohammad.shenasa@gmail.com

Card Electrophysiol Clin 13 (2021) 211–219
https://doi.org/10.1016/j.ccep.2020.10.002

reflects atrial dromotropic disturbance. It is defined by manual annotation of the earliest onset and latest offset of the P wave in the 12-lead ECG. Prolonged PWD is indicative of underlying atrial disease with hemodynamic changes leading to elevated intraatrial pressure, atrial wall stress, atrial fibrosis, and abnormal electrical coupling between atrial cardiomyocytes through gap junctions Cx40 and Cx43,[5] causing dromotropic disturbance.[6] The vulnerability to arrhythmias is determined by the combined presence of an arrhythmogenic substrate and initiating triggers, which most frequently originate from firing foci in the pulmonary veins and/or superior vena cava. Triggers for AF include sleep deprivation, physical illness, strong emotions, recent surgery, premature menopause, exhaustive exercise, nasal decongestants, cocaine, recreational drug and alcohol, excess caffeine intake, low carbohydrate diets, caffeinated drinks, and dehydration, and so forth.

Congenital short QT syndrome (SQTS) is a genetic example of a very short, effective refractory period with high AF tendency (**Fig. 1**).

Left Atrial Enlargement

Electrocardiographic criteria for left atrial enlargement (LAE) are as follows: duration of the negative (terminal) portion of the P wave in lead V_1 >40 milliseconds, depth of the negative (terminal) portion of the P wave in lead V_1 ≥1 mm, total PWD in lead II >110 milliseconds, and bimodal P wave in lead II with interpeak notch duration greater than 40 milliseconds (**Fig. 2**).

Macruz and colleagues[8] proposed a simple formula for electrocardiographic recognition of right, left, and biatrial atrial enlargement. It is based on the measurement of the PR interval, PWD, and PR segment. According to these investigators, the normal ratio of the PWD to the PR segment (PWD/PRs) as measured in standard lead II is between 1.0 and 1.6, with an average value of 1.2. In cases of right atrial enlargement, there is no significant prolongation of the PWD, but the PR interval increases, and therefore, the PR segment ratio falls below the normal range. LAE, on the other hand, does not affect the PR interval, but the P-wave lengthens at the expense of the PR segment. The result is a ratio above the normal upper limit of 1.6. In biatrial enlargement, both the PR

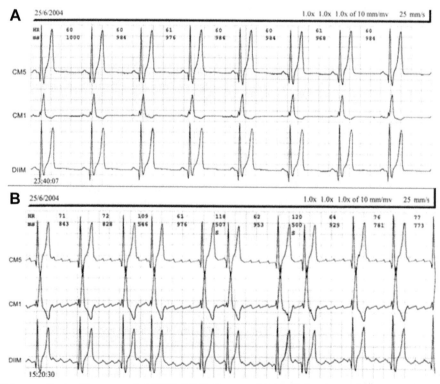

Fig. 1. ECG in a patient with congenital SQTS. (*A*) Holter monitoring strip: sinus rhythm, tall/peaked, narrow-based T waves and very short QT interval. (*B*) Eight hours later, the patient had a transient paroxysmal AF.

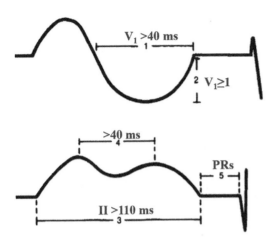

Fig. 2. ECG criteria for LAE: duration of negative portion of P wave in lead V1 >40 milliseconds (*1*); depth of negative portion of P wave in lead V1 ≥1 mm; P-terminal force (1 × 2) ≥, negative P-terminal force in lead V1 ≥0.04 mm/s (Morris index)[7]; total PWD in lead II (*3*) greater than 110 milliseconds; bimodal P wave in lead II with interpeak notch duration (*4*) >40 milliseconds; and total PWD (*3*): PRs = PR segment (*5*).

interval and the P-wave are prolonged, and the PWD to PR segment ratio is normal.

The Concept of Interatrial Block and Its Association with Atrial Fibrillation

Interatrial block (IAB) is a conduction delay between the right atrium (RA) and left atrium (LA)

with higher prevalence in the elderly and in patients with structural heart disease (**Fig. 3**).

Prolonged PR Interval

The PR interval is measured from the beginning of the P-wave to the beginning of the QRS complex, and it reflects the time it takes for the electrical impulse to travel from the sinus node through the atrioventricular (AV) node to the ventricles (**Fig. 4**).

PR-INTERVAL COMPONENTS
Association Between PR-Interval Prolongation and the Risk of Atrial Fibrillation

PR-interval prolongation is associated with an increased risk for AF (see **Fig. 4**). Schumacher and colleagues[10] studied the association between PR-interval prolongation and LA remodeling measured as low-voltage areas during catheter ablation of AF. Besides persistent AF and LA size, PR-interval prolongation might be useful for the prediction of electroanatomical substrate in AF patients.

The Framingham Heart Study (FHS) and the Atherosclerosis Risk in Communities (ARIC) Study investigated the association between PR-interval prolongation and the risk of AF.[11,12] In the FHS, the risk of AF was found to be significantly higher in subjects with a PR interval greater than 200 milliseconds compared with subjects without first-degree AV block. In addition, each 1 standard deviation (20 milliseconds) increment in PR-interval duration was associated with a hazard ratio of

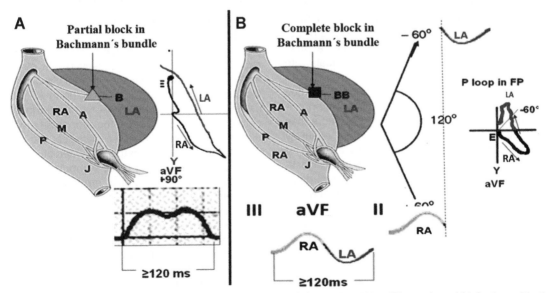

Fig. 3. (*A*) Partial IAB:PWD ≥120 milliseconds. (*B*) Advanced IAB:PWD ≥120 milliseconds and biphasic positive/negative P wave in the inferior leads. LA activation occurs retrogradely (caudocephalic). FP, frontal plane.

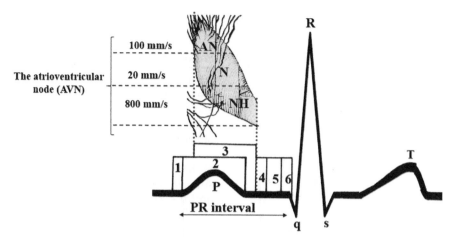

Fig. 4. (*1*) Sinoatrial (SA) node[9]; (*2*) atria; (*3*) AV node; (*4*) His bundle branch; (*5*) Right and left bundle branch and their fascicles; (*6*) Purkinje fibers. AN, atrionodal portion of AV node; N, nodal portion of AV node; NH, Nodo-Hissian portion of the AV node.

1.11 (95%confidence interval: 1.02–1.22; *P* = .02) for AF.[11]

As in the FHS, PR-interval duration was examined as both a continuous linear and a categorical variable (first-degree AV block vs no AV block) in the ARIC study. The former was significantly associated with a risk of incident AF, while the latter did not reach statistical significance. In both the FHS and the ARIC study, the reported associations were adjusted for several potential confounders, including age, gender, hypertension, body mass index, diabetes, and smoking status.

The Health ABC study demonstrated a linear increase in the risk of AF with longer PR intervals.[13]

In a Finnish cohort study comprising more than 10,000 individuals and 30 years of follow-up, there was not even a trend toward an increased risk of AF for individuals with PR interval greater than 200 milliseconds compared with individuals with a normal PR interval.[14]

In the Copenhagen ECG study, almost 300,000 individuals were followed for a median of approximately 6 years, and during this period, more than 11,000 subjects developed AF. The relatively strong statistical power in this study allowed for a more flexible and nonlinear approach for investigating the association between PR-interval duration and AF. It was found that both women with a short PR interval and women with a long PR interval have an increased risk of AF compared with the reference group (a PR interval of 148–157 milliseconds). Regarding men, a long PR interval was statistically significantly associated with an increased risk of AF, whereas the association between shorter PR intervals and AF did not reach statistical significance.[15] Results from the Cohorts for

Heart and Aging Research in Genomic Epidemiology-AF Consortium (which included data from the ARIC, Cardiovascular Health Study [CHS], and FHS cohorts) are in line with the results from the Copenhagen ECG Study and point to an increased risk of AF for short PR intervals. In this study, PR intervals less than 120 milliseconds conferred an increased risk of AF compared with PR intervals in the range 120 to 199 milliseconds. The investigators did not find a statistically significant association for PR intervals greater than 199 milliseconds.[16]

Risk Prediction of Atrial Fibrillation

In a clinical setting, an AF risk score can serve as a tool in determining an individual's risk of developing AF. AF risk models have been developed and validated.[16] In the FHS-derived risk model for AF, the predictive value of several clinical risk factors for the assessment of long-term AF was investigated. Known risk factors for AF were incorporated into the risk score if they improved model discrimination (estimated by c-statistics) and calibration (χ^2 test) in a setting of internal cross-validation. As a result of these computations, the PR interval was incorporated into the risk model in the way that 0 points were given for a PR interval less than 160 milliseconds, 1 point for 160 to 199 milliseconds, and 2 points for a PR interval $\geq$200 milliseconds. Later, the FHS-derived risk algorithm was externally validated in 2 independent cohorts: the Age, Gene/Environment Susceptibility-Reykjavik Study (AGES), and the CHS cohorts with a subdivision of the CHS cohort based on ethnicity (CHS whites; CHS African

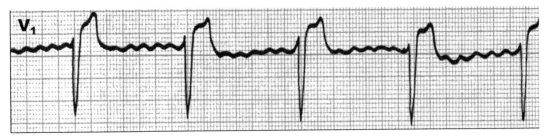

Fig. 5. Coarse "f" waves, regular QRS complexes, and very low HR in complete AV block.

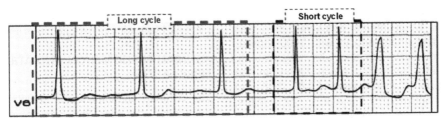

Fig. 6. A long strip of V6 of a patient in AF. Aberration occurs when a short cycle follows a long one. The 2 last QRS complexes are aberrant with a left bundle branch block pattern: Gouaux-Ashman or Ashman phenomenon.

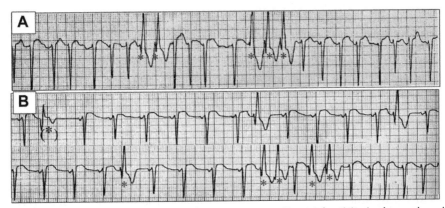

Fig. 7. (*A*) The rhythm is AF with a high ventricular response rate. No atrial activity is observed, and QRS complexes are of irregular presentation with marked variation in timely occurrence. The QRS complexes indicated by asterisks show triphasic rsR′ pattern of the right bundle branch block (RBBB) type, the first r deflection has the same direction as that of the predominant beats, and there is no compensatory pause. These 3 elements confirm the presence of aberrant conduction. (*B*) The same tracing in sinus rhythm. The second beat (*asterisk*) is a premature ventricular contraction (PVC) because the first deflection (Q) presents an opposite direction compared with the prevailing complexes (r) and because there is complete compensatory pause. In addition, repolarization reveals an "injury current" and transmural ischemia with ST elevation. The beats indicated by red asterisks are supraventricular extrasystoles with aberrant conduction, because they have a triphasic RBBB pattern of variable width.

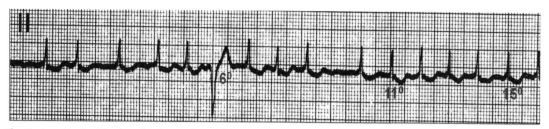

Fig. 8. A patient with chronic obstructive pulmonary disease and regular digoxin medication. There is AF. The sixth beat is a PVC. Beats 11 to 15 have regular RR intervals, which in the presence of AF suggests digitalis intoxication.

Americans). Although the FHS-derived AF risk score was still of value in risk prediction of AF, the score had a considerably lower discriminative value in the external validation cohorts compared with the FHS derivation cohort. Whereas the c-statistic decreased from 0.78 to 0.76 in the original FHS cohort when internal cross-validation was applied (using bootstrapping with 1000 replications of individuals sampled with replacement), the c-statistic decreased much further in the external cohorts, where values of 0.67, 0.68, and 0.66 were obtained in the AGES, CHS whites, and CHS African Americans cohorts, respectively.[17] A statistically significant association between a linear increase in PR-interval and the risk of incident AF was found in the AGES, CHS whites, and FHS cohorts. However, the association did not reach statistical significance in the CHS African American cohort.

Another AF risk score was developed based on the ARIC study cohort. Selection of prediction variables was based on Cox regression and the use of backward stepwise elimination, whereby variables were eliminated in case of an association less than $P<.10$. As a result of this, the PR interval was not included in the final risk model. C-statistics for the final model was 0.76 when internal validation was not applied and 0.77 when interval validation was applied. In the same study, the investigators tested the FHS-derived risk score and found a c-statistic of 0.68, which is in accordance with previous external validations of the FHS-derived AF risk score.[18]

ELECTROCARDIOGRAPHIC CHARACTERIZATION OF ATRIAL FIBRILLATION

Absence of the P wave, presence of small waves of high frequency (between 350 and 700 bpm) with irregular voltage, variable morphology, and duration, called "f" waves. The complete variability in shape and timing of the atrial complexes rules out flutter. Sometimes f waves are clearly discernible, but

they may be completely absent, at least temporarily. F waves are best identified in leads V_1 or V_1 and V_2 because these leads are close to the atria and because the direction of the waves usually heads to the front and the right. The ventricular rhythm in AF is irregular except when associated with complete AV block without capture beats (**Fig. 5**).

ASHMAN PHENOMENON AND ATRIAL FIBRILLATION

The Ashman phenomenon is an intraventricular conduction disorder that occurs in the His-Purkinje system, caused by a change in heart rate (HR). It is dependent on the effects of HR on the electrophysiological properties of the heart and may be modulated by metabolic, electrolytic, and drug-induced alterations, which alter the duration of the refractory period of the ventricular branches of the conduction system.[19] The Ashman phenomenon is commonly observed in AF, atrial tachycardia, and premature atrial contractions. Aberrant conduction occurs when a short cycle follows a long one (**Fig. 6**).

Fig. 7 illustrates the phenomenon of *aberrant conduction and extrasystoles during AF with high ventricular rate*.

Fig. 8 illustrates ECG aspects of *AF in digitalis intoxication*.

Fig. 9 shows *AF in the context of preexcitation*.

ECHOCARDIOGRAPHIC ABNORMALITIES IN PATIENTS WITH ATRIAL FIBRILLATION
Transthoracic Echocardiography

Transthoracic echocardiography (TTE), including 2-dimensional imaging and Doppler assessment of the valves, is recommended for all subjects with AF.[20] TTE allows measurement of LA dimensions and volumes, left ventricular (LV) dimensions and volumes, LV ejection fraction, LV diastolic function, and valvular function. Harmonic imaging, alone or with microbubble contrast agents, allows enhanced endocardial border definition for assessment of LV volumes and function. Color M

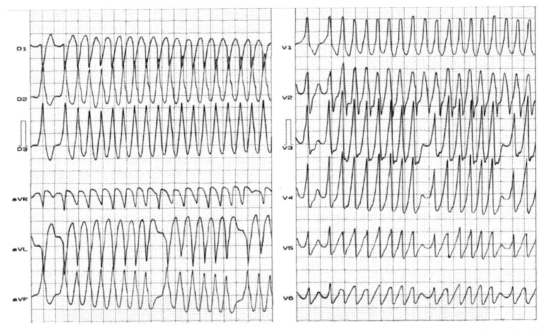

Fig. 9. AF in preexcitation due to an accessory pathway with short refractory period: irregular RR intervals, QRS width with variable duration, and fast ventricular rate ($\approx$300 bpm).

mode and tissue Doppler imaging allow more accurate assessment of the diastolic function and for the estimation of filling pressures. Assessment of systolic and diastolic LV function in AF may be challenging because of irregular RR interval and fast ventricular rate. TTE provides suboptimal visualization of the atrial appendages and has inadequate sensitivity and specificity for diagnosing LAA thrombus[21] (**Fig. 10**).

Transesophageal Echocardiography

Transesophageal echocardiography (TEE) allows for high-resolution exploration of the posterior cardiac structures, including the atria, atrial septum, pulmonary veins, and the atrial appendages for thrombus detection. Also, alternative thromboembolic sources can be identified, including complex atheromas of the aorta. In AF, TEE is performed in patients at high risk of thromboembolism, those being considered for early cardioversion, or those with a secondary indication such as valvular disease.[20] Structures evaluated with TEE include LA and left atrial appendage (LAA): structure, function, spontaneous echo contrast and thrombus, RA, and right atrial appendage structure, function and thrombus, pulmonary vein anatomy/flow, atrial septum (patent foramen ovale, and so forth),

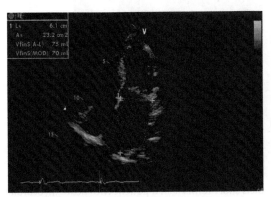

Fig. 10. Mitral stenosis. Volume measurement of LA by Simpson method.

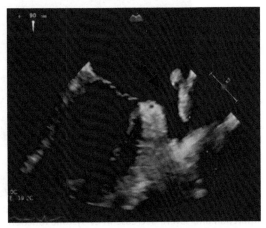

Fig. 11. TEE to 90°. LAA free of thrombi (arrow).

ascending aorta and arch atheroma, valvular function (**Fig. 11**).

Intracardiac Echocardiography

Intracardiac echocardiography (ICE) is performed with a transducer placed in the RA via a 6 to 10F sheath in the femoral vein. Modified from intravascular ultrasound probes, these steerable monoplane transducers produce ultrasound waves mechanically or via phased array. The latter offer the same modalities as TEE, including color, pulsed wave, and continuous-wave Doppler, to allow assessment of intracardiac flow in addition to 2-dimensional visualization of structures.

ICE can play a key role in the guidance of cardiac interventions and is used for radiofrequency ablation procedures,[22] for percutaneous closure of patent foramen ovale, or for atrial septal defects. Structures evaluated include LA/LAA structure and function, LA/LAA thrombus, atrial septum, and pulmonary vein anatomy and flow.

Speckle Tracking Bidimensional Echocardiography

Through longitudinal atrial strain, reservoir, conduction, and pump functions can be measured, which are inversely correlated with the degree of fibrosis estimated by late gadolinium enhancement. A low strain value guides us toward a fibrous atria, not included and with decreased contractile capacity (**Fig. 12**). However, in the latest guidelines by the American Society of Echocardiography and

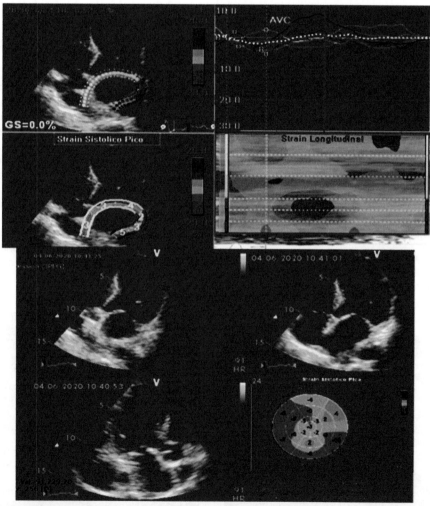

Fig. 12. (*A*) Strain of LA. Severe contractile deficit that predicts short-term AF in a patient with acute myocardial infarction and severe decrease in LV systolic function. (*B*) Longitudinal global strain of left ventricle in the same patient. Ejection fraction by Simpson: 28%. AVC, aortic valve closure; GS, global longitudinal strain.

the European Association of Cardiovascular Imaging for diastolic evaluation and the quantification of chamber function and size, the estimation of atrial strain has not been included (see **Fig. 12**).

DISCLOSURE

The authors have nothing to disclose.

CLINICS CARE POINTS

- Biphasic P-wave (+/-) in the inferior leads is a risk marker for future atrial fibrillation.
- Prolonged HV interval is an indicative of poor prognosis in cases of first degree atrioventricular block.
- On the other hand, PR interval <120 ms is also a risk marker of atrial fibrillation.

REFERENCES

1. Zoni-Berisso M, Lercari F, Carazza T, et al. Epidemiology of atrial fibrillation: European perspective. Clin Epidemiol 2014;6:213–20.
2. Chen LY, Sotoodehnia N, Buzkova P, et al. Atrial fibrillation and the risk of sudden cardiac death: the atherosclerosis risk in communities study and cardiovascular health study. JAMA Intern Med 2013;173:29–35.
3. Kannel WB, Wolf PA, Benjamin EJ, et al. Prevalence, incidence, prognosis, and predisposing conditions for atrial fibrillation: population-based estimates. Am J Cardiol 1998;82:2N–9N.
4. Wang TJ, Larson MG, Levy D, et al. Temporal relations of atrial fibrillation and congestive heart failure and their joint influence on mortality: the Framingham Heart Study. Circulation 2003;107:2920–5.
5. van Veen AA, van Rijen HV, Opthof T. Cardiac gap junction channels: modulation of expression and channel properties. Cardiovasc Res 2001;51:217–29.
6. van der Velden HM, Jongsma HJ. Cardiac gap junctions and connexins: their role in atrial fibrillation and potential as therapeutic targets. Cardiovasc Res 2002;54:270–9.
7. Morris JJ Jr, Estes EH Jr, Whalen RE, et al. P-wave analysis in valvular heart disease. Circulation 1964;29:242–52.
8. Macruz R, Perloff JK, Case RB. A method for the electrocardiographic recognition of atrial enlargement. Circulation 1958;17:882–9.
9. de CA, de AD. Spread of activity through the atrioventricular node. Circ Res 1960;8:801–9.
10. Schumacher K, Buttner P, Dagres N, et al. Association between PR interval prolongation and electro-anatomical substrate in patients with atrial fibrillation. PLoS One 2018;13:e0206933.
11. Cheng S, Keyes MJ, Larson MG, et al. Long-term outcomes in individuals with prolonged PR interval or first-degree atrioventricular block. JAMA 2009;301:2571–7.
12. Soliman EZ, Prineas RJ, Case LD, et al. Ethnic distribution of ECG predictors of atrial fibrillation and its impact on understanding the ethnic distribution of ischemic stroke in the Atherosclerosis Risk in Communities (ARIC) study. Stroke 2009;40:1204–11.
13. Magnani JW, Wang N, Nelson KP, et al. Electrocardiographic PR interval and adverse outcomes in older adults: the Health, Aging, and Body Composition Study. Circ Arrhythm Electrophysiol 2013;6:84–90.
14. Aro AL, Anttonen O, Kerola T, et al. Prognostic significance of prolonged PR interval in the general population. Eur Heart J 2014;35:123–9.
15. Nielsen JB, Pietersen A, Graff C, et al. Risk of atrial fibrillation as a function of the electrocardiographic PR interval: results from the Copenhagen ECG Study. Heart Rhythm 2013;10:1249–56.
16. Alonso A, Krijthe BP, Aspelund T, et al. Simple risk model predicts incidence of atrial fibrillation in a racially and geographically diverse population: the CHARGE-AF consortium. J Am Heart Assoc 2013;2:e000102.
17. Schnabel RB, Aspelund T, Li G, et al. Validation of an atrial fibrillation risk algorithm in whites and African Americans. Arch Intern Med 2010;170:1909–17.
18. Chamberlain AM, Agarwal SK, Folsom AR, et al. A clinical risk score for atrial fibrillation in a biracial prospective cohort (from the Atherosclerosis Risk in Communities [ARIC] study). Am J Cardiol 2011;107:85–91.
19. Gouaux JL, Ashman R. Auricular fibrillation with aberration simulating ventricular paroxysmal tachycardia. Am Heart J 1947;34:366–73.
20. January CT, Samuel Wann L, Calkins H, et al. 2019 AHA/ACC/HRS focused update of the 2014 AHA/ACC/HRS guideline for the management of patients with atrial fibrillation: a report of the American College of Cardiology/American Heart Association Task Force on Clinical Practice Guidelines and the Heart Rhythm Society in Collaboration with the Society of Thoracic Surgeons. Circulation 2019;140:e125–51.
21. Omran H, Jung W, Rabahieh R, et al. Imaging of thrombi and assessment of left atrial appendage function: a prospective study comparing transthoracic and transoesophageal echocardiography. Heart 1999;81:192–8.
22. Cooper JM, Epstein LM. Use of intracardiac echocardiography to guide ablation of atrial fibrillation. Circulation 2001;104:3010–3.

Biomarkers in Atrial Fibrillation
Pathogenesis and Clinical Implications

Jean Jacques Noubiap, MD, MMed[a], Prashanthan Sanders, MBBS, PhD[a,b], Stanley Nattel, MD[c], Dennis H. Lau, MBBS, PhD[a,b,*]

KEYWORDS

• Atrial fibrillation • Biomarkers • Stroke • Troponin • BNP • Inflammation • Oxidative stress
• Atrial fibrosis

KEY POINTS

• Biomarkers can be derived from mechanistic pathways underlying structural and electrical atrial re-modeling, atrial dysfunction, and procoagulant state in atrial fibrillation (AF).
• Such biomarkers have the potential to improve early identification of AF phenotype and to aid in clinical risk stratification in patients with AF.
• Natriuretic peptides, cardiac troponins, and growth differentiation factor-15 have been included in novel biomarker–based risk scores to predict adverse outcomes in patients with AF.
• Biomarkers may also have a role in predicting outcomes of rhythm-control therapies and may help in the development of new therapeutics.

INTRODUCTION

Atrial fibrillation (AF) is the most common sustained arrhythmia. Individuals with AF have a 5-fold increased risk of stroke, 3-fold increased risk of heart failure, and almost 2-fold increased risk of overall mortality.[1,2] Although the exact mechanisms underlying AF are not fully understood, significant advances have been made in elucidating its pathogenesis. The milieu leading to AF in each individual is often driven by risk factors that induce pathophysiologic mechanisms such as inflammation, oxidative stress, cardiomyocyte damage, atrial fibrosis, and thrombogenesis. The effects of these risk factors are modulated by the background influence of aging and underlying genetic predisposition. Various molecules involved in these mechanisms have the potential to indicate the risk of AF occurrence, progression, and complications, including thromboembolism and death. This article summarizes data on the association between key biomarkers (**Fig. 1**, **Table 1**) and incident AF, as well as adverse clinical events in patients with AF, and highlights the potential implications of these biomarkers in clinical practice.

Inflammation

A large number of studies have suggested a pivotal role of inflammation in the development and perpetuation of AF. Inflammation is directly involved in several pathologic processes underlying the atrial substrate for AF, including oxidative stress, myocyte injury, and fibrosis. Inflammation seems to have prognostic implications in patients with AF, because it has been linked to mortality and adverse cerebrovascular and coronary events. The link between inflammation and AF is detailed in Masahide Harada and Stanley Nattel's article, "Implications of Inflammation and Fibrosis

a Centre for Heart Rhythm Disorders, University of Adelaide, Adelaide, Australia; b Department of Cardiology, Royal Adelaide Hospital, Adelaide, Australia; c Department of Medicine, Montreal Heart Institute and Université de Montréal, Montréal, Canada
* Corresponding author. Department of Cardiology, Royal Adelaide Hospital, Centre for Heart Rhythm Disorders, Port Road, Adelaide South Australia 5000, Australia.
E-mail address: dennis.h.lau@adelaide.edu.au

Card Electrophysiol Clin 13 (2021) 221–233
https://doi.org/10.1016/j.ccep.2020.10.006
1877-9182/21/© 2020 Elsevier Inc. All rights reserved.

cardiacEP.theclinics.com

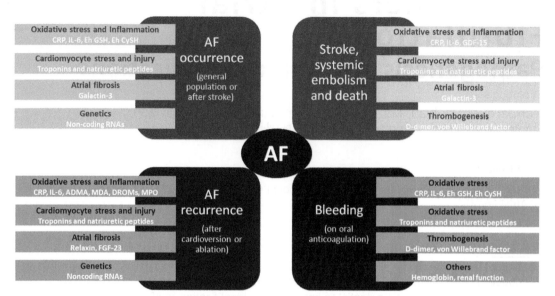

Fig. 1. Summary of biomarkers according to mechanistic pathways and clinical utility. ADMA, asymmetric dimethylarginine; CRP, C-reactive protein; DROMs, derivatives of reactive oxidative metabolites; Eh CySH, reduced cysteine; Eh GSH, reduced glutathione, FGF-23, fibroblast growth factor 23; GDF-15, growth differentiation factor 15; IL-6, interleukin 6; MDA, malondialdehyde; MPO, myeloperoxidase.

in Atrial Fibrillation Pathophysiology," elsewhere in this issue.

C-reactive protein

C-reactive protein (CRP) is an acute-phase protein produced by the liver in response to inflammatory cytokines. CRP has been shown to be associated with incident AF as well as the progression from paroxysmal to permanent AF.[3,4] Moreover, CRP levels have been shown to be positively correlated with AF recurrence after catheter ablation or electrical cardioversion.[5] A systematic review and meta-analysis has shown that an increase between baseline and postoperative CRP levels is associated with the onset of AF following cardiac surgery.[6] In terms of adverse outcomes, CRP and high-sensitivity CRP (hsCRP) have been associated with risk of stroke, myocardial infarction, bleeding, and cardiovascular death in patients with AF.[7,8]

Table 1
Biomarkers with a potential role in atrial fibrillation

Mechanism	Biomarkers
Inflammation	C-reactive protein, IL-2, IL-6, IL-8, IL-10, IL-17A, IL-18, IL-27, IL-37, TNF-α, MCP-1, GDF-15
Oxidative stress	NOX2, NOX4, small G-protein Rac1, asymmetric dimethylarginine, Eh GSH, Eh CySH, isoprostanes, biopyrrin, MDA, nitrotyrosine, DROMs, GDF-15
Cardiomyocyte stress	BNP, NT-proBNP
Cardiomyocyte injury	Cardiac troponin T and I
Atrial fibrosis	Relaxin, galectin-3, FGF-23, PIIINP, ICTP
Thrombogenesis	D-dimer, vWF, PAI-1, TAT
Epigenetic regulation	MicroRNAs, long noncoding RNAs

Abbreviations: BNP, B-type natriuretic peptide; DROMs, derivatives of reactive oxidative metabolites; Eh CySH; reduced cysteine; Eh GSH, reduced glutathione; FGF-23, fibroblast growth factor-23; GDF-15, growth differentiation factor 15; ICTP, type I collagen carboxy-terminal telopeptide; IL, interleukin; MCP-1, monocyte chemoattractant protein-1; MDA, malondialdehyde; NT-proBNP, N-terminal pro–B-type natriuretic peptide; PAI-1, plasminogen activator inhibitor-1; PIIINP, procollagen type III N-terminal propeptide; TAT, thrombin-antithrombin; TNF, tumor necrosis factor; vWF, von Willebrand factor.

Interleukins

Interleukins (ILs) are cytokines produced by various types of cells, mostly leukocytes, that participate in the regulation of immune responses, inflammatory reactions, hematopoiesis, and thrombogenesis. Interleukin (IL)-6 is the most investigated interleukin in association with AF and outcomes. Increased serum IL-6 levels were reported to be associated with an increased risk of AF, and with AF recurrence after catheter ablation or electrical cardioversion.[9] Increased serum IL-6 levels were also shown to be predictors of thromboembolic events, major bleeding, and vascular death.[7,8,10]

Oxidative Stress

Oxidative stress refers to the consequences of the production of excess reactive oxygen species, with the potential to damage cell components, including proteins, lipids, and DNA. Oxidative stress results from an imbalance between oxidant production and the removal of oxidant species by endogenous antioxidant defenses. Oxidative stress is implicated in atrial fibrosis and AF, with an interplay of other mechanisms, including inflammation and the renin-angiotensin system.[11] Numerous mechanistic pathways linking oxidative stress to AF have been identified. These pathways include the xanthine oxidase pathway, nicotinamide adenine dinucleotide phosphate (NADPH) oxidase (through the NADPH oxidase [NOX] 2 and 4, small G-protein Rac1), mitochondrial damage (via the nuclear factor-kappa B, lectinlike oxidized low-density lipoprotein receptor-1 [LOX-1], intercellular adhesion molecule-1 [ICAM-1], heme oxygenase-1), calcium overload, and disrupted electrical activity.[11]

In a cohort study with long follow-up (median 6.3 years), the redox state of the glutathione-related thiol/disulfide pools was associated with prevalent and incident AF.[12] Similarly, high asymmetric dimethylarginine (ADMA) levels were associated with an increased risk of AF recurrence within 1 month after electrical cardioversion,[13] whereas malondialdehyde (MDA) and nitrotyrosine predicted 1-year sinus rhythm maintenance following cardioversion.[14] Plasma derivatives of reactive oxygen metabolites (DROMs) and myeloperoxidase (MPO) have also been shown to be independent predictors of AF recurrence after catheter ablation.[15] The Apixaban for the Prevention of Stroke in Subjects with Atrial Fibrillation (ARISTOTLE) biomarker substudy examined the correlation between growth differentiation factor 15 (GDF-15) plasma concentrations and outcomes in a large cohort of patients with AF.[16] GDF-15, a

marker of oxidative stress and inflammation, was independently related to the risk of major bleeding, death, and stroke. Specifically, compared with patients within the lowest quartile of GDF-15 levels, those in the highest quartile had a 2-fold higher risk of stroke or systemic embolism, a 3.5-fold higher risk of major bleeding, and a 4-fold to 5-fold higher risk of all-cause and cardiac mortality. These associations between baseline GDF-15 level and adverse outcomes remained stable over time and significant after adjustment for clinical risk factors and the CHA_2DS_2-VASc (cardiac failure or dysfunction; hypertension; age ≥ 75, 65–74, <65 years; diabetes mellitus; previous stroke; vascular disease; and sex) score.[16]

Cardiomyocyte Stress and Injury

Troponin

Troponins (subunits I, T, and C) are a group of proteins found in skeletal and heart (cardiac) muscle fibers that, together with tropomyosin, regulate the interaction between actin and myosin filaments leading to muscular contraction. Cardiac troponin is a sensitive and specific marker of myocardial damage and a powerful diagnostic and prognostic tool in acute coronary syndrome. Recent systematic review and meta-analysis found troponin T (TnT) but not troponin I (TnI), to be associated with both incident AF and AF recurrences after radiofrequency ablation.[17] Further, high-sensitivity cardiac TnT (hsTnT) and TnI (hsTnI) have been shown to correlate with incident AF and AF-related hospitalization risks, although they did not improve risk stratification.[18,19] Interesting, early positive cardiac troponins may help to identify (among patients with acute stroke) those who have a cardioembolic source subtype that might benefit from oral anticoagulation.[20]

Pertaining to adverse events, the first major study to show the potential prognostic importance of troponin in patients with AF was the Randomized Evaluation of Long-Term Anticoagulant Therapy (RE-LY) biomarker substudy. The study was performed in 6189 patients with AF and 1 or more risk factor for stroke, and treated with either warfarin or dabigatran, and showed that nearly half of the patients had detectable levels of TnI (≥ 0.01 µg/L).[21] Furthermore, persistent increase (over 3 months) of TnI level was associated with a higher risk of thromboembolic events and cardiovascular mortality, compared with none or transient increase.[21] In hospitalized patients with AF, others have shown that circulating TnI levels were associated with mortality and major adverse cardiac events, with cumulative 3-year event-free survival rates of 78% in patients with nondetectable TnI, 62% in those with a minor increase, and 57% in the those with a significant increase in TnI level (log-rank $P<.001$).[22] A more recent retrospective cohort study of 957 patients with newly diagnosed AF reported increased mortality and readmission rates for heart failure and revascularization associated with increased hsTnI level.[23] Similar results were observed with TnT. In the ARISTOTLE biomarker study performed in 14,892 patients with AF with increased stroke risk treated with either apixaban or warfarin, hsTnT level was independently associated with an increased risk of stroke, cardiac death, and major bleeding.[24] Consistent findings have been reported in a cohort of 930 patients with AF who were effectively anticoagulated (International Normalized Ratios 2.0–3.0) for at least 6 months, with increased hsTnT level being associated with increased rates of cardiovascular events and death.[10] A study using electronic health records from 5 tertiary centers in the United Kingdom also reported the association of increased troponin levels with increased mortality.[25]

B-type natriuretic peptide

B-type natriuretic peptide (BNP) is a hormone secreted by cardiomyocytes in response to stretch in the setting of volume or pressure overload. It is synthesized as a precursor protein, pro-BNP, which is then cleaved into the bioactive BNP and the amino terminal N-terminal proBNP (NT-proBNP). Levels of BNP are increased in various cardiac conditions, including left ventricular hypertrophy, cardiomyopathy, heart failure, and acute coronary events. The Cardiovascular Health Study (CHS) was one of the first large community-based cohort studies to establish that NT-proBNP was associated with incident-AF occurrence in a community-based population of older adults independent of established risk factors.[26] An association between preoperative BNP and postoperative AF in patients undergoing thoracic surgery has also been shown in a meta-analysis.[27] Furthermore, other investigators have shown that BNP level is increased in patients with AF, and that this increase normalizes after restoration of sinus rhythm, indicating a potential predictive role for AF recurrences after rhythm-control intervention.[28,29]

Biomarker substudies of 2 large randomized controlled trials provided firm evidence regarding the prognostic value of NT-proBNP in patients with AF. In the RE-LY biomarker substudy, which analyzed data from 6189 patients with AF, in comparison with normal NT-proBNP levels, the highest quartile of NT-proBNP levels was associated with a 2-fold and 5-fold increased risk of stroke or systemic embolism and cardiovascular death respectively.[21] The ARISTOLE biomarker substudy, involving 14,892 patients with AF, confirmed the association between increased NT-proBNP levels and stroke or systemic embolism and cardiac death.[30] More recently, the US multicenter nationwide Outcomes Registry for Better Informed Treatment of Atrial Fibrillation II (ORBIT-AF II) showed among 13,375 patients with AF that BNP levels were associated with the risk of AF progression as well as a composite of major adverse cardiovascular or neurologic events.[31]

Atrial Fibrosis

Atrial fibrosis is a key structural abnormality in different substrates for AF involving different signaling pathways.[32,33] Atrial structural remodeling includes apoptosis of cardiomyocytes, proliferation of fibroblasts, differentiation to myofibroblasts, and increased production of extracellular matrix. All these pathologic processes seem to be driven by an overlap of myocyte injury, oxidative stress, and inflammation, among other things.[32] Ultimately, fibrosis of myocardial tissue can result in conduction slowing and increased conduction heterogeneity that favor wavefront reentry and perpetuation of AF. Studies on some biomarkers of atrial fibrosis have yielded promising results, highlighting their potential value to guide AF management.

Relaxin

Relaxin is a hormone that downregulates the deposition of collagen and other extracellular matrix proteins, reducing oxidative stress and inflammatory response. Therefore, it has antiinflammatory and antifibrotic properties. Relaxin has been shown to reduce the susceptibility to AF in a murine hypertensive model by reversing atrial fibrosis, improving atrial conduction, and increasing sodium current density in cardiomyocytes.[34] Clinical studies have shown that relaxin concentration was higher in patients with AF than those in sinus rhythm and that higher circulating relaxin level was associated with higher AF recurrence after catheter ablation and greater risk of heart failure.[35,36]

Galectin-3

Galectin-3 is an inflammatory β-galactoside–binding lectin secreted by activated macrophages that, when bound to the matrix, exerts matricellular functions. It has been associated with atrial fibrosis in patients with AF, and has emerged as a potential prognostic marker in AF. Galactin-3 levels were shown to independently correlate with the extent of left atrial fibrosis detected with MRI and assessed from atrial appendage tissue samples.[37] There is evidence suggesting an association between galactin-3 levels and incident AF, AF burden, and AF recurrence following rhythm-control therapies.[37,38] Serum galectin-3 is also a potential marker of thrombogenicity in AF. Studies have shown that serum galectin-3 levels correlate with left atrial appendage remodeling and predict left atrial appendage thrombus formation in patients with AF.[39,40]

Fibroblast growth factor-23

Fibroblast growth factor-23 (FGF-23) is a bone-derived hormone that plays a central role in phosphate homeostasis, vitamin D metabolism, and bone mineralization. Meta-analytical data suggest that higher FGF-23 levels are associated with increased risk of stroke, myocardial infarction, heart failure, cardiovascular mortality, and all-cause mortality.[41] In addition, higher serum FGF-23 levels were associated with incident AF in the Multi-Ethnic Study of Atherosclerosis (MESA) and the CHS.[42] However, in the Atherosclerosis Risk in Communities (ARIC) study, a larger community-based cohort, baseline FGF-23 levels were not associated with AF risk independently of renal function.[43] In the Chronic Renal Insufficiency Cohort (CRIC) study, FGF-23 was independently associated with prevalent and incident AF in patients with mild to severe chronic kidney disease.[44] These data suggest that serum FGF-23 level may be used as a biomarker of AF risk in patients with renal dysfunction. Findings from recent mechanistic studies suggested both profibrotic and proarrhythmic roles of FGF-23,[45,46] although there are limited data on the link between FGF-23 and AF outcomes following rhythm-control intervention.[47,48]

Thrombogenesis

D-dimer

D-dimer is a fibrin degradation product, a small protein fragment present in the blood after a blood clot is degraded by fibrinolysis. D-dimer is therefore a marker of fibrin turnover, and increased D-dimer plasma levels suggest the presence of hypercoagulability or prothrombotic state. A recent meta-analysis found high plasma D-dimer level to be associated with left atrial spontaneous echo contrast and left atrial thrombus.[49] In a RE-LY substudy, the risk of stroke or systemic embolism and of cardiovascular death was 3-fold and 3.5-fold higher in patients with AF in the highest quartile of D-dimer levels compared with those in the lowest quartile.[50] Similarly, in the ARISTOTLE substudy, higher baseline D-dimer levels were associated with an increased risk of stroke, bleeding, and death.[51] Further, a recent study that enrolled 1441 patients with AF-related stroke and atherosclerosis showed that high D-dimer levels (≥ 2 μg/mL) were significantly associated with higher risk of recurrent ischemic stroke.[52]

von Willebrand factor

von Willebrand factor (vWF) is a blood glycoprotein synthesized by endothelial cells that plays a pivotal role in hemostasis after vascular injury through platelet adhesion and aggregation. A recent meta-analysis of prospective cohort studies showed that high vWF levels were associated with increased risks of all-cause death (relative risk [RR], 1.56; 95% confidence interval [CI], 1.16–2.11), cardiovascular death (RR, 1.91; 95% CI, 1.20–3.03), major adverse cardiac events (RR, 1.83; 95% CI, 1.28–2.62), stroke (RR, 1.69; 95% CI, 1.08–2.64), and bleeding (RR, 2.01; 95% CI, 1.65–2.45) in patients with AF.[53] This finding suggests that vWF may also be a clinically useful risk marker in AF.

Noncoding RNAs

Noncoding RNAs are functional RNA molecules that are transcribed from DNA but not translated into proteins. They are derived from noncoding genes, which represent about 98% of the human genome and were previously considered as genetic junk or transcriptional noise because of presumed noninvolvement in cellular function. However, in recent years, noncoding RNAs have emerged as crucial regulators of cellular processes and key contributors in the pathogenesis of several disease states. Noncoding RNAs are mainly classified as either linear RNAs or circular RNAs. Linear RNAs can be subclassified based on the length of transcripts (<200 nucleotides vs ≥ 200 nucleotides) into microRNAs (miRNAs) or long noncoding RNAs. MiRNAs have been the most studied and have to date the strongest evidence on the pathogenic link between noncoding RNAs and AF, although there are increasing data regarding lncNRAs.[54,55] The focus here is on miRNAs.

Table 2 summarizes the data from human studies on several key miRNAs thought to be involved in AF. Several miRNAs might contribute to electrical remodeling in AF by affecting the conductance of L-type Ca^{2+} current (I_{CaL}) and of inward rectifier current (IK_1), as well as triggering changes in the electrical properties of Ca^{2+}-activated K^+ channels and connexin 40 and 43. These miRNAs include miR-1, which promotes cardiomyocyte arrhythmogenicity; miR-26, which regulates IK_1 in both cardiomyocytes[54] and

Table 2
MicroRNAs involved in the pathogenesis of atrial fibrillation

MicroRNA	Source	Target Gene	Remodeling Mechanism	Regulatory Mechanism
miR-1	Right atrial appendage	KCNE1, KCNB2, KCNJ2, HCN2, HCN4	Structural	Up
miR-1	Plasma	KCNE1, KCNB2, KCNJ2, HCN2, HCN4	Electrical	Down
miR-21	Atrial tissue	Spry1, Rac1-GTPase, CTGF	Structural	Up
miR-26a	Right atrial appendage	KCNJ2, NFAT	Electrical	Down
miR-26a	Right atrial appendage	TRPC3	Structural	Down
miR-26a	Right atrial appendage	KIR2.1, KCNJ2	Electrical/structural	Down
miR-29b	Rapid pacing model	COL1A1, COL3A1, fibrillin	Structural	Down
miR-30d	Right atrial appendage	KCNJ3/Kir3.1	Electrical	Up
miR-30	Atrial tissue	I_{KACh}, snail 1	Electrical/structural	Down
miR-31	Right atrial tissue	nNOS	Electrical	Up
miR-34	Right atrial tissue	Ank-B	Structural	Up
miR-106	Atrial tissue, plasma	RYR2, klf2a	Electrical	Down
miR-125	Atrial tissue/plasma	IL-6R, TNFa	Structural	Down
miR-126	Serum	EGFL7	Structural	Down
miR-133	Right atrial appendage	TGF-β1, TGF-β receptor-II	Structural	Down
miR-138-5p	Right atrial appendage	CYP11B2	Structural	Down
miR-146	Left atrial appendage	TIMP-4	Structural	Up
miR-150	Serum, plasma	IL-6, IL-18, TNF-a/b	Structural	Down
miR-199a	Right atrial appendage	SIRT1	Structural	Down
miR-206	Rapid pacing model	SOD1	Electrical	Up
miR-208a	Plasma	CACNA1C, CACNB2, MYH7, Cx40	Electrical/structural	Up
miR-208b	Right atrial appendage	CACNA1C, CACNB1, SERCA2	Electrical	Up
miR-328	Rapid pacing model	CACNA1C, CACNB1	Electrical	Up
miR-409	Plasma	SMAD2, ITGB3, ACE, CDKN2B	Structural	Down
miR-432	Plasma	SMAD2, ITGB3, ACE, CDKN2B	Structural	Down
miR-499	Right atrial appendage	CACNA1C, CACNB2	Electrical	Up
miR-483	Plasma	IGF2	Structural	Up
miR-590	Right atrial appendage	TGF-β1, TGF-β receptor-II	Structural	Down

Abbreviations: IGF2, insulinlike growth factor 2; TGF, transforming growth factor; TNF, tumor necrosis factor.

fibroblasts[56]; miR-499, which contributes to the remodeling of L-type Ca^{2+} currents; and miR-328, which plays a pivotal role in cardiomyocyte calcium handling and electrical remodeling.[54,57,58] Both miR-208 and miR-106 expression have been shown to have an impact on calcium handling in cardiomyocytes through the downregulation of the sarcoplasmic reticulum Ca^{2+} adenosine triphosphates type 2a (SERCA2a) protein and the upregulation of RYR2 protein, respectively. These proteins are involved in Ca^{2+} transport between the cytosol and the sarcoplasmic reticulum.[57,58]

MiRNAs are also involved in atrial structural remodeling by regulating the genes that encode proteins forming the extracellular matrix. For instance, the upregulation of miR-21 promotes atrial remodeling and fibrosis by activating the mitogen-activated protein kinase/extracellular signal-regulated kinase (MAPK/ERK) and the phosphoinositide 3-kinase (PI3K) signaling pathways. MiR-29b upregulates the collagen-1A1, collagen-3A1, and fibrillin genes leading to increased production of the extracellular matrix proteins.[57,58] MiR-26 controls fibroblast function by regulating calcium entry in fibroblasts, via effects on both IK_1[56] and transient-receptor potential channel-3[59] expression. In addition, miR-126, miR-150, miR-483, miR-409, and miR432 are involved in various cellular processes, including inflammation, oxidative stress, platelet function and aggression, angiogenesis, and ultimately atrial fibrosis.[57] A few miRNAs have been shown to contribute to the occurrence and progression of AF via autonomic remodeling. For instance, miR-30 and miR-206 cause autonomic nerve remodeling by downregulating acetylcholine-dependent potassium current, and enhancing the production of reactive oxygen species, respectively.[57,58]

The involvement of these miRNAs in the pathogenesis of AF underpins their potential as biomarkers to predict the development or recurrence of AF. For instance, miR-1 and miR-483 were suggested to potentially predict postoperative AF, whereas miR-125 may play a role in postablation AF recurrence.[57] There have been conflicting results in different studies about the specific miRNA plasma concentrations associated with AF outcomes. One concern is that the amounts of circulating miRNA derived from the atria are very small relative to their production in other tissues.

Clinical Implications

AF accounts for up to a third of ischemic strokes. Biomarkers that can improve stratification of AF risk in high-risk individuals or those with embolic stroke of unknown source have potential clinical value in both primary and secondary stroke prevention. For example, such biomarkers may guide patient selection for more prolonged electrocardiogram (ECG) monitoring or implantation of an insertable cardiac monitor to maximize cost-effectiveness, especially in the context of limited resources.[60] Natriuretic peptides such as BNP and NT-proBNP are the most promising biomarkers to improve the prediction of AF detection after ischemic stroke. It has been suggested that BNP values of greater than 100 pg/mL and NT-proBNP values greater than 400 pg/mL have a predictive value for the occurrence of AF in patients with stroke.[61] A subanalysis of the Find-AF$_{RANDOMISED}$ trial showed that BNP measured early after ischemic stroke identified a subgroup of patients with stroke at increased risk for AF, in whom enhanced and prolonged Holter-ECG is very useful, with significantly reduced number needed to screen.[62] A BNP-based prediction model is being investigated for post–thoracic surgery AF, and this may improve management and reduce complications in this patient group.[63]

Natriuretic peptides have also shown a potential benefit in improving community screening of AF. The CHARGE-AF consortium of community-based cohort studies reported that adding BNP to the CHARGE-AF risk score, which is purely based on clinical factors, substantially improved its predictive performance.[64] In the STROKESTOP II study, NT-proBNP–stratified systematic screening for AF increased the detection of AF in high-risk elderly from the community (from 8.1% to 10.5%), with 94.5% of the participants with newly diagnosed AF accepting the initiation of oral anticoagulation.[65] A recent study using data-driven discovery through logistic regression and machine learning identified BNP and FGF-23, along with 3 clinical risk factors (age, sex, and body mass index), as robustly associated with AF.[66] These biomarkers could therefore be used to risk stratify patients and select those who are more likely to develop AF for more targeted electrocardiographic screening; however, the added value of biomarker guidance can only be determined by well-designed prospective studies.

The ARISTOTLE and RE-LY biomarker substudies have shown associations between NT-proBNP, TnI (RE-LY)/TnT (ARISTOTLE) levels and increased adverse outcomes in patients with AF.[21,24] These findings underpinned the development of the first hybrid score, the ABC-stroke (age, biomarkers [high-sensitivity troponin and NT-proBNP], and clinical history of prior stroke/transient ischemic attack) risk score.[67] The ABC-stroke risk score has been externally validated in independent cohorts (**Table 3**). Similar scores for the prediction of major bleeding and death have also been proposed, the ABC-bleeding (age, biomarkers [growth differentiation factor-15, hsTnT, and hemoglobin], and clinical history of previous bleeding)[68] and the ABC-death (age, biomarkers [growth differentiation factor-15, hsTnT, and NT-proBNP], and clinical history of heart failure)[69] risk scores (see **Table 3**). Specifically, the ABC-stroke score and the ABC-bleeding score were shown to outperform the CHA_2DS_2-VASc and HAS-BLED (hypertension, abnormal renal/liver function, stroke, bleeding history or predisposition, labile International Normalized Ratio, elderly, drugs/alcohol concomitantly) scores, respectively.[67,68,70–72] However, 1 real-world study showed better performance of the HAS-BLED score,[73] and network meta-analysis revealed

Table 3
Studies comparing the predictive performance of the biomarker-based ABC scores with clinical risk scores

Study	Biomarker-Based Score	End Point	Comparator	Cohort (External)	C Statistics
Hijazi et al,[67] 2016	ABC-stroke score	Stroke	CHA_2DS_2-VASc	STABILITY trial: 1400 participants with AF or atrial flutter (689 on oral anticoagulation) with a median follow-up was 3.4 y and a total of 48 events	ABC-stroke score: 0.66 (0.58–0.74) CHA_2DS_2-VASc: 0.58 (0.49–0.67)
Oldgren et al,[70] 2016	ABC-stroke score	Stroke and systemic embolism	CHA_2DS_2-VASc, ATRIA	RE-LY trial: 8356 patients with AF randomized to dabigatran vs warfarin, median follow-up of 1.9 y, and a total of 219 events	ABC-stroke score: 0.65 (0.61–0.69) CHA_2DS_2-VASc: 0.60 (0.57–0.64) ATRIA: 0.61 (0.58–0.65)
Rivera-Caravaca et al,[72] 2017	ABC-stroke score	Ischemic stroke	CHA_2DS_2-VASc	Murcia AF Project: 1125 consecutive patients with AF stable on vitamin K antagonists, median follow-up of 6.5 y, and a total of 114 events	ABC-stroke score: 0.662 (0.633–0.690) CHA_2DS_2-VASc: 0.620 (0.590–0.648)
Berg et al,[71] 2019	ABC-stroke score	Stroke and systemic embolism	CHA_2DS_2-VASc	ENGAGE AF-TIMI 48: 8705 patients with AF and $CHADS_2$ score ≥2 randomized to edoxaban vs warfarin, median follow-up of 2.8 y, and a total of 139 events	ABC-stroke score: 0.66 (0.63–0.68) CHA_2DS_2-VASc: 0.59 (0.57–0.62)
Berg et al,[71] 2019	ABC-bleeding score	Major bleeding	HAS-BLED	ENGAGE AF-TIMI 48: 8705 patients with AF and $CHADS_2$ score ≥2 randomized to edoxaban vs warfarin, median follow-up of 2.8 y, and a total of 251 events	ABC-bleeding: 0.67 (0.65–0.70) HAS-BLED: 0.62 (0.60–0.64)

Study	Score	Outcome	Comparators	Population	Results
Hijazi et al,[68] 2016	ABC-bleeding score	Major bleeding	HAS-BLED, ORBIT	RE-LY trial: 8468 patients with AF randomized to dabigatran vs warfarin, median follow-up of 1.9 y, and a total of 463 events	ABC-bleeding: 0·71 (0·68–0·73) ORBIT: 0·68 (0·65–0·70) HAS-BLED: 0·62 (0·59–0·64)
Esteve-Pastor et al,[73] 2017	ABC-bleeding score	Major bleeding	HAS-BLED	Murcia AF Project: 1120 consecutive patients with AF stable on vitamin K antagonists, median follow-up of 6.5 y, and a total of 207 events	ABC-bleeding: 0.518 (0.488–0.548) HAS-BLED: 0.583 (0.554–0.612)
Hijazi et al,[69] 2018	ABC-death score	Death	CHA_2DS_2-VASc	RE-LY trial: 8548 patients with AF randomized to dabigatran vs warfarin, median follow-up of 1.9 y, and a total of 594 events	ABC-death: 0.74 (0.72–0.76) CHA_2DS_2-VASc: 0.58 (0.56–0.61)

ABC-bleeding score: age, biomarkers (growth differentiation factor-15, hsTnT, and hemoglobin), and clinical history (previous bleeding). ABC-death score: age, biomarkers (growth differentiation factor-15, hsTnT, NT-proBNP), clinical history of heart failure. ATRIA: Anticoagulation and Risk Factors in Atrial Fibrillation): prior stroke, age categories (≥85, 75–84, 65–74, <65 y), sex, diabetes mellitus, congestive heart failure. HAS-BLED: hypertension, abnormal renal/liver function, stroke, bleeding history or predisposition, labile International Normalized Ratio, elderly (>65 y), drugs/alcohol concomitantly.

that, although the ABC-bleeding score has a high sensitivity, the HAS-BLED is a more balanced bleeding risk assessment tool with higher specificity.[74]

FUTURE DIRECTIONS

Despite the significant limitations of current clinical risk scores for ischemic stroke and systemic embolism prediction in nonvalvular AF, the CHA_2DS_2-VASc score remain the mainstay tool in clinical practice. Further research in this field will test the added value of incorporation of biomarkers as discussed in this article, and other patient-specific indices such as measures of atrial fibrosis/function, left atrial appendage morphology, and electrocardiographic markers to improve risk stratification in specific AF populations.[75] Such studies must also incorporate cost-effectiveness data to justify the need for additional testing, beyond simple clinical risk scores.

SUMMARY

Many biomarkers have been shown to correlate with AF outcomes and have the potential to aid in clinical risk assessment. A multimarker strategy incorporating various epigenetic, inflammatory, oxidative stress, atrial fibrosis, and cardiomyocyte stress and injury biomarkers into a single point-of-care test in combination with clinical predictors might help to improve AF screening and risk stratification in patients with AF. However, considerably more work is needed to delineate the ideal combination of biomarkers and clinical risk factors that can be implemented into routine patient care in a clinically useful and cost-effective manner.

DISCLOSURE

Dr J.J. Noubiap is supported by a postgraduate scholarship from the University of Adelaide (UoA). Dr P. Sanders is supported by a practitioner fellowship from the National Health and Medical Research Council of Australia and the National Heart Foundation of Australia. Dr D.H. Lau is supported by a midcareer fellowship from The Hospital Research Foundation.

CONFLICTS OF INTEREST

Dr P. Sanders reports having served on the advisory board of Medtronic, Abbott Medical, Boston Scientific, Pacemate, and CathRx. Dr P. Sanders reports that the UoA has received on his behalf lecture and/or consulting fees from Medtronic, Abbott Medical, Bayer, and Boston Scientific. Dr P. Sanders reports that the UoA has received on his behalf research funding from Medtronic, Abbott Medical, Boston Scientific, and Microport. Dr D.H. Lau reports that the UoA has received on his behalf lecture and/or consulting fees from Abbott Medical, Bayer, Biotronik, Boehringer Ingelheim, Medtronic, Microport, and Pfizer. J.J. Noubiap and S. Nattel report no conflicts.

REFERENCES

1. Wang TJ, Larson MG, Levy D, et al. Temporal relations of atrial fibrillation and congestive heart failure and their joint influence on mortality: the Framingham Heart Study. Circulation 2003;107(23):2920–5.
2. Wolf PA, Abbott RD, Kannel WB. Atrial fibrillation as an independent risk factor for stroke: the Framingham Study. Stroke 1991;22(8):983–8.
3. Wu L, Emmens RW, van Wezenbeek J, et al. Atrial inflammation in different atrial fibrillation subtypes and its relation with clinical risk factors. Clin Res Cardiol 2020;109(10):1271–81.
4. Kwon CH, Kang JG, Lee HJ, et al. C-reactive protein and risk of atrial fibrillation in East Asians. Europace 2017;19(10):1643–9.
5. Jiang Z, Dai L, Song Z, et al. Association between C-reactive protein and atrial fibrillation recurrence after catheter ablation: a meta-analysis. Clin Cardiol 2013;36(9):548–54.
6. Weymann A, Popov AF, Sabashnikov A, et al. Baseline and postoperative levels of C-reactive protein and interleukins as inflammatory predictors of atrial fibrillation following cardiac surgery: a systematic review and meta-analysis. Kardiol Pol 2018;76(2):440–51.
7. Harada M, Van Wagoner DR, Nattel S. Role of inflammation in atrial fibrillation pathophysiology and management. Circ J 2015;79(3):495–502.
8. Aulin J, Siegbahn A, Hijazi Z, et al. Interleukin-6 and C-reactive protein and risk for death and cardiovascular events in patients with atrial fibrillation. Am Heart J 2015;170(6):1151–60.
9. Wu N, Xu B, Xiang Y, et al. Association of inflammatory factors with occurrence and recurrence of atrial fibrillation: a meta-analysis. Int J Cardiol 2013;169(1):62–72.
10. Roldan V, Marin F, Diaz J, et al. High sensitivity cardiac troponin T and interleukin-6 predict adverse cardiovascular events and mortality in anticoagulated patients with atrial fibrillation. J Thromb Haemost 2012;10(8):1500–7.
11. Ren X, Wang X, Yuan M, et al. Mechanisms and treatments of oxidative stress in atrial fibrillation. Curr Pharm Des 2018;24(26):3062–71.
12. Samman Tahhan A, Sandesara PB, Hayek SS, et al. Association between oxidative stress and atrial fibrillation. Heart Rhythm 2017;14(12):1849–55.

13. Xia W, Qu X, Yu Y, et al. Asymmetric dimethylarginine concentration and early recurrence of atrial fibrillation after electrical cardioversion. Pacing Clin Electrophysiol 2008;31(8):1036–40.
14. Leftheriotis DI, Fountoulaki KT, Flevari PG, et al. The predictive value of inflammatory and oxidative markers following the successful cardioversion of persistent lone atrial fibrillation. Int J Cardiol 2009;135(3):361–9.
15. Shimano M, Shibata R, Inden Y, et al. Reactive oxidative metabolites are associated with atrial conduction disturbance in patients with atrial fibrillation. Heart Rhythm 2009;6(7):935–40.
16. Wallentin L, Hijazi Z, Andersson U, et al. Growth differentiation factor 15, a marker of oxidative stress and inflammation, for risk assessment in patients with atrial fibrillation: insights from the Apixaban for Reduction in Stroke and Other Thromboembolic Events in Atrial Fibrillation (ARISTOTLE) trial. Circulation 2014;130(21):1847–58.
17. Bai Y, Guo SD, Liu Y, et al. Relationship of troponin to incident atrial fibrillation occurrence, recurrence after radiofrequency ablation and prognosis: a systematic review, meta-analysis and meta-regression. Biomarkers 2018;23(6):512–7.
18. Filion KB, Agarwal SK, Ballantyne CM, et al. High-sensitivity cardiac troponin T and the risk of incident atrial fibrillation: the Atherosclerosis Risk in Communities (ARIC) study. Am Heart J 2015;169(1):31–8.e3.
19. Zhu K, Hung J, Divitini M, et al. High-sensitivity cardiac troponin I and risk of incident atrial fibrillation hospitalisation in an Australian community-based cohort: the Busselton health study. Clin Biochem 2018;58:20–5.
20. Yaghi S, Chang AD, Ricci BA, et al. Early elevated troponin levels after ischemic stroke suggests a cardioembolic source. Stroke 2018;49(1):121–6.
21. Hijazi Z, Oldgren J, Andersson U, et al. Cardiac biomarkers are associated with an increased risk of stroke and death in patients with atrial fibrillation: a Randomized Evaluation of Long-term Anticoagulation Therapy (RE-LY) substudy. Circulation 2012;125(13):1605–16.
22. van den Bos EJ, Constantinescu AA, van Domburg RT, et al. Minor elevations in troponin I are associated with mortality and adverse cardiac events in patients with atrial fibrillation. Eur Heart J 2011;32(5):611–7.
23. Kim BS, Kwon CH, Chang H, et al. Usefulness of high-sensitivity troponin I to predict outcome in patients with newly detected atrial fibrillation. Am J Cardiol 2020;125(5):744–50.
24. Hijazi Z, Wallentin L, Siegbahn A, et al. High-sensitivity troponin T and risk stratification in patients with atrial fibrillation during treatment with apixaban or warfarin. J Am Coll Cardiol 2014;63(1):52–61.
25. Kaura A, Arnold AD, Panoulas V, et al. Prognostic significance of troponin level in 3121 patients presenting with atrial fibrillation (The NIHR Health Informatics Collaborative TROP-AF study). J Am Heart Assoc 2020;9(7):e013684.
26. Patton KK, Ellinor PT, Heckbert SR, et al. N-terminal pro-B-type natriuretic peptide is a major predictor of the development of atrial fibrillation: the Cardiovascular Health Study. Circulation 2009;120(18):1768–74.
27. Simmers D, Potgieter D, Ryan L, et al. The use of preoperative B-type natriuretic peptide as a predictor of atrial fibrillation after thoracic surgery: systematic review and meta-analysis. J Cardiothorac Vasc Anesth 2015;29(2):389–95.
28. Yamada T, Murakami Y, Okada T, et al. Plasma atrial natriuretic Peptide and brain natriuretic Peptide levels after radiofrequency catheter ablation of atrial fibrillation. Am J Cardiol 2006;97(12):1741–4.
29. Miake J, Kato M, Ogura K, et al. Pre-ablation levels of brain natriuretic peptide are independently associated with the recurrence of atrial fibrillation after radiofrequency catheter ablation in patients with nonvalvular atrial fibrillation. Heart Vessels 2019;34(3):517–26.
30. Hijazi Z, Wallentin L, Siegbahn A, et al. N-terminal pro-B-type natriuretic peptide for risk assessment in patients with atrial fibrillation: insights from the ARISTOTLE Trial (Apixaban for the Prevention of Stroke in Subjects with Atrial Fibrillation). J Am Coll Cardiol 2013;61(22):2274–84.
31. Inohara T, Kim S, Pieper K, et al. B-type natriuretic peptide, disease progression and clinical outcomes in atrial fibrillation. Heart 2019;105(5):370–7.
32. Nattel S. Molecular and cellular mechanisms of atrial fibrosis in atrial fibrillation. JACC Clin Electrophysiol 2017;3(5):425–35.
33. Thanigaimani S, Lau DH, Agbaedeng T, et al. Molecular mechanisms of atrial fibrosis: implications for the clinic. Expert Rev Cardiovasc Ther 2017;15(4):247–56.
34. Parikh A, Patel D, McTiernan CF, et al. Relaxin suppresses atrial fibrillation by reversing fibrosis and myocyte hypertrophy and increasing conduction velocity and sodium current in spontaneously hypertensive rat hearts. Circ Res 2013;113(3):313–21.
35. Qu X, Chen L, Sun L, et al. Serum relaxin level predicts recurrence of atrial fibrillation after radiofrequency catheter ablation. Heart Vessels 2019;34(9):1543–51.
36. Zhou H, Qu X, Gao Z, et al. Relaxin level in patients with atrial fibrillation and association with heart failure occurrence: a STROBE compliant article. Medicine (Baltimore) 2016;95(21):e3664.
37. Hernandez-Romero D, Vilchez JA, Lahoz A, et al. Galectin-3 as a marker of interstitial atrial

remodelling involved in atrial fibrillation. Sci Rep 2017;7:40378.

38. Gong M, Cheung A, Wang QS, et al. Galectin-3 and risk of atrial fibrillation: a systematic review and meta-analysis. J Clin Lab Anal 2020;34(3):e23104.

39. Kocyigit D, Gurses KM, Yalcin MU, et al. Serum galectin-3 level as a marker of thrombogenicity in atrial fibrillation. J Clin Lab Anal 2017;31(6):22120.

40. Tang Z, Zeng L, Lin Y, et al. Circulating galectin-3 is associated with left atrial appendage remodelling and thrombus formation in patients with atrial fibrillation. Heart Lung Circ 2019;28(6):923–31.

41. Marthi A, Donovan K, Haynes R, et al. Fibroblast growth factor-23 and risks of cardiovascular and noncardiovascular diseases: a meta-analysis. J Am Soc Nephrol 2018;29(7):2015–27.

42. Mathew JS, Sachs MC, Katz R, et al. Fibroblast growth factor-23 and incident atrial fibrillation: the multi-ethnic study of atherosclerosis (MESA) and the cardiovascular health study (CHS). Circulation 2014;130(4):298–307.

43. Alonso A, Misialek JR, Eckfeldt JH, et al. Circulating fibroblast growth factor-23 and the incidence of atrial fibrillation: the Atherosclerosis Risk in Communities study. J Am Heart Assoc 2014;3(5):e001082.

44. Mehta R, Cai X, Lee J, et al. Association of fibroblast growth factor 23 with atrial fibrillation in chronic kidney disease, from the chronic renal insufficiency cohort study. JAMA Cardiol 2016;1(5):548–56.

45. Dong Q, Li S, Wang W, et al. FGF23 regulates atrial fibrosis in atrial fibrillation by mediating the STAT3 and SMAD3 pathways. J Cell Physiol 2019; 234(11):19502–10.

46. Huang SY, Chen YC, Kao YH, et al. Fibroblast growth factor 23 dysregulates late sodium current and calcium homeostasis with enhanced arrhythmogenesis in pulmonary vein cardiomyocytes. Oncotarget 2016;7(43):69231–42.

47. Begg GA, Lip GY, Plein S, et al. Circulating biomarkers of fibrosis and cardioversion of atrial fibrillation: a prospective, controlled cohort study. Clin Biochem 2017;50(1–2):11–5.

48. Mizia-Stec K, Wieczorek J, Polak M, et al. Lower soluble Klotho and higher fibroblast growth factor 23 serum levels are associated with episodes of atrial fibrillation. Cytokine 2018;111:106–11.

49. Wan H, Wu S, Yang Y, et al. Plasma fibrin D-dimer and the risk of left atrial thrombus: a systematic review and meta-analysis. PLoS One 2017;12(2): e0172272.

50. Siegbahn A, Oldgren J, Andersson U, et al. D-dimer and factor VIIa in atrial fibrillation - prognostic values for cardiovascular events and effects of anticoagulation therapy. A RE-LY substudy. Thromb Haemost 2016;115(5):921–30.

51. Christersson C, Wallentin L, Andersson U, et al. D-dimer and risk of thromboembolic and bleeding events in patients with atrial fibrillation–observations from the ARISTOTLE trial. J Thromb Haemost 2014; 12(9):1401–12.

52. Choi KH, Seo WK, Park MS, et al. Baseline D-dimer levels as a risk assessment biomarker for recurrent stroke in patients with combined atrial fibrillation and atherosclerosis. J Clin Med 2019;8(9):1457.

53. Ye YZ, Chang YF, Wang BZ, et al. Prognostic value of von Willebrand factor for patients with atrial fibrillation: a meta-analysis of prospective cohort studies. Postgrad Med J 2019;96(1135):267–76.

54. Luo X, Yang B, Nattel S. MicroRNAs and atrial fibrillation: mechanisms and translational potential. Nat Rev Cardiol 2015;12(2):80–90.

55. Babapoor-Farrokhran S, Gill D, Rasekhi RT. The role of long noncoding RNAs in atrial fibrillation. Heart Rhythm 2020;17(6):1043–9.

56. Qi XY, Huang H, Ordog B, et al. Fibroblast inward-rectifier potassium current upregulation in profibrillatory atrial remodeling. Circ Res 2015;116(5):836–45.

57. Komal S, Yin JJ, Wang SH, et al. MicroRNAs: emerging biomarkers for atrial fibrillation. J Cardiol 2019;74(6):475–82.

58. Zhou D, Yang K, Hu J, et al. Noncoding RNAs in atrial fibrillation: current status and prospect. J Cardiovasc Pharmacol 2020;75(1):10–7.

59. Harada M, Luo X, Qi XY, et al. Transient receptor potential canonical-3 channel-dependent fibroblast regulation in atrial fibrillation. Circulation 2012; 126(17):2051–64.

60. Schnabel RB, Haeusler KG, Healey JS, et al. Searching for atrial fibrillation poststroke: a white paper of the AF-SCREEN international collaboration. Circulation 2019;140(22):1834–50.

61. Wachter R, Lahno R, Haase B, et al. Natriuretic peptides for the detection of paroxysmal atrial fibrillation in patients with cerebral ischemia–the Find-AF study. PLoS One 2012;7(4):e34351.

62. Wasser K, Weber-Kruger M, Groschel S, et al. Brain natriuretic peptide and discovery of atrial fibrillation after stroke: a subanalysis of the find-AFRANDOMISED trial. Stroke 2020;51(2):395–401.

63. Amar D, Zhang H, Tan KS, et al. A brain natriuretic peptide-based prediction model for atrial fibrillation after thoracic surgery: development and internal validation. J Thorac Cardiovasc Surg 2019;157(6): 2493–9.e1.

64. Sinner MF, Stepas KA, Moser CB, et al. B-type natriuretic peptide and C-reactive protein in the prediction of atrial fibrillation risk: the CHARGE-AF Consortium of community-based cohort studies. Europace 2014;16(10):1426–33.

65. Kemp Gudmundsdottir K, Fredriksson T, Svennberg E, et al. Stepwise mass screening for atrial fibrillation using N-terminal B-type natriuretic peptide: the STROKESTOP II study. Europace 2020;22(1):24–32.

66. Chua W, Purmah Y, Cardoso VR, et al. Data-driven discovery and validation of circulating blood-based biomarkers associated with prevalent atrial fibrillation. Eur Heart J 2019;40(16):1268–76.

67. Hijazi Z, Lindback J, Alexander JH, et al. The ABC (age, biomarkers, clinical history) stroke risk score: a biomarker-based risk score for predicting stroke in atrial fibrillation. Eur Heart J 2016;37(20):1582–90.

68. Hijazi Z, Oldgren J, Lindback J, et al. The novel biomarker-based ABC (age, biomarkers, clinical history)-bleeding risk score for patients with atrial fibrillation: a derivation and validation study. Lancet 2016;387(10035):2302–11.

69. Hijazi Z, Oldgren J, Lindback J, et al. A biomarker-based risk score to predict death in patients with atrial fibrillation: the ABC (age, biomarkers, clinical history) death risk score. Eur Heart J 2018;39(6):477–85.

70. Oldgren J, Hijazi Z, Lindback J, et al. Performance and validation of a novel biomarker-based stroke risk score for atrial fibrillation. Circulation 2016; 134(22):1697–707.

71. Berg DD, Ruff CT, Jarolim P, et al. Performance of the ABC scores for assessing the risk of stroke or systemic embolism and bleeding in patients with atrial fibrillation in ENGAGE AF-TIMI 48. Circulation 2019;139(6):760–71.

72. Rivera-Caravaca JM, Roldán V, Esteve-Pastor MA, et al. Long-Term stroke risk prediction in patients with atrial fibrillation: comparison of the ABC-stroke and CHA(2)DS(2)-VASc scores. J Am Heart Assoc 2017;6(7):e006490.

73. Esteve-Pastor MA, Rivera-Caravaca JM, Roldan V, et al. Long-term bleeding risk prediction in 'real world' patients with atrial fibrillation: comparison of the HAS-BLED and ABC-Bleeding risk scores. The Murcia Atrial Fibrillation Project. Thromb Haemost 2017;117(10):1848–58.

74. Chang G, Xie Q, Ma L, et al. Accuracy of HAS-BLED and other bleeding risk assessment tools in predicting major bleeding events in atrial fibrillation: a network meta-analysis. J Thromb Haemost 2020; 18(4):791–801.

75. Alkhouli M, Friedman PA. Ischemic stroke risk in patients with nonvalvular atrial fibrillation: JACC review topic of the week. J Am Coll Cardiol 2019;74(24): 3050–65.

Is Screening for Atrial Fibrillation and Its Risk Factors Useful and Cost-Effective?

Roopinder K. Sandhu, MD, MPH[a], Jeff S. Healey, MD, MSc[b],*

KEYWORDS

• Atrial fibrillation • Risk factors • Screening • Cost-effectiveness

KEY POINTS

- Atrial fibrillation (AF) screening initiatives are possible because of the availability of effective, safe, convenient stroke prevention therapy, well-defined stroke risk schemes, and advancements in simple technologies for AF monitoring.
- Screening for silent AF provides an important opportunity to simultaneously identify known cardiovascular risk factors caused by AF and its complications. Treatment of modifiable risk factors is important for those with known AF.
- Early work demonstrates integrated screening programs are cost-effective; however; more research is needed evaluating effect on outcomes, health care utilization, and costs in different health care systems.

INTRODUCTION

Over the last decade, there has been growing interest in atrial fibrillation (AF) screening initiatives given the availability of effective, safe, convenient stroke prevention therapy,[1] well-defined stroke risk schemes,[2,3] and advancements in simple technologies for AF monitoring.[4–6] However, ongoing research must define the optimal population, setting, screening technique, and method to link AF detection to the initiation of appropriate oral anticoagulation therapy.[5] Randomized trials of AF screening and economic analyses are also required to evaluate the true impact of screening and to determine its cost-effectiveness.[7,8]

Screening for silent AF also provides an important opportunity to simultaneously identify known risk factors that cause AF and its complications.[9,10] Cohort studies have shown that the presence of combined risk factors including cigarette smoking, diabetes, hypertension, and coronary heart disease explained 44% of the AF burden in men and 58% of the burden in women,[11] and the presence of at least 1 borderline or elevated risk factor levels (presence of heart failure or coronary heart disease, elevated systolic or diastolic blood pressure [BP], body mass index, fasting serum glucose, current smoker) was attributed to 56.5% of all AF cases.[9] The same risk factors are those that predict the adverse outcomes of AF, specifically stroke and heart failure.[2,12–14] Aggressive risk factor modification and early initiation of AF therapies may be a key to reducing AF burden

[a] Mazankowski Alberta Heart Institute, University of Alberta, 8440-112 Street, 2C2 WMC, Edmonton, Alberta T6G 2B7, Canada; [b] Population Health Research Institute, McMaster University, 237 Barton Street, C3-121, Hamilton, Ontario L8L 2X2, Canada
* Corresponding author. Hamilton Health Sciences, General Site, Room C3-121, DBCVSRI Building, 30 Birge Street, Hamilton, Ontario L8L 0A6, Canada.
E-mail address: Jeff.Healey@phri.ca

and subsequent AF-related morbidity, mortality, and costs.[15,16]

HOW AND IN WHOM TO SCREEN FOR ATRIAL FIBRILLATION?

The 2 main considerations for an AF screening program are: who to screen? and how to screen? It is well recognized that AF is more common among older individuals, so the detection rate will be higher as one selects an older population.[6,10,17] Younger populations can be enriched by including those with cardiovascular conditions predisposing to AF, or by using biomarkers such as left atrial enlargement or elevated NT-ProBNP.[18,19] The more AF that is detected, the more likely screening will prove cost-effective.[7] The method of screening is also relevant, as methods using single timepoint ECG are widely available and inexpensive yet will detect less AF.[5,20,21] More sensitive methods including continuous ambulatory or implantable monitoring will detect more AF, but with greater cost, less convenience and less availability.[18] Short-lasting, low-burden AF also appears to carry a lower stroke risk,[22] and anticoagulation may not prevent stroke in these patients to the same extent as higher-burden AF.[23,24]

Several guidelines and consensus documents recommend opportunistic AF screening with pulse palpation for patients 65 years of age or older during routine BP measurement in primary care clinics.[5,25,26] Pulse palpitations are inexpensive and have good diagnostic accuracy with a sensitivity and specificity, respectively of 0.92 (95% confidence interval [CI] 0.85–0.96) and 0.82 (95% CI 0.76–88) compared with a gold standard 12-lead electrocardiogram (ECG).[20,27] The lower specificity means there is a significant risk of false-positive screening and need for downstream confirmatory testing in nearly 1 out of 5 individuals screened.[5] In addition, pulse palpation needs to be performed during the visit as part of a physical examination, which is not always routinely done.

Ambulatory electrocardiographic monitoring greatly minimizes the need for downstream testing and can be accomplished with intermittent 30-second monitoring with a handheld device[19,21] or watch,[17] or using continuous monitoring with a Holter or patch device for a variable length of time.[28] There are several ongoing trials using all of these different techniques.[5] There will likely not be 1 best method, as the optimal screening method will likely depend on the population screened and the health care setting of the screening program. Direct, consumer-facing screening methods, such as the recent Apple

watch study,[17,29] have the advantage of reaching a large number of motivated individuals and having no initial costs to the health care system. However, many participants were actually at low risk of AF, thus increasing the likelihood of false-positive screening and reducing the anticipated cost-effectiveness of the strategy. The latter is also challenged by the difficulties in connecting positive screening results with downstream testing and treatment.[17]

As an alternative, AF can be detected using automated oscillometric BP devices, which have the added advantages of being widely used in the community and of measuring BP at the same time.[30] The algorithm for AF detection is based on the last 10 pulses during cuff deflation, calculating an irregularity index defined as the standard deviation of the time intervals between successive heartbeats divided by the mean of the intervals calculated; threshold exceeding 0.06 indicates AF.[31] The device automatically performs 3 sequential BP measurements in accordance with AHA and ESC guideline recommendations,[32] provides an average BP, and denotes AF, if present.

A meta-analysis of 6 clinical trials (n = 2332) has been conducted evaluating the diagnostic accuracy of AF detection with automated BP measurement and in a random effects model found a pooled estimate for sensitivity of 0.98 (95% CI, 0.95–1.00) and specificity 0.92 (95% CI, 0.88–0.96).[33] A higher sensitivity for the accuracy of an AF diagnosis was achieved with 2 of 3 reading for AF (0.98, 95% CI 0.95–1.0) compared with 3 of 3 (0.90, 95% CI 0.87–0.93) readings but with slightly lower specificity (0.94, 95% CI, 0.88–0.99 vs 0.95, 95% CI 0.86–1.00).[33]

INTEGRATING ATRIAL FIBRILLATION SCREENING WITH OTHER HEALTH MAINTENANCE PROGRAMS?

Any new screening program has costs, not only financial but also the time that they require from patients and health care providers. Public health and primary care providers have a finite capacity to provide health maintenance across a range of areas; thus priorities need to be set and efficiencies found. One initial success with AF screening was combining this with annual influenza vaccinations. Both targeted an older, at-risk population and took advantage of the required postvaccination observation period to conduct AF screening.[34,35] This strategy changes focus from population-based screening, to opportunistic case finding among individuals presenting to a health care provider for another reason.[5] Another good example is to screen for AF among patients with hypertension, which is both a leading cause of AF, and of stroke among individuals with AF.[9]

In 20 13, the United Kingdom (UK) National Institute for Health Care Excellence (NICE) recommended the automated oscillometric BP monitor WatchBP Home A (Microlife AG, Widnau, Switzerland) with AF detecting algorithm for routine office BP measurement in patients at least 65 years of age in the primary care setting.[36] An estimated 45% cost savings (£12M) and 11% reduction in the number of strokes compared with pulse palpation were reported. In a study of 6 UK primary care practices of patients at least 75 years of age (n = 1000) evaluating the performance of the Watch BP Home A device and 2 single-lead ECG devices (Omron model HCG-801 and Merlin ECG event recorder) compared with 12-lead ECG, the sensitivity for AF detection was high for all 3 devices (>94%), but the WatchBP had the highest specificity.[27] A recent study conducted in 22 Canadian primary care clinics of patients at least 65 years of age (n = 2054) who underwent screening using pulse check, single-lead ECG device (HeartCheck, CardioComm Solutions, Inc.) and the WatchBP Home A device showed superior specificity for AF detection compared with pulse check.[37] In an economic evaluation comparing the different strategies simultaneously, the most cost-effective AF screening strategy test was pulse check, single-lead ECG device, BP monitor, and then no screening.[38]

IS THERE A BENEFIT IN SCREENING FOR CARDIOVASCULAR RISK FACTORS IN INDIVIDUALS WITH ATRIAL FIBRILLATION?

Hypertension is recognized as the most important modifiable risk factor of AF, accounting for 22% of incident AF cases[39,40] and a comorbidity present in 90% of participants in AF trials.[41,42] Hypertension is also under-recognized and undertreated in patients with AF, with between 30% and 40% of patients in AF stroke prevention trials having BP values of at least 140/90 mm Hg.[41] In a recent Canadian cohort study of AF screening, such suboptimal BP control was documented in nearly 50% of individuals in whom new AF was detected by screening.[10] As the treatment of hypertension is also an effective way to prevent both ischemic and hemorrhagic stroke and to prevent heart failure,[43] combining AF and BP screening AF holds potential to improve the efficiency and cost-effectiveness of both programs.

SLEEP APNEA

Obstructive sleep apnea (OSA) is highly prevalent in obesity and an established risk factor for the development of AF. There are studies demonstrating the association between OSA and AF is independent of obesity.[44,45] The known association between OSA and AF begs the questions of screening for silent AF in individuals with OSA, and vice versa. Few studies have investigated the prevalence of AF in sleep apnea.[46–49] In the Sleep Heart Health study, AF was found in 4.8% of 228 individuals with severe disordered breathing compared to 0.9% of 338 individuals without assessed from single-lead ECG obtained during the sleep period. The prevalence of AF was found to be much higher in a population, which included both central and OSA matched for age, sex, and body mass index (BMI) (27% vs 1.7%) using a single-lead ECG obtained during the night of the study.[48] Two studies evaluated incident AF using cardiac monitors.[46,49] In a small, prospective observation study (n = 20) randomly selected patients with severe OSA (apnea-hypopnea index ≥30) without known AF were provided a 7-day event monitor (eCardio, Houston, Texas), and clinically meaningful silent AF defined at 5 minutes was not detected.[46] The prevalence of AF was investigated among 201 patients without known AF referred for suspected OSA with a 12-lead ECG at hospital and a handheld ECG recordings (twice daily and with symptoms) at home for a 2-week period (Zenicor-EKG, Sweden). AF was found in 6.5% of patients, and OSA was present in all. Screening for AF in larger studies, standard definition for clinically meaningful AF and longer duration of monitoring using newer technology is needed to determine feasibility and effectiveness in a sleep apnea population. The results from the Arrhythmia Detection in OSA (ADIOS) study, which completed recruitment of patients with OSA who underwent 30-day cardiac monitoring using the Lifestar Act III device, will be an important step forward (ClinicalTrials.gov Identifier: NCT02743520).

MULTIPLE RISK FACTORS

The Program for the Identification of 'Actionable' AF (PIAAF) performed a stroke risk screening program in participants at least 65 years of age attending community pharmacies in Canada. AF was assessed using a handheld ECG device; BP was measured using an automated BP machine, and diabetes risk was estimated using he Canadian Diabetes Risk Assessment questionnaire. Among the 1145 participants, AF was identified in 2.5%; a BP of greater than 140/90 was identified in 55%, and 44% of participants were found to be at high risk for diabetes.[10] This information was provided to a primary care physician; at 3 months, 50% had an improvement in BP, and 71% had confirmatory diabetes testing; however, only 17% were started on OAC therapy. The PIAAF-Pharmacy study was cost-effective, yielding an incremental cost per quality-adjusted life-years (QALYs) of $CDN 7480.[38]

IS THERE A BENEFIT IN SCREENING FOR CARDIOVASCULAR RISK FACTORS IN INDIVIDUAL WITH KNOWN ATRIAL FIBRILLATION AND OBESITY?

BMI is a well-established risk factor for development of incident AF[50] and an independent predictor of progression from paroxysmal to sustained forms of AF.[51] More recently, evidence has been accumulating that comprehensive interventions aimed at modifying risk factors of AF particularly, weight loss alongside improved glycemic control, achieving hypertension targets, lipid lowering strategies, lifestyle interventions, and improving cardiorespiratory fitness reduce AF recurrence and AF burden and improve underlying conditions.[52,53]

Most intervention data are from the Australian group led by Pathak and colleagues,[52] who found in patients with symptomatic paroxysmal and persistent AF and a BMI of at least 27 kg/m^2, a structured weight management program resulting in weight loss of at least10% in addition to screening and managing hypertension, glucose intolerance, sleep apnea and smoking to guideline targets was associated with a sixfold greater probability of AF-free survival compared to less weight loss over a 5-year follow up period. Weight reduction and aggressive risk factor management were also shown to reduce AF frequency, duration, symptoms, and symptom severity after AF ablation.[52] However, fluctuations in weight increased risk of AF recurrence. Similar results were reported from a retrospective Italian study in patients with paroxysmal or permanent AF and a BMI greater than 25 kg/m.^{2} A higher and increasing BMI had a greater risk of AF recurrence during long-term follow up.[54] In a setting with appropriate resources/supports and a motivated patient, 88% of patients were shown to reverse progression of AF type to paroxysmal or no AF.[55] The cost-effectiveness of such intense risk factor management was found to lessen the need for medications and procedures and reduce health care utilization.[56] The cost-saving benefit amounted to US$12,094 and an increase of 0.193 QALYs.

FUTURE DIRECTIONS

Several risk factors and cardiovascular conditions have been identified as independently associated with the development and progression of AF and AF-related complications. Although there are risk factors such as advancing age, sex, ethnicity, or genetic predisposition, which cannot be modified, most are modifiable or have established treatments. Recent guideline documents for the management of patients with AF from the European Heart Association[57] and American Heart Association/American College of Cardiology/Heart Rhythm Society[58] highlight the importance of identifying and treating modifiable risk factors of AF, but data evaluating whether systematic screening of modifiable risk factors and conditions in clinical practice are largely speculative. To better address the complexities involved in AF management, an integrated, structured approach to AF care has been proposed that includes patient involvement and a multidisciplinary team including primary care, specialists, and allied health professionals to support lifestyle interventions and treatment of risk factors along with AF-specific therapy.[59] Data evaluating the benefit of integrated AF care are sparse. Observational studies have found integrated AF care reduces hospitalizations, stroke[60] and may lower a composite outcome of death, cardiovascular hospitalization, and AF-related emergency department (ED) visits.[61] A single randomized clinical trial demonstrated an increase in evidence-based treatments and a 35% reduction in the composite outcome of cardiovascular hospitalizations and death at almost 2 years and contributed to 0.009 QALY gains with a reduced cost of €1109 per patient and a gain of 0.02 life-years with a reduced cost of €735 per patient compared to usual care.[62]

There is an opportunity to identify unrecognized risk factors and cardiovascular conditions when screening for silent AF. An integrated screening program may further reduce AF-related complications, health care utilization, and costs, but robust studies are needed to define optimal screening methods, populations, and settings in different health care systems.

CLINICS CARE POINTS

- Identification and treatment of modifiable risk factors is important for patients with known AF.
- AF screening initiatives may provide an opportunity to identify unrecognized risk factors and cardiovascular conditions are associated with AF.
- Future research is needed to identify optimal population, setting, and methods for a comprehensive screening program.

DISCLOSURE

Dr R.K. Sandhu reports research grants from BMS/Pfizer and Servier, and Dr J.S. Healey reports research grants and speaking fees from BMS/Pfizer, Bayer, Servier, Medtronic, Boston Scientific, and St. Jude Medical.

REFERENCES

1. Ruff CT, Giugliano RP, Braunwald E, et al. Comparison of the efficacy and safety of new oral anticoagulants with warfarin in patients with atrial fibrillation: a meta-analysis of randomised trials. Lancet 2014; 383:955–62.

2. Gage BF, Waterman AD, Shannon W, et al. Validation of clinical classification schemes for predicting stroke: results from the National Registry of Atrial Fibrillation. JAMA 2001;285:2864–70.

3. Potpara TS, Polovina MM, Marinkovic JM, et al. A comparison of clinical characteristics and long-term prognosis in asymptomatic and symptomatic patients with first-diagnosed atrial fibrillation: the Belgrade Atrial Fibrillation Study. Int J Cardiol 2013;168:4744–9.

4. Freedman B, Potpara TS, Lip GY. Stroke prevention in atrial fibrillation. Lancet 2016;388:806–17.

5. Freedman B, Camm J, Calkins H, et al. Screening for atrial fibrillation: a report of the AF-SCREEN International Collaboration. Circulation 2017;135:1851–67.

6. Engdahl J, Andersson L, Mirskaya M, et al. Stepwise screening of atrial fibrillation in a 75-year-old population: implications for stroke prevention. Circulation 2013;127:930–7.

7. Aronsson M, Svennberg E, Rosenqvist M, et al. Cost-effectiveness of mass screening for untreated atrial fibrillation using intermittent ECG recording. Europace 2015;17:1023–9.

8. Curry SJ, Krist AH, Owens DK, et al. Screening for atrial fibrillation with electrocardiography: US preventive Services Task Force Recommendation Statement. JAMA 2018;320:478–84.

9. Huxley RR, Lopez FL, Folsom AR, et al. Absolute and attributable risks of atrial fibrillation in relation to optimal and borderline risk factors: the Atherosclerosis Risk in Communities (ARIC) study. Circulation 2011;123:1501–8.

10. Sandhu RK, Dolovich L, Deif B, et al. High prevalence of modifiable stroke risk factors identified in a pharmacy-based screening programme. Open Heart 2016;3:e000515.

11. Benjamin EJ, Levy D, Vaziri SM, et al. Independent risk factors for atrial fibrillation in a population-based cohort. The Framingham Heart Study. JAMA 1994;271:840–4.

12. Potpara TS, Polovina MM, Licina MM, et al. Predictors and prognostic implications of incident heart failure following the first diagnosis of atrial fibrillation in patients with structurally normal hearts: the Belgrade Atrial Fibrillation Study. Eur J Heart Fail 2013;15:415–24.

13. Wong JA, Conen D, Van Gelder IC, et al. Progression of device-detected subclinical atrial fibrillation and the risk of heart failure. J Am Coll Cardiol 2018;71:2603–11.

14. Healey JS, Oldgren J, Ezekowitz M, et al. Occurrence of death and stroke in patients in 47 countries 1 year after presenting with atrial fibrillation: a cohort study. Lancet 2016;388:1161–9.

15. Chung MK, Eckhardt LL, Chen LY, et al. Lifestyle and risk factor modification for reduction of atrial fibrillation: a scientific statement from the American Heart Association. Circulation 2020;141:e750–72.

16. Kirchhof P, Camm AJ, Goette A, et al. Early rhythm-control therapy in patients with atrial fibrillation. N Engl J Med 2020;383(14):1305–16.

17. Perez MV, Mahaffey KW, Hedlin H, et al. Large-scale assessment of a smartwatch to identify atrial fibrillation. N Engl J Med 2019;381:1909–17.

18. Healey JS, Alings M, Ha A, et al. Subclinical atrial fibrillation in older patients. Circulation 2017;136: 1276–83.

19. Svennberg E, Engdahl J, Al-Khalili F, et al. Mass screening for untreated atrial fibrillation: the STRO-KESTOP study. Circulation 2015;131:2176–84.

20. Lowres N, Neubeck L, Salkeld G, et al. Feasibility and cost-effectiveness of stroke prevention through community screening for atrial fibrillation using iPhone ECG in pharmacies. The SEARCH-AF study. Thromb Haemost 2014;111:1167–76.

21. Halcox JPJ, Wareham K, Cardew A, et al. Assessment of remote heart rhythm sampling using the AliveCor heart monitor to screen for atrial fibrillation: the REHEARSE-AF study. Circulation 2017;136: 1784–94.

22. Van Gelder IC, Healey JS, Crijns HJ, et al. Duration of device-detected subclinical atrial fibrillation and occurrence of stroke in ASSERT. Eur Heart J 2017; 38(17):1339–44.

23. Lopes RD, Alings M, Connolly SJ, et al. Rationale and design of the Apixaban for the reduction of thrombo-embolism in patients with device-detected sub-clinical atrial fibrillation (ARTESiA) trial. Am Heart J 2017;189:137–45.

24. Kirchhof P, Blank BF, Calvert M, et al. Probing oral anticoagulation in patients with atrial high rate episodes: rationale and design of the Non-vitamin K antagonist Oral anticoagulants in patients with Atrial High rate episodes (NOAH-AFNET 6) trial. Am Heart J 2017;190:12–8.

25. Camm AJ, Kirchhof P, Lip GY, et al. Guidelines for the management of atrial fibrillation: the task force for the management of atrial fibrillation of the European Society of Cardiology (ESC). Eur Heart J 2010;31:2369–429.

26. Mairesse GH, Moran P, Van Gelder IC, et al. Screening for atrial fibrillation: a European Heart Rhythm Association (EHRA) consensus document

endorsed by the Heart Rhythm Society (HRS), Asia Pacific Heart Rhythm Society (APHRS), and Sociedad Latinoamericana de Estimulación Cardíaca y Electrofisiología (SOLAECE). Europace 2017;19:1589–623.

27. Kearley K, Selwood M, Van den Bruel A, et al. Triage tests for identifying atrial fibrillation in primary care: a diagnostic accuracy study comparing single-lead ECG and modified BP monitors. BMJ Open 2014;4:e004565.

28. Tung CE, Su D, Turakhia MP, et al. Diagnostic yield of extended cardiac patch monitoring in patients with stroke or TIA. Front Neurol 2014;5:266.

29. Turakhia MP, Desai M, Hedlin H, et al. Rationale and design of a large-scale, app-based study to identify cardiac arrhythmias using a smartwatch: the Apple Heart Study. Am Heart J 2019;207:66–75.

30. Marazzi G, Iellamo F, Volterrani M, et al. Comparison of Microlife BP A200 Plus and Omron M6 blood pressure monitors to detect atrial fibrillation in hypertensive patients. Adv Ther 2012;29:64–70 [Erratum appears in Adv Ther 2014;31(12):1317].

31. Wiesel J, Fitzig L, Herschman Y, et al. Detection of atrial fibrillation using a modified Microlife blood pressure monitor. Am J Hypertens 2009;22:848–52.

32. Muntner P, Shimbo D, Carey RM, et al. Measurement of blood pressure in humans: a scientific statement from the American Heart Association. Hypertension 2019;73:e35–66.

33. Verberk WJ, Omboni S, Kollias A, et al. Screening for atrial fibrillation with automated blood pressure measurement: research evidence and practice recommendations. Int J Cardiol 2016;203:465–73.

34. Orchard J, Lowres N, Freedman B, et al. Screening for atrial fibrillation during influenza vaccinations by primary care nurses using a smartphone electrocardiograph (iECG): a feasibility study. Eur J Prev Cardiol 2016;23(2 suppl):13–20.

35. Kaasenbrood F, Hollander M, Rutten FH, et al. Yield of screening for atrial fibrillation in primary care with a hand-held, single-lead electrocardiogram device during influenza vaccination. Europace 2016;18:1514–20.

36. Willits I, Keltie K, Craig J, et al. WatchBP Home A for opportunistically detecting atrial fibrillation during diagnosis and monitoring of hypertension: a NICE Medical Technology Guidance. Appl Health Econ Health Pol 2014;12:255–65.

37. Quinn FR, Gladstone DJ, Ivers NM, et al. Diagnostic accuracy and yield of screening tests for atrial fibrillation in the family practice setting: a multicentre cohort study. CMAJ Open 2018;6:E308–15.

38. Tarride JE, Quinn FR, Blackhouse G, et al. Is screening for atrial fibrillation in Canadian family practices cost-effective in patients 65 years and older? Can J Cardiol 2018;34:1522–5.

39. Huxley RR, Lopez FL, Folsom AR, et al. Absolute and attributable risks of atrial fibrillation in relation to optimal and borderline risk factors: the Atherosclerosis Risk in Communities (ARIC) study. Circulation 2011;123:1501–8.

40. Oldgren J, Healey JS, Ezekowitz M, et al. Variations in cause and management of atrial fibrillation in a prospective registry of 15,400 emergency department patients in 46 countries: the RE-LY Atrial Fibrillation Registry. Circulation 2014;129:1568–76.

41. Yusuf S, Healey JS, Pogue J, et al. Irbesartan in patients with atrial fibrillation. N Engl J Med 2011;364:928–38.

42. Connolly SJ, Ezekowitz MD, Yusuf S, et al. Dabigatran versus warfarin in patients with atrial fibrillation. N Engl J Med 2009;361:1139–51.

43. Healey JS, Wharton S, Al-Kaabi S, et al. Stroke prevention in patients with atrial fibrillation: the diagnosis and management of hypertension by specialists. Can J Cardiol 2006;22:485–8.

44. Gami AS, Pressman G, Caples SM, et al. Association of atrial fibrillation and obstructive sleep apnea. Circulation 2004;110:364–7.

45. Gami AS, Hodge DO, Herges RM, et al. Obstructive sleep apnea, obesity, and the risk of incident atrial fibrillation. J Am Coll Cardiol 2007;49:565–71.

46. Chanda A, Wolff A, McPherson C, et al. Utility of extended cardiac monitoring to detect atrial fibrillation in patients with severe obstructive sleep apnea. Sleep Breath 2015;19:407–10.

47. Mehra R, Benjamin EJ, Shahar E, et al. Association of nocturnal arrhythmias with sleep-disordered breathing: the sleep heart health study. Am J Respir Crit Care Med 2006;173:910–6.

48. Leung RS, Huber MA, Rogge T, et al. Association between atrial fibrillation and central sleep apnea. Sleep 2005;28:1543–6.

49. Hendrikx T, Sundqvist M, Sandström H, et al. Atrial fibrillation among patients under investigation for suspected obstructive sleep apnea. PLoS One 2017;12:e0171575.

50. Tedrow UB, Conen D, Ridker PM, et al. The long- and short-term impact of elevated body mass index on the risk of new atrial fibrillation the WHS (women's health study). J Am Coll Cardiol 2010;55:2319–27.

51. Sandhu RK, Conen D, Tedrow UB, et al. Predisposing factors associated with development of persistent compared with paroxysmal atrial fibrillation. J Am Heart Assoc 2014;3:e000916.

52. Pathak RK, Middeldorp ME, Meredith M, et al. Long-term effect of goal-directed weight management in an atrial fibrillation cohort: a long-term follow-up study (LEGACY). J Am Coll Cardiol 2015;65:2159–69.

53. Brandes A, Smit MD, Nguyen BO, et al. Risk factor management in atrial fibrillation. Arrhythm Electrophysiol Rev 2018;7:118–27.

54. Fioravanti F, Brisinda D, Sorbo AR, et al. BMI reduction decreases AF recurrence rate in a Mediterranean cohort. J Am Coll Cardiol 2015;66: 2264–5.

55. Middeldorp ME, Pathak RK, Meredith M, et al. PREVEntion and regReSsive Effect of weight-loss and risk factor modification on Atrial Fibrillation: the REVERSE-AF study. Europace 2018;20:1929–35.

56. Pathak RK, Evans M, Middeldorp ME, et al. Cost-effectiveness and clinical effectiveness of the risk factor management clinic in atrial fibrillation: the CENT study. JACC Clin Electrophysiol 2017;3: 436–47.

57. European Heart Rhythm Association, European Association for Cardio-Thoracic Surgery, Camm AJ, Kirchhof P, Lip GY, et al. Guidelines for the management of atrial fibrillation: the task force for the management of atrial fibrillation of the European Society of Cardiology (ESC). Europace 2010;12: 1360–420.

58. Andrade JG, Verma A, Mitchell LB, et al. 2018 focused update of the Canadian Cardiovascular Society guidelines for the management of atrial fibrillation. Can J Cardiol 2018;34:1371–92.

59. Tran HN, Tafreshi J, Hernandez EA, et al. A multidisciplinary atrial fibrillation clinic. Curr Cardiol Rev 2013;9:55–62.

60. Conti A, Canuti E, Mariannini Y, et al. Clinical management of atrial fibrillation: early interventions, observation, and structured follow-up reduce hospitalizations. Am J Emerg Med 2012;30:1962–9.

61. Carter L, Gardner M, Magee K, et al. An integrated management approach to atrial fibrillation. J Am Heart Assoc 2016;5.

62. Hendriks JM, de Wit R, Crijns HJ, et al. Nurse-led care vs. usual care for patients with atrial fibrillation: results of a randomized trial of integrated chronic care vs. routine clinical care in ambulatory patients with atrial fibrillation. Eur Heart J 2012;33: 2692–9.

Atrial Fibrillation and Stroke

Hani Essa, MRes, Mrcp[a], Andrew M. Hill, MSc, FRCP[a,b], Gregory Y.H. Lip, MD FRCP[a,c],*

KEYWORDS

• Atrial fibrillation • Stroke • Cardioembolic • Embolic stroke • AF • Warfarin

KEY POINTS

- Atrial fibrillation is the most common cardiac arrythmia and the most common preventable cause of cardioembolic stroke, accounting for 23.7% of all stokes.
- The principal guiding management of stroke in atrial fibrillation is prevention of cardioembolic stroke and systemic thromboembolism via oral anticoagulation.
- Oral anticoagulation is effective in the prevention of strokes secondary to atrial fibrillation, reducing overall stroke numbers by approximately 64%.

INTRODUCTION

Atrial fibrillation (AF) is the most common cardiac arrythmia[1] and is one of the major causes of stroke, heart failure, sudden death, and cardiovascular morbidity in the world. It is estimated that 25% of adults in Europe and the United States eventually will develop AF.[2,3] The incidence of AF is increasing due to a combination of improved detection rates,[4] increasing age, and comorbidities predisposing to AF.[5] The focus of this article is to review the literature with regard to AF and stroke and its investigations and management.

In 1814, a thrombus was demonstrated inside the left atrium in a patient with AF,[6] and in 1847 Virchow published his triad of predisposing factors to thrombus formation: this triad refers to abnormalities of blood flow, abnormalities of vessel well, and abnormal blood constituents.[7] In 1930, it was demonstrated on studies via autopsy that AF leads to cardiac thrombi,[8] whereas in 1978, epidemiologic data from the Framingham study reported an increased risk of stroke in patients with AF.[9]

Cohort studies previously demonstrated that approximately 20% to 30% of patients presenting with an ischemic stroke have AF diagnosed before, during, or after the initial event.[4,10]

Large vessel occlusions (LVOs) are ischemic strokes affecting the proximal middle cerebral artery or basilar system. LVO strokes are more likely to have AF prestroke,[11] and LVO stroke is associated with a greater probability of identifying poststroke AF.[12] LVOs are associated with larger neurologic deficits and significantly worse rates of disability and stroke than non-LVO strokes.[13] This is reflected in clinical audit outcome data: AF-associated stroke carries a 46% chance of significant disability (modified Rankin Scale score at hospital discharge of 3–5) and a 25% chance of death versus a 40% chance of significant disability and 13.5% chance of death in the overall stroke population.[14]

Atrial Fibrillation after Stroke—Evidence for the Neurogenic Hypothesis

Acute subarachnoid hemorrhage results in myocardial injury and stunning.[15] Extrapolating this knowledge to stroke, some reports suggest that some AF may represent the consequence of

[a] Liverpool Centre for Cardiovascular Science, University of Liverpool and Liverpool Heart and Chest Hospital, Thomas Drive, Liverpool L14 3PE, UK; [b] Department of Medicine for Older People, St Helens and Knowsley Teaching Hospitals NHS Trust, Marshalls Cross Road, St Helens, Liverpool WA9 3DA, UK; [c] Aalborg Thrombosis Research Unit, Department of Clinical Medicine, Aalborg University, Sondra Skovvej, 15, Aalborg 9000, Denmark

* Corresponding author. Liverpool Centre for Cardiovascular Science, University of Liverpool and Liverpool Heart and Chest Hospital, Thomas Drive, Liverpool L14 3PE, United Kingdom.
E-mail address: gregory.lip@liverpool.ac.uk

Card Electrophysiol Clin 13 (2021) 243–255
https://doi.org/10.1016/j.ccep.2020.11.003

brain damage that is induced by the ischemic stroke rather than its cause per se.[16] In this scenario, AF may be induced by imbalances of sympathetic and parasympathetic activity with resulting myocardial changes poststroke, giving rise to the so-called neurogenic AF theory.[17] This was explored in a network mendelian randomization study exploring the causal pathway from ischemic stroke to AF.[18,19] One retrospective study suggested that that AF discovered after stroke confers a lower risk of future stroke compared with preexisting AF, which could be related to a different underlying etiology of AF post stroke[17]; however, other studies have failed to validate these findings.[20]

The risk of thromboembolic disease generally is similar between paroxysmal and persistent AF.[21,22] These findings are not consistently reported, however, across all studies, given that risk is driven by the presence of stroke risk factors.[23,24] Also, paroxysmal AF is heterogeneous given that there is a wide range in arrhythmia burden.

Even a single brief episode of AF is linked to higher rates of stroke in patients above 65 year old[25]; however, these findings are not evident in younger, lower-risk patients.[26] There also is the perception that a rhythm control strategy should reduce stasis and result in a lower stroke burden if the main etiology of the cardioembolic events is stasis, but the risks of stroke with a rhythm control strategy are the same as with a rate control strategy.[27] AF recurrences after rhythm control are common and often asymptomatic. Hence, the theory of stasis resulting in thrombosis and resultant cardioembolic events is simplistic. The etiology of stroke in AF is more complex than this.[28]

DIAGNOSIS, RISK ASSESSMENT, AND MANAGEMENT
Diagnosis of Atrial Fibrillation Poststroke and Embolic Stroke of Undetermined Source

In patients presenting with acute ischemic stroke it is essential that careful evaluation is undertaken to elucidate the underlying etiology so that appropriate secondary prevention can be started. Electrocardiogram monitoring poststroke has been demonstrated to pick up AF in between 11.5%[4] and 23.7%[29] of patients, depending on the methodology utilized by the metanalysis. The chances of picking up AF appear to increase with increasing duration of monitoring, so clinicians need to look harder, look longer, and look using more sophisticated methods to improve the diagnosis rate.[30–32]

In patients with implantable cardioverter-defibrillators, subclinical episodes of AF are picked up in the absence of clinical symptoms of AF.[33] The role of emerging technologies, such as smartwatches, as an investigative tool to diagnose asymptomatic AF via long-term monitoring has been demonstrated.[34,35] The role of this in the diagnostics pathway is as yet unclear, but the capability of the technology potentially can revolutionize the process with large-scale screening.

Embolic stroke of undetermined source (ESUS) is defined as a stroke in which the cause cannot be identified after extensive investigations.[36] This represents as many as 20% of all strokes.[33] There has been an argument that all ESUS is undiscovered AF that would benefit from oral anticoagulation (OAC). Prospective data have demonstrated that aggressive investigation of ESUS can pick up AF in 12.4% of patients after the index stroke.[37] This has resulted in 2 separate randomized controlled trials (RCTs) investigating both rivaroxaban[38] and dabigatran[39] compared with standard antiplatelet therapy in the treatment of ESUS. Both failed to demonstrate any benefit of an OAC over standard aspirin therapy.

Stratification of Stroke Risk in Atrial Fibrillation

The proportion of stroke associated with AF increases progressively with age, ranging from 6.7% in individuals aged 50 years to 59 years to 36.2% in those aged 80 years to 89 years.[9,40] There are many stroke risk factors and the more common and validated ones have been used to formulate stroke risk stratification schemes, and, of the most popular ones, the most validated are the $CHADS_2$ (Congestive cardiac failure, hypertension, Age $\geq$ 75, Diabetes mellitus history, Stroke or transient ischemic attack symptoms previously) and CHA_2DS_2 -VASc scores (congestive cardiac failure, hypertension, Age $\geq$ 75, diabetes Mellitus, prior stroke, previous transient ischemic event/stroke/thromboembolism, vascular disease, age 65-74 years, female sex)[41,42] The CHA_2DS_2-VASc score is shown in **Table 1** and has been extensively validated[43–45] and adopted in guidelines.[46–48] Typical of a score based on clinical factors, CHA_2DS_2-VASc score has only modest predictive value for identifying high-risk patients who sustain events and, even then, is a mere simplification of a more complex scenario. These risk factors are dynamic, and stroke risk in AF is altered by increasing age and incident risk factors.[49] Also, individual risk factors within the points of the CHA_2DS_2-VASc score do not carry equal

Table 1
CHA$_2$DS$_2$–VASc risk stratification tool breakdown for assessment of stroke risk in patients with underlying atrial fibrillation

CHA$_2$ DS$_2$–VASc Risk Factor	Score

Congestive heart failure
  Signs/symptoms of heart failure or objective
    evidence of reduced left vntricular ejection
    fraction
	+ 1 point

Hypertension
  Current hypertensive therapy or resting blood
    pressure >140/90 mm hg on at least 2 occasions
	+ 1 point

Age 75 or older	+ 2 points

Diabetes mellitus
  Current diabetes therapy or based on hemoglobin
    A$_{1c}$
	+ 1 point

Previous stroke, transient ischemic attack, or thromboembolism	+ 1 point

Vascular disease
  Previous myocardial infarction, peripheral artery
    disease, or aortic plaque
	+ 1 point

Age 65–74	+ 1 point
Sex category Female	+ 1 point

Abbreviations: CHA2DS2-VASc, congestive cardiac failure, hypertension, Age ≥ 75, diabetes Mellitus, prior stroke, previous transient ischemic event/stroke/thromboembolism, vascular disease, age 65-74 years, female sex. Each factor earns 1 point except for Age ≥ 75 and a history of transient ischemic event/stroke/thromboembolism which earn 2 points.

weight for stroke risk and how they change over time.[50,51] There are other possible risk factors for stroke in AF that are not accounted for in the CHA$_2$DS$_2$-VASc scoring system. More complex risk stratification schemes have been proposed (some including biomarkers), which may offer statistically significant improvements but are less practical for use in everyday clinical practice.[52]

Medical Management in Prevention of Stroke in Atrial Fibrillation

OAC therapy has been proved to prevent a vast majority cardioembolic events in AF patients and prolong life, as shown in clinical trials and observational cohorts.[53–55]

The vitamin K antagonists (VKAs), for example, warfarin, have been the main OAC for more than 50 years, and in the historical AF trials, warfarin was associated with a 64% reduction in stroke and 26% reduction in all-cause mortality compared with control or placebo.[54] The efficacy and safety of the VKAs are dependent on the quality of anticoagulation control, as reflected by time in therapeutic range, with a target international normalized ratio (INR) 2.0 of 3.0.[56] There is limited evidence supporting a lower target INR range, which often is promoted in some countries.[57,58]

Measures to improve adherence and persistence with treatment and updates of guideline-based management should be promoted.[59,60] These are important because OAC cessation and nonpersistence are associated with worse outcomes.[61]

More recently, the non-VKA OACs (NOACs), also called direct oral anticoagulants (DOACs), have been introduced and offer improved effectiveness, safety and convenience compared with the VKAs based on their RCTs[62–65] (**Table 2**) and large postmarketing real-world observational studies.[66–69] The NOACs include a direct thrombin inhibitor (dabigatran) and the oral factor Xa inhibitors (rivaroxaban, apixaban, and edoxaban) (**Fig. 1**).

A metanalysis of 71,683 participants in the pivotal phase 3 RCTs demonstrated that the DOACs reduced stroke or systemic embolic events by 19% compared with warfarin (relative risk [RR] 0.81; 95% CI, 0.73–0.91; P<0.0001), mainly driven by a reduction in hemorrhagic stroke (RR 0.49; 95% CI, 0.38–0.64; P<0.0001).[70] DOACs reduced all-cause mortality (RR 0.90; 95% CI, 0.85–0.95; P = 0.0003) and intracranial hemorrhage (RR 0.48; 95% CI, 0.39–0.59; P<0.0001) but increased gastrointestinal bleeding (RR 1.25; 95% CI, 1.01–1.55; P = 0.04), compared with warfarin.

Table 2
Evidence table for the direct oral anticoagulants

Active-drug cells show "% per year (effect estimate, 95% CI)"; Warfarin cells show "% per Year". Effect estimates are Relative Risk for Dabigatran (RE-LY) and Hazard Ratio for the other trials.

Trial, Year	Dabigatran 110 mg BD (RE-LY,[58] 2009)	Dabigatran 150 mg BD	Warfarin as per INR	Rivaroxaban 20 mg OD (ROCKET-AF,[60] 2011)	Warfarin as per INR	Apixaban 5 mg BD (ARISTOTLE,[59] 2011)	Warfarin as per INR	Edoxaban 60 mg OD	Edoxaban 30 mg OD (ENGAGE AF TIMI 48,[61] 2014)	Warfarin as per INR
Number of patients	6015	6076	6022	7131	7133	9088	9052	7035	7034	7036
Follow-up period (years)	2			1.9		1.8			2.8	
Age, years	71.5 ± 8.7 (Mean ± SD)			73 (65–78) [median (interquartile range)]		70 (63–76) [median (interquartile range)]			72 (64–78) [median (interquartile range)]	
Mean CHA$_2$DS$_2$-VASc	2.1			3.5		2.1			2.8	
Stroke/systemic embolism	1.53%[a] (0.91, 0.74–1.11)	1.11%[a] (0.66, 0.53–0.82)	1.69%	2.1 (0.88, 0.75–1.03)	2.4%	1.27%[a] (0.79, 0.66–0.95)	1.6%	1.57% (0.87, 0.73–1.04)	2.04% (1.13, 0.96–1.34)	1.8%
Major bleeding	2.71%[a] (0.80, 0.69–0.93)	3.11% (0.93, 0.81–1.07)	3.36%	3.60% (1.04; 0.90–2.30; P = .58)	3.45%	2.13%[a] (0.69, 0.60–0.80)	3.09%	2.75%[a] (0.80, 0.71–0.91)	1.61%[a] (0.47, 0.41–0.55)	3.43%
Intracerebral bleeding	0.23%[a] (0.31, 0.12–0.47)	0.30%[a] (0.42, 0.29–0.61)	0.74%	0.49%[a] (0.67; 0.47–0.93)	0.74%	0.33%[a] (0.42, 0.30–0.58)	0.8%	0.39%[a] (0.47, 0.34–0.63)	0.26%[a] (0.30, 0.21–0.43)	0.85%
Death	3.75% (0.91, 0.80–1.03)	3.64% (0.88, 0.77–1.00)	4.13%	1.87% (0.85; 0.70–1.02)	2.21%	3.52%[a] (0.89, 0.80–0.99)	3.94%	3.99% (0.92, 0.83–1.01)	3.80% (0.87, 0.79–0.96)	4.35%

Abbreviations: ARISTOTLE, Apixaban for Reduction in Stroke and Other Thromboembolic Events in Atrial Fibrillation) trial[59]; ENGAGE AF-TIMI 48, Effective Anticoagulation With Factor Xa Next Generation in Atrial Fibrillation–Thrombolysis In Myocardial Infarction Study 48[61]; RE-LY, Randomized Evaluation of Long-Term Anticoagulation Therapy)[58]; ROCKET AF, Rivaroxaban Once Daily Oral Direct Factor Xa Inhibition Compared With Vitamin K Antagonism for Prevention of Stroke And Embolism Trial in Atrial Fibrillation;[60] SD, standard deviation; OD, once daily; BD, twice daily; INR, international normalized ratio.

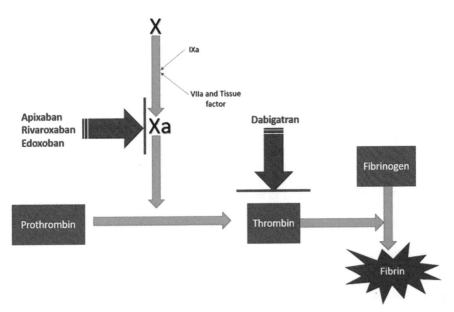

Fig. 1. Mechanism of action of direct oral anticoagulants.

Individually, each of the RCTs had a proportion of AF patients with prior stroke, and meta-analyses of these secondary prevention patients have been reported.[70,71] There was a significant reduction in the rate of stroke or systemic embolism (RR 0.86; 95% CI, 0.77–0.97), mainly from a reduction in hemorrhagic stroke (RR 0.45; 95% CI, 0.33–0.61) but not ischemic stroke (RR 0.98; 95% CI, 0.85–1.13). Major bleeding was lowered (RR 0.86; 95% CI, 0.77–0.96), and there was a nonsignificant trend to a lower rate of all-case death (RR 0.89; 95% CI, 0.82–0.97).

In patients with AF who were unable or unwilling to take a VKA, apixaban was compared with aspirin in the Apixaban vs Aspirin to Reduce the Risk of Stroke (AVERROES) trial.[72] The trial was stopped early, because apixaban was more effective than aspirin for the prevention of stroke and systemic embolic events, with similar risks for major bleeding and intracranial hemorrhage. The results were consistent in the secondary prevention cohort from AVERROES.[73]

Aside from the RCT data, so-called real-world registries and observational cohorts have been published, comparing NOACs to warfarin and to each other. The largest of the retrospective data sets published was the Anticoagulants for Reduction in Stroke: Observational Pooled Analysis on Health Outcomes and Experience of Patients (ARISTOPHANES) study,[67] which showed that the NOACs had lower rates of stroke/systemic embolism and variable comparative rates of major bleeding versus warfarin. Similar data have been published from Europe,[66,69] Korea, and Taiwan.[74,75]

Appropriate strategies for ensuring patients with known AF are on anticoagulation if appropriate remains one of the biggest challenges in stroke prevention. Sentinel Stroke National Audit Programme, a prospective audit of stroke care in England, Wales, and Northern Ireland, with 98% national case ascertainment, have shown that in 2018/2019, 64% of patients with known AF are on an anticoagulant at the time of their stroke (an improvement from 38% in 2013/2014).[76]

Nonmedical Management in the Prevention of Stroke in Atrial Fibrillation

Left atrial appendage occlusion

More than 90% of stroke-causing cardioembolic clots are formed in the left atrial appendage[77] (LAA), whereas in AF related to valvular heart disease (VHD), this is approximately 57%.[77] There has been a growth in LAA occlusion/closure/exclusion strategies seeking to provide an alternative treatment modality, especially where OACs are intolerable or pose too high a bleeding risk. Also, in patients with known AF, noncompliance rates are high, with only approximately 50% actually taking OACs.[78] Furthermore, the rates of life-threatening bleeds on warfarin have been shown to vary from 1.3% to 7.2% per year.[79] When compared with warfarin, DOACs have a lower but nonetheless still significant bleeding risk.[80] Therefore, there is an unmet need for the prevention of stroke in patients with AF unable to tolerate OAC for a variety of reasons.

There are 2 RCTs comparing percutaneous left atrial appendage occlusion (LAAO) to an OAC;

both are for the Watchman device: the Watchman (Boston scientific, United states) Left Atrial Appendage System for Embolic Protection in Patients With Atrial Fibrillation (PROTECT AF)[81] was a multicenter RCT of 707 patients allocated to LAA closure with the Watchman device or warfarin as per INR. The mean follow-up period was 18 months and the primary outcome was a composite outcome of stroke, cardiovascular or unexplained death, or systemic embolism. The primary composite endpoints (event/patient year [PY]) were 21/694.1 versus 18/370.8 (RR 0.62; 95% CI, 0.35–1.25), respectively, with a trend to more ischemic strokes; however, primary safety events (major bleeding, pericardial effusion, and device embolization) were more frequent in the intervention group than in the control group.

The Prospective Randomized Evaluation of the Watchman Left Atrial Appendage Closure Device In Patients with AF Versus Long Term Warfarin Therapy (PREVAIL)[82] trial was a multicenter RCT of 407 participants allocating patients to the Watchman device or warfarin as per INR. The mean follow-up was 11.8 months was and the primary endpoint was a composite of stroke, systemic embolism, and cardiovascular/unexplained death. At 18 months, the primary outcome occurred was not significantly different (rate ratio 1.07; 95% CI, 0.57–1.89). In both the PREVAIL and PROTECT AF trials, LAA occlusion was noninferior to warfarin in the prevention of stroke in patients with AF with possibly lower bleeding rate. A patient-level meta-analysis[83] of the 2 trials and their associated registries demonstrated that over a mean follow-up period of 2.69 years, patients receiving LAA occlusion with the Watchman device had fewer hemorrhagic strokes (0.15 events/100 PY vs 0.96 events/100 PY; hazard ratio [HR] 0.22; P = .004), cardiovascular/unexplained death (1.1 events/100 PY vs 2.3 events/100 PY; HR 0.48; P = .006), and nonprocedural bleeding (6.0% events/100 PY vs 11.3% events/100 PY; HR 0.51; P = .006) compared with warfarin. Overall all-cause stroke and embolism were similar between both strategies; however, ischemic strokes were more common in the device group (1.6 events/100 PY vs 0.9 events/100 PY and 0.2 events/100 PY vs 1.0 events/100 PY; HRs 1.95 and 0.22, respectively; P = .05 and P = .004, respectively). These trials suffer methodological shortcoming, limiting widespread adoption so far, and have been subject to critical discussions.[84,85]

The PRAGUE-17[86] trial was an RCT of 415 patients with AF randomized to DOAC or LAA (via the Watchman or Amplatzer device (Abbot, United States), with a mean duration of follow-up on 20.8 months. The results are not yet unpublished,

with some provisional data presented in the 2019 European society of cardiology meeting. The primary net outcome of cardiovascular death, stroke/transient ischemic attack, systemic embolism, clinically significant bleeding, or significant procedure/device-related complication was similar between the 2 treatment groups (HR 0.84; P for noninferiority = 0.004).

Surgical left atrial appendage occlusion

Excision of the LAA during cardiac surgery or utilizing a minimally invasive approach is another prophylactic technique for prevention of thromboembolic disease in AF. Multiple procedures and techniques historically have been used, including oversewing, excision, ligation, and stapling.[87]

Most data on surgical LAA are observational. A 2015[88] meta-analysis of 7 studies with 3653 patients evaluating surgical LAAO versus LAA preservation in patients with AF showed a significant reduction in the risk of stroke (odds ratio [OR] 0.46; 95% CI, 0.27–0.79; P = .005) and death (OR 0.38; 95% CI, 0.22–0.64; P = .0003) in favor of surgical LAA. In 2017, a national observational case-control study of 1304 patients compared LAAO with those who did not undergo LAAO concomitantly in cardiac surgery and found that LAAO was associated with a significant reduction of in-hospital stroke events (2.5% vs 4.6%, respectively; P = .04) and in-hospital mortality (1.5% vs 4.9%, respectively; P = .001).[89]

Gillinov and colleagues,[90] however, reported a small RCT of 260 patients with mitral valve disease and AF undergoing valvular surgery who were randomized to surgical LAAO or no procedure, with no difference in primary endpoints (composite of death, stroke, increasing heart failure symptoms, hospitalization for heart failure, and mitral valve reoperation), which occurred in 20.5% versus 23.3% (P = .58) in the control versus surgical LAAO groups, respectively. An ongoing RCT, the LAAOS III, is looking at 4700 patients with AF undergoing cardiac surgery randomized to LAAO or no procedure.[91]

Atrial Fibrillation with Valvular Heart Disease and Stroke

The management of AF traditionally was subdivided into nonvalvular and valvular AF, with the latter having either rheumatic valvular disease (predominantly mitral stenosis) or mechanical heart valves.[92] Valvular AF has been correlated with substantially higher burden of cardioembolic disease.[9,93,94]

More recently, the definition of valvular AF is subject to marked heterogeneity in the literature.

A survey of European cardiologists demonstrated that just 57% felt that the definition in guidelines is sufficiently clear.[95] A 2017 European consensus commented that the term VHD is outdated and proposed a new classification on the basis of a more functional evaluated heart valves, rheumatic or artificial (EHRA) categorization in relation to the type of OAC used in patients with AF.[96] This categorization defines EHRA type 1 patients as those with AF and VHD requiring therapy with VKA. The VHD considered in this category are only mechanical prosthetic valves or rheumatic mitral stenosis with moderate–severe dysfunction. EHRA type 2 patients are those with AF and all other types of valve disease, who can be anticoagulated with either a VKA or a NOAC.

The landmark trials comparing DOACs and warfarin in AF all have excluded AF patients with EHRA type I VHD. One phase II trial of dabigatran (RE-ALIGN) demonstrated an increased rate of cardioembolic and bleeding events compared with warfarin in patients with mechanical heart valves.[97] A metanalysis of 13,585 patients from the 4 phase III AF trials comparing NOACS versus warfarin in patients with coexisting VHD demonstrated similar overall efficacy and safety in AF patients with or without VHD.[98] Patients with mitral stenosis never have been randomized to alternative treatment apart from warfarin and currently there is no evidence to suggest a differential response.[99]

Bleeding Risk Stratification in Atrial Fibrillation

Anticoagulation is not without its risks, mainly that of increased bleeding rates. Patient-specific risks and benefits of anticoagulation must be weighed carefully in all patients who are potential candidates for long-term anticoagulation therapy.

A meta-analysis[100] of 8 RCTs with 55,789 patients reported that annual rates of major bleeding varied from 1.4% to 3.5% among patients with AF treated with warfarin. The risk of intracerebral hemorrhage (ICH) was reported to be 0.61%: a disproportionately large amount of overall morbidity and mortality of bleeding events on an OAC. On discharge, 75% of ICH patients had severe disability or death, compared with only 3% of those with extracranial hemorrhage.[101]

ICHs represent approximately 11% of strokes. Prognosis is significantly worse than for cerebral infarctions, with mortality rates of approximately 33%, with only one-third returning to functional independence and with outcomes significantly worse for those on an anticoagulant at event onset.[102]

Multiple scoring systems exist to attempt to weigh this risk[103]; the most validated is the hypertension, abnormal renal/liver function, stroke, bleeding history or predisposition, labile INR, elderly (>65 years), drugs/alcohol concomitantly (1 point each) (HAS-BLED) score.[42,104] As a clinical risk score, it performs modestly in predicting events and has been validated to predict bleeding in all parts of the patient journey, when first diagnosed on aspirin or no antithrombotic therapy and when on VKA or NOACs. Although bleeding and stroke risks track each other, numerous studies show that a formal bleeding risk score outperforms stroke risk scores, such as CHADS$_2$ and CHA$_2$DS$_2$-VASc, for predicting bleeding risk.[104–107] More complicated bleeding risk scores, or those incorporating biomarkers, have not shown practical advantage in real-world

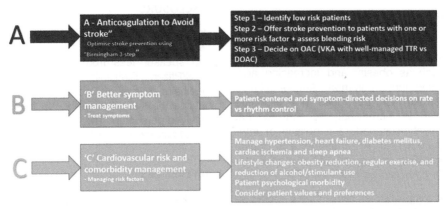

Fig. 2. The Atrial fibrillation Better Care (ABC) pathway for holistic management. Step A is to identify which patients are at risk of stroke and require oral anticoagulation (OAC). Step B is to focus on better symptom control for patients and 3 C is to manage cardiovascular risk and comorbidities. VKA; Vitamin K antagonist, TTR; Time in therapeutic range, DOAC; Direct oral anticoagulant.

clinical practice[108–110] nor have they been adequately validated in all steps of the patient journey.[111]

Bleeding risk assessment often is misused by the ill-informed. A high bleeding risk score generally should not result in withholding OAC. Rather, appropriate use of a bleeding risk score, such as HAS-BLED, is to mitigate the modifiable bleeding risk factors and to flag high bleeding risk patients for early review and follow-up. In the mobile atrial fibrillation application (mAFA)-II trial, dynamic risk monitoring using the HAS-BLED score, together with holistic mobile application-based management using mAFA-II reduced bleeding events, facilitated mitigation of modifiable bleeding risks, resulting in lowered major bleeding events and increased uptake of OACs over 12 months compared with usual care.[112]

Stroke Despite Anticoagulation

Patients with AF still may suffer strokes despite being on OAC, and a common reason for this often is subtherapeutic anticoagulation.[113] Patients who have strokes while on OAC therapy are at higher risk of future stroke compared with those who are OAC-naive (8.9% vs 3.9%, respectively).[114] Patients who have a stroke despite appropriate anticoagulation present a clinical challenge, and it is unknown if switching OAC (VKA to DOAC, DOAC to VKA, or DOAC to other DOAC) confers any advantages. The stroke may occur through other mechanisms (eg, noncardioembolic stroke),[115] and it is important to ensure that patients are compliant with their treatment and taking guideline-adherent dosing. Also, uncontrolled blood pressure or carotid stenosis should be managed.

SUMMARY

AF is the most common cardiac arrythmia, and its prevalence is expected to increase as risk factors, such as obesity and increasing age, are becoming more common. Anticoagulation reduces stroke risk but does not eliminate it.[113] It also is increasingly recognized that stroke prevention is part of a holistic or integrated approach to AF management, which can be simplified as the atrial fibrillation better care (ABC) pathway, as follows[48,116]:

- A: anticoagulation to avoid stroke—anticoagulation with NOAC or well-managed warfarin
- B: better symptom management with patient-centered, symptom-directed shared decisions for rate or rhythm control
- C: cardiovascular risk and comorbidity management (blood pressure, sleep apnea, and so forth) plus lifestyle changes (weight reduction, regular exercise, reducing alcohol/stimulants, psychological morbidity, smoking cessation, and so forth)

The value of compliance with ABC pathway (**Fig. 2**) in reducing adverse AF-related clinical outcomes has been investigated in post hoc analyses of clinical trials,[117,118] observational cohorts,[119,120] and a prospective cluster RCT, the mAFA-II trial.[121,122]

CLINICS CARE POINTS

- AF is the most common cardiac arrythmia and cause of preventable stroke.
- Anticoagulation is the mainstream of stroke prevention in AF.
- A decision to anticoagulate should utilize a validated risk stratification tool for stroke and bleeding, such as CHA_2DS_2-VASc and HAS-BLED.
- DOACs are as effective as warfarin in preventing ischemic events and have a lower rate of intracerebral bleeding. There are no trials directly comparing the individual DOACs against each other.
- The management of recurrent strokes despite anticoagulation in AF is unclear and warrants further research.
- Stroke prevention is 1 component of a holistic and integrated approach to AF management, the ABC pathway.

DISCLOSURE

Dr H. Essa and Dr A.M. Hill have nothing to declare. Professor G.Y.H. Lip reports consultancy and speaker fees from Bayer, Bayer/Janssen, BMS/Pfizer, Biotronik, Medtronic, Boehringer Ingelheim, Microlife, Roche, and Daiichi-Sankyo outside the submitted work. No fees have been received personally. The authors declare no sources of funding were utilised for this review.

REFERENCES

1. Rahman F, Kwan GF, Benjamin EJ. Global epidemiology of atrial fibrillation. Nat Rev Cardiol 2014; 11(11):639–54.
2. Heeringa J, van der Kuip DA, Hofman A, et al. Prevalence, incidence and lifetime risk of atrial

fibrillation: the Rotterdam study. Eur Heart J 2006; 27(8):949–53.

3. Lloyd-Jones DM, Wang TJ, Leip EP, et al. Lifetime risk for development of atrial fibrillation: the Framingham heart study. Circulation 2004;110(9): 1042–6.

4. Kishore A, Vail A, Majid A, et al. Detection of atrial fibrillation after ischemic stroke or transient ischemic attack: a systematic review and meta-analysis. Stroke 2014;45(2):520–6.

5. Schnabel RB, Yin X, Gona P, et al. 50 year trends in atrial fibrillation prevalence, incidence, risk factors, and mortality in the Framingham heart study: a cohort study. Lancet 2015;386(9989):154–62.

6. Wood W. History and dissection of a case, in which a foreign body was found within the heart. Edinb Med Surg J 1814;10(37):50–4.

7. Watson T, Shantsila E, Lip GY. Mechanisms of thrombogenesis in atrial fibrillation: Virchow's triad revisited. Lancet 2009 Jan 10;373(9658):155–66. https://doi.org/10.1016/S0140-6736(09)60040-4.

8. Harvey EA, Levine SA. A study of uninfected mural thrombi of the heart. Am J Med Sci 1930;180: 365–71.

9. Wolf PA, Dawber TR, Thomas HE Jr, et al. Epidemiologic assessment of chronic atrial fibrillation and risk of stroke: the Framingham study. Neurology 1978;28(10):973–7.

10. Grond M, Jauss M, Hamann G, et al. Improved detection of silent atrial fibrillation using 72-hour Holter ECG in patients with ischemic stroke: a prospective multicenter cohort study. Stroke 2013; 44(12):3357–64.

11. Inoue M, Noda R, Yamaguchi, et al. Specific factors to predict large vessel occlusion in acute stroke patients. J Stroke Cerebrovasc Dis 2018; 27(4):886–91.

12. Pagola J, Juega J, Francisco-Pascual J, et al. Large vessel occlusion is independently associated with atrial fibrillation detection. Eur J Neurol 2020. https://doi.org/10.1111/ene.14281.

13. Smith WS, Lev MH, English JD, et al. Significance of large vessel intracranial occlusion causing acute ischemic stroke and TIA. Stroke 2009;40(12): 3834–40.

14. Stroke sentinel national audit. Atrial fibrillation outcome data, 2018-19 annual clinical audit results. Kings college london and the health quality improvement programme. Available at. https://www.strokeaudit.org/Documents/National/Clinical/Apr2018Mar2019/Apr2018Mar2019-CCGAFReport .aspx. Accessed May 18, 2020.

15. Kono T, Morita H, Kuroiwa T, et al. Left ventricular wall motion abnormalities in patients with subarachnoid hemorrhage: neurogenic stunned myocardium. J Am Coll Cardiol 1994;24(3):636–40.

16. Gonzalez Toledo ME, Klein FR, Riccio PM, et al. Atrial fibrillation detected after acute ischemic stroke: evidence supporting the neurogenic hypothesis. J Stroke Cerebrovasc Dis 2013;22(8): e486–91.

17. Sposato LA, Riccio PM, Hachinski V. Poststroke atrial fibrillation: cause or consequence? Critical review of current views. Neurology 2014;82(13):1180–6.

18. Hou L, Xu M, Yu Y, et al. Exploring the causal pathway from ischemic stroke to atrial fibrillation: a network Mendelian randomization study. Mol Med 2020;26(1):7.

19. Sposato LA, Cerasuolo JO, Cipriano LE, et al. Atrial fibrillation detected after stroke is related to a low risk of ischemic stroke recurrence. Neurology 2018;90(11):e924–31.

20. Yang XM, Rao ZZ, Gu HQ, et al. Atrial fibrillation known before or detected after stroke share similar risk of ischemic stroke recurrence and death. Stroke 2019;50(5):1124–9.

21. Hohnloser SH, Pajitnev D, Pogue J, et al. Incidence of stroke in paroxysmal versus sustained atrial fibrillation in patients taking oral anticoagulation or combined antiplatelet therapy: an ACTIVE W Substudy. J Am Coll Cardiol 2007;50(22):2156–61.

22. Hart RG, Pearce LA, Rothbart RM, et al. Stroke with intermittent atrial fibrillation: incidence and predictors during aspirin therapy. Stroke prevention in atrial fibrillation investigators. J Am Coll Cardiol 2000;35(1):183–7.

23. Inoue H, Atarashi H, Okumura K, et al. Thromboembolic events in paroxysmal vs. permanent nonvalvular atrial fibrillation. Subanalysis of the J-RHYTHM Registry. Circ J 2014;78(10):2388–93.

24. Senoo K, Lip GY, Lane DA, et al. Residual risk of stroke and death in anticoagulated patients according to the type of atrial fibrillation: AMADEUS trial. Stroke 2015;46(9):2523–8.

25. Healey JS, Connolly SJ, Gold MR, et al. Subclinical atrial fibrillation and the risk of stroke. N Engl J Med 2012;366(2):120–9.

26. Chao TF, Liu CJ, Chen SJ, et al. Atrial fibrillation and the risk of ischemic stroke: does it still matter in patients with a CHA2DS2-VASc score of 0 or 1? Stroke 2012;43(10):2551–5.

27. Al-Khatib SM, Allen LaPointe NM, Chatterjee R, et al. Rate- and rhythm-control therapies in patients with atrial fibrillation: a systematic review. Ann Intern Med 2014;160(11):760–73.

28. Kamel H, Okin PM, Elkind MS, et al. Atrial fibrillation and mechanisms of stroke: time for a new model. Stroke 2016;47(3):895–900.

29. Sposato LA, Cipriano LE, Saposnik G, et al. Diagnosis of atrial fibrillation after stroke and transient ischaemic attack: a systematic review and meta-analysis. Lancet Neurol 2015;14(4):377–87.

30. Steinhubl SR, Waalen J, Edwards AM, et al. Effect of a home-based wearable continuous ECG monitoring patch on detection of undiagnosed atrial fibrillation: the mSToPS randomized clinical trial. JAMA 2018;320(2):146–55.

31. Israel C, Kitsiou A, Kalyani M, et al. Detection of atrial fibrillation in patients with embolic stroke of undetermined source by prolonged monitoring with implantable loop recorders. Thromb Haemost 2017;117(10):1962–9.

32. Wachter R, Freedman B. The role of atrial fibrillation in patients with an embolic stroke of unknown source (ESUS). Thromb Haemost 2017;117(10): 1833–5.

33. Glotzer TV, Daoud EG, Wyse DG, et al. The relationship between daily atrial tachyarrhythmia burden from implantable device diagnostics and stroke risk: the TRENDS study. Circ Arrhythm Electrophysiol 2009;2(5):474–80.

34. Guo Y, Wang H, Zhang H, et al. Mobile photoplethysmographic technology to detect atrial fibrillation. J Am Coll Cardiol 2019;74(19):2365–75.

35. Perez MV, Mahaffey KW, Hedlin H, et al. Large-scale assessment of a smartwatch to identify atrial fibrillation. N Engl J Med 2019;381(20):1909–17.

36. Hart RG, Diener HC, Coutts SB, et al. Embolic strokes of undetermined source: the case for a new clinical construct. Lancet Neurol 2014;13(4): 429–38.

37. Sanna T, Diener HC, Passman RS, et al. Cryptogenic stroke and underlying atrial fibrillation. N Engl J Med 2014;370(26):2478–86.

38. Hart RG, Sharma M, Mundl H, et al. Rivaroxaban for stroke prevention after embolic stroke of undetermined source. N Engl J Med 2018;378(23): 2191–201.

39. Diener HC, Sacco RL, Easton JD, et al. Dabigatran for prevention of stroke after embolic stroke of undetermined source. N Engl J Med 2019;380(20): 1906–17.

40. Arboix A, Cendros V, Besa M, et al. Trends in risk factors, stroke subtypes and outcome. Nineteen-year data from the sagrat cor hospital of barcelona stroke registry. Cerebrovasc Dis 2008;26(5): 509–16.

41. Lip GY, Nieuwlaat R, Pisters R, et al. Refining clinical risk stratification for predicting stroke and thromboembolism in atrial fibrillation using a novel risk factor-based approach: the euro heart survey on atrial fibrillation. Chest 2010;137(2):263–72.

42. Borre ED, Goode A, Raitz G, et al. Predicting thromboembolic and bleeding event risk in patients with non-valvular atrial fibrillation: a systematic review. Thromb Haemost 2018;118(12):2171–87.

43. Ntaios G, Lip GY, Makaritsis K, et al. CHADS(2), CHA(2)S(2)DS(2)-VASc, and long-term stroke outcome in patients without atrial fibrillation. Neurology 2013;80(11):1009–17.

44. Friberg L, Rosenqvist M, Lip GY. Evaluation of risk stratification schemes for ischaemic stroke and bleeding in 182 678 patients with atrial fibrillation: the Swedish atrial fibrillation cohort study. Eur Heart J 2012;33(12):1500–10.

45. Olesen JB, Lip GY, Hansen ML, et al. Validation of risk stratification schemes for predicting stroke and thromboembolism in patients with atrial fibrillation: nationwide cohort study. BMJ 2011;342:d124.

46. Kirchhof P, Benussi S, Kotecha D, et al. 2016 ESC Guidelines for the management of atrial fibrillation developed in collaboration with EACTS. Eur J Cardiothorac Surg 2016;50(5):e1–88.

47. January CT, Wann LS, Calkins H, et al. 2019 AHA/ACC/HRS Focused Update of the 2014 AHA/ACC/HRS guideline for the management of patients with atrial fibrillation: a report of the american college of cardiology/American heart association task force on clinical practice guidelines and the heart rhythm society in collaboration with the society of thoracic surgeons. Circulation 2019;140(2):e125–51.

48. Lip GYH, Banerjee A, Boriani G, et al. Antithrombotic therapy for atrial fibrillation: CHEST guideline and expert panel report. Chest 2018;154(5): 1121–201.

49. Fauchier L, Bodin A, Bisson A, et al. Incident comorbidities, aging and the risk of stroke in 608,108 patients with atrial fibrillation: a nationwide analysis. J Clin Med 2020;9(4):1234.

50. Chao TF, Liao JN, Tuan TC, et al. Incident Comorbidities in patients with atrial fibrillation initially with a CHA2DS2-VASc Score of 0 (Males) or 1 (Females): implications for reassessment of stroke risk in initially 'low-risk' patients. Thromb Haemost 2019;119(7):1162–70.

51. Yoon M, Yang PS, Jang E, et al. Dynamic changes of CHA2DS2-VASc score and the risk of ischaemic stroke in asian patients with atrial fibrillation: a nationwide cohort study. Thromb Haemost 2018; 118(7):1296–304.

52. Proietti M, Mujovic N, Potpara TS. Optimizing stroke and bleeding risk assessment in patients with atrial fibrillation: a balance of evidence, practicality and precision. Thromb Haemost 2018; 118(12):2014–7.

53. Lip GY, Laroche C, Ioachim PM, et al. Prognosis and treatment of atrial fibrillation patients by European cardiologists: one year follow-up of the EURObservational research programme-atrial fibrillation general registry pilot phase (EORP-AF Pilot registry). Eur Heart J 2014;35(47):3365–76.

54. Hart RG, Pearce LA, Aguilar MI. Meta-analysis: antithrombotic therapy to prevent stroke in patients who have nonvalvular atrial fibrillation. Ann Intern Med 2007;146(12):857–67.

55. Lip G, Freedman B, De Caterina R, et al. Stroke prevention in atrial fibrillation: past, present and future. Comparing the guidelines and practical decision-making. Thromb Haemost 2017;117(7):1230–9.

56. Wan Y, Heneghan C, Perera R, et al. Anticoagulation control and prediction of adverse events in patients with atrial fibrillation: a systematic review. Circ Cardiovasc Qual Outcomes 2008;1(2):84–91.

57. Chao TF, Guo Y. Should we adopt a standard international normalized ratio range of 2.0 to 3.0 for asian patients with atrial fibrillation? an appeal for evidence-based management, not eminence-based recommendations. Thromb Haemost 2020;120(3):366–8.

58. Pandey AK, Xu K, Zhang L, et al. Lower versus standard INR targets in atrial fibrillation: a systematic review and meta-analysis of randomized controlled trials. Thromb Haemost 2020;120(3):484–94.

59. Pritchett RV, Bem D, Turner GM, et al. Improving the prescription of oral anticoagulants in atrial fibrillation: a systematic review. Thromb Haemost 2019;119(2):294–307.

60. Hylek EM. Treatment persistence in atrial fibrillation: the next major hurdle. Thromb Haemost 2018;118(12):2018–9.

61. Gallego P, Roldan V, Marin F, et al. Cessation of oral anticoagulation in relation to mortality and the risk of thrombotic events in patients with atrial fibrillation. Thromb Haemost 2013;110(6):1189–98.

62. Connolly SJ, Ezekowitz MD, Yusuf S, et al. Dabigatran versus warfarin in patients with atrial fibrillation. N Engl J Med 2009;361(12):1139–51.

63. Granger CB, Alexander JH, McMurray JJ, et al. Apixaban versus warfarin in patients with atrial fibrillation. N Engl J Med 2011;365(11):981–92.

64. Patel MR, Mahaffey KW, Garg J, et al. Rivaroxaban versus warfarin in nonvalvular atrial fibrillation. N Engl J Med 2011;365(10):883–91.

65. Giugliano RP, Ruff CT, Braunwald E, et al. Edoxaban versus warfarin in patients with atrial fibrillation. N Engl J Med 2013;369(22):2093–104.

66. Hohmann C, Hohnloser SH, Jacob J, et al. Non-Vitamin K oral anticoagulants in comparison to phenprocoumon in geriatric and non-geriatric patients with non-valvular atrial fibrillation. Thromb Haemost 2019;119(6):971–80.

67. Lip GYH, Keshishian A, Li X, et al. Effectiveness and safety of oral anticoagulants among nonvalvular atrial fibrillation patients. Stroke 2018;49(12):2933–44.

68. Camm AJ, Coleman CI, Larsen TB, et al. Understanding the value of real-world evidence: focus on stroke prevention in atrial fibrillation with rivaroxaban. Thromb Haemost 2018;118(S 01):S45–60.

69. Hohnloser SH, Basic E, Hohmann C, et al. Effectiveness and safety of non-vitamin k oral anticoagulants in comparison to phenprocoumon: data from 61,000 patients with atrial fibrillation. Thromb Haemost 2018;118(3):526–38.

70. Ruff CT, Giugliano RP, Braunwald E, et al. Comparison of the efficacy and safety of new oral anticoagulants with warfarin in patients with atrial fibrillation: a meta-analysis of randomised trials. Lancet 2014;383(9921):955–62.

71. Ntaios G, Papavasileiou V, Diener HC, et al. Nonvitamin-K-antagonist oral anticoagulants versus warfarin in patients with atrial fibrillation and previous stroke or transient ischemic attack: an updated systematic review and meta-analysis of randomized controlled trials. Int J Stroke 2017;12(6):589–96.

72. Connolly SJ, Eikelboom J, Joyner C, et al. Apixaban in patients with atrial fibrillation. N Engl J Med 2011;364(9):806–17.

73. Diener HC, Eikelboom J, Connolly SJ, et al. Apixaban versus aspirin in patients with atrial fibrillation and previous stroke or transient ischaemic attack: a predefined subgroup analysis from AVERROES, a randomised trial. Lancet Neurol 2012;11(3):225–31.

74. Park J, Lee SR, Choi EK, et al. Effectiveness and safety of direct oral anticoagulant for secondary prevention in asians with atrial fibrillation. J Clin Med 2019;8(12):2228.

75. Chan YH, Lee HF, See LC, et al. Effectiveness and safety of four direct oral anticoagulants in asian patients with nonvalvular atrial fibrillation. Chest 2019;156(3):529–43.

76. Moving the dial of stroke care: the sixth SSNAP annual report. Kings college london and the health quality improvement programme. Available at: https://www.strokeaudit.org/Documents/National/Clinical/Apr2018Mar2019/Apr2018Mar2019-AnnualReport.aspx. Accessed May 16, 2020.

77. Blackshear JL, Odell JA. Appendage obliteration to reduce stroke in cardiac surgical patients with atrial fibrillation. Ann Thorac Surg 1996;61(2):755–9.

78. Waldo AL, Becker RC, Tapson VF, et al. Hospitalized patients with atrial fibrillation and a high risk of stroke are not being provided with adequate anticoagulation. J Am Coll Cardiol 2005;46(9):1729–36.

79. Lip GY, Andreotti F, Fauchier L, et al. Bleeding risk assessment and management in atrial fibrillation patients: a position document from the European heart rhythm association, endorsed by the european society of cardiology working group on thrombosis. Europace 2011;13(5):723–46.

80. Eikelboom J, Merli G. Bleeding with direct oral anticoagulants vs warfarin: clinical experience. Am J Med 2016;129(11s):S33–40.

81. Holmes DR, Reddy VY, Turi ZG, et al. Percutaneous closure of the left atrial appendage versus warfarin therapy for prevention of stroke in patients with atrial fibrillation: a randomised non-inferiority trial. Lancet 2009;374(9689):534–42.

82. Holmes DR Jr, Kar S, Price MJ, et al. Prospective randomized evaluation of the watchman left atrial appendage closure device in patients with atrial fibrillation versus long-term warfarin therapy: the PREVAIL trial. J Am Coll Cardiol 2014;64(1):1–12.

83. Holmes DR Jr, Doshi SK, Kar S, et al. Left atrial appendage closure as an alternative to warfarin for stroke prevention in atrial fibrillation: a patient-level meta-analysis. J Am Coll Cardiol 2015; 65(24):2614–23.

84. Mandrola J, Foy A, Naccarelli G. Percutaneous left atrial appendage closure is not ready for routine clinical use. Heart Rhythm 2018;15(2):298–301.

85. Glikson M, Wolff R, Hindricks G, et al. EHRA/EAPCI expert consensus statement on catheter-based left atrial appendage occlusion - an update. Europace 2019. https://doi.org/10.1093/europace/euz258.

86. Percutaneous left atrial appendage closure vs. novel anticoagulation agents in high-risk atrial fibrillation patients - American college of cardiology. Available at: http://www.acc.org/latest-in-cardiology/clinical-trials/2019/08/30/22/20/prague%2017. Accessed April 15, 2020.

87. Alsagheir A, Koziarz A, Belley-Cote EP, et al. Left atrial appendage occlusion: a narrative review. J Cardiothorac Vasc Anesth 2019;33(6):1753–65.

88. Ibrahim AM, Tandan N, Koester C, et al. Meta-analysis evaluating outcomes of surgical left atrial appendage occlusion during cardiac surgery. Am J Cardiol 2019;124(8):1218–25.

89. Elbadawi A, Olorunfemi O, Ogunbayo GO, et al. Cardiovascular outcomes with surgical left atrial appendage exclusion in patients with atrial fibrillation who underwent valvular heart surgery (from the national inpatient sample database). Am J Cardiol 2017;119(12):2056–60.

90. Gillinov AM, Gelijns AC, Parides MK, et al. Surgical ablation of atrial fibrillation during mitral-valve surgery. N Engl J Med 2015;372(15):1399–409.

91. Whitlock R, Healey J, Vincent J, et al. Rationale and design of the left atrial appendage occlusion study (LAAOS) III. Ann Cardiothorac Surg 2014;3(1): 45–54.

92. Halperin JL, Hart RG. Atrial fibrillation and stroke: new ideas, persisting dilemmas. Stroke 1988; 19(8):937–41.

93. Abernathy WS, Willis PW 3rd. Thromboembolic complications of rheumatic heart disease. Cardiovasc Clin 1973;5(2):131–75.

94. Olesen KH. The natural history of 271 patients with mitral stenosis under medical treatment. Br Heart J 1962;24:349–57.

95. Molteni M, Polo Friz H, Primitz L, et al. The definition of valvular and non-valvular atrial fibrillation: results of a physicians' survey. Europace 2014;16(12): 1720–5.

96. Lip GYH, Collet JP, Caterina R, et al. Antithrombotic therapy in atrial fibrillation associated with valvular heart disease: a joint consensus document from the European heart rhythm association (EHRA) and European society of cardiology working group on thrombosis, endorsed by the ESC working group on valvular heart disease, cardiac arrhythmia society of southern Africa (CASSA), heart rhythm society (HRS), Asia pacific heart rhythm society (APHRS), South African heart (SA Heart) Association and sociedad latinoamericana de estimulacion cardiaca y electrofisiologia (SOL-EACE). Europace 2017;19(11):1757–8.

97. Kearon C, Akl EA, Comerota AJ, et al. Antithrombotic therapy for VTE disease: antithrombotic therapy and prevention of thrombosis, 9th ed: American college of chest physicians evidence-based clinical practice guidelines. Chest 2012; 141(2 Suppl):e419S–96S.

98. Renda G, Ricci F, Giugliano RP, et al. Non-Vitamin K antagonist oral anticoagulants in patients with atrial fibrillation and valvular heart disease. J Am Coll Cardiol 2017;69(11):1363–71.

99. De Caterina R, Camm AJ. What is 'valvular' atrial fibrillation? A reappraisal. Eur Heart J 2014; 35(47):3328–35.

100. Agarwal S, Hachamovitch R, Menon V. Current trial-associated outcomes with warfarin in prevention of stroke in patients with nonvalvular atrial fibrillation: a meta-analysis. Arch Intern Med 2012;172(8): 623–31 [discussion 631–23].

101. Fang MC, Go AS, Chang Y, et al. Death and disability from warfarin-associated intracranial and extracranial hemorrhages. Am J Med 2007; 120(8):700–5.

102. Zulkifly H, Lip GYH, Lane DA. Bleeding risk scores in atrial fibrillation and venous thromboembolism. Am J Cardiol 2017;120(7):1139–45.

103. Intercollegiate stroke working party. National Clinical guideline for stroke. 2016. Royal college of physicians, London. Available at: https://www.strokeaudit.org/SupportFiles/Documents/Guidelines/2016-National-Clinical-Guideline-for-Stroke-5t-(1).aspx. Accessed May 17, 2020.

104. Pisters R, Lane DA, Nieuwlaat R, et al. A novel user-friendly score (HAS-BLED) to assess 1-year risk of major bleeding in patients with atrial fibrillation: the Euro Heart Survey. Chest 2010;138(5):1093–100.

105. Lane DA, Lip GY. Use of the CHA(2)DS(2)-VASc and HAS-BLED scores to aid decision making for thromboprophylaxis in nonvalvular atrial fibrillation. Circulation 2012;126(7):860–5.

106. Roldan V, Marin F, Manzano-Fernandez S, et al. The HAS-BLED score has better prediction accuracy for major bleeding than CHADS2 or CHA2DS2-VASc scores in anticoagulated patients with atrial fibrillation. J Am Coll Cardiol 2013;62(23):2199–204.

107. Apostolakis S, Lane DA, Buller H, et al. Comparison of the CHADS2, CHA2DS2-VASc and HAS-BLED scores for the prediction of clinically relevant bleeding in anticoagulated patients with atrial fibrillation: the AMADEUS trial. Thromb Haemost 2013;110(5):1074–9.

108. Esteve-Pastor MA, Rivera-Caravaca JM, Roldan V, et al. Long-term bleeding risk prediction in 'real world' patients with atrial fibrillation: comparison of the HAS-BLED and ABC-Bleeding risk scores. The Murcia Atrial Fibrillation Project. Thromb Haemost 2017;117(10):1848–58.

109. Proietti M, Rivera-Caravaca JM, Esteve-Pastor MA, et al. Predicting bleeding events in anticoagulated patients with atrial fibrillation: a comparison between the HAS-BLED and GARFIELD-AF bleeding scores. J Am Heart Assoc 2018;7(18):e009766.

110. Rivera-Caravaca JM, Marin F, Vilchez JA, et al. Refining stroke and bleeding prediction in atrial fibrillation by adding consecutive biomarkers to clinical risk scores. Stroke 2019;50(6):1372–9.

111. Esteve-Pastor MA, Roldan V, Rivera-Caravaca JM, et al. The use of biomarkers in clinical management guidelines: a critical appraisal. Thromb Haemost 2019;119(12):1901–19.

112. Guo Y, Lane DA, Chen Y, et al. Regular bleeding risk assessment associated with reduction in bleeding outcomes: the mAFA-II randomized trial. Am J Med 2020;133(10):1195–202.e2.

113. Xian Y, O'Brien EC, Liang L, et al. Association of preceding antithrombotic treatment with acute ischemic stroke severity and in-hospital outcomes among patients with atrial fibrillation. JAMA 2017;317(10):1057–67.

114. Seiffge DJ, De Marchis GM, Koga M, et al. Ischemic stroke despite oral anticoagulant therapy in patients with atrial fibrillation. Ann Neurol 2020;87(5):677–87.

115. Freedman B, Martinez C, Katholing A, et al. Residual risk of stroke and death in anticoagulant-treated patients with atrial fibrillation. JAMA Cardiol 2016;1(3):366–8.

116. Lip GYH. The ABC pathway: an integrated approach to improve AF management. Nat Rev Cardiol 2017;14(11):627–8.

117. Proietti M, Raparelli V, Olshansky B, et al. Polypharmacy and major adverse events in atrial fibrillation: observations from the AFFIRM trial. Clin Res Cardiol 2016;105(5):412–20.

118. Proietti M, Romiti GF, Olshansky B, et al. Comprehensive management with the ABC (Atrial Fibrillation Better Care) pathway in clinically complex patients with atrial fibrillation: a post hoc ancillary analysis from the AFFIRM trial. J Am Heart Assoc 2020;9(10):e014932.

119. Gumprecht J, Domek M, Proietti M, et al. Compliance of atrial fibrillation treatment with the atrial fibrillation better care (ABC) pathway improves the clinical outcomes in the middle east population: a report from the gulf survey of atrial fibrillation events (SAFE) registry. J Clin Med 2020;9(5):1286.

120. Pastori D, Pignatelli P, Menichelli D, et al. Integrated care management of patients with atrial fibrillation and risk of cardiovascular events: the ABC (atrial fibrillation better care) pathway in the ATHERO-AF study cohort. Mayo Clin Proc 2019;94(7):1261–7.

121. Guo Y, Lane DA, Wang L, et al. Mobile health technology to improve care for patients with atrial fibrillation. J Am Coll Cardiol 2020;75(13):1523–34.

122. Guo Y, Lane DA, Wang L, et al. Mobile health (mHealth) technology for improved screening, patient involvement and optimising integrated care in atrial fibrillation: the mAFA (mAF-App) II randomised trial. Int J Clin Pract 2019;73(7):e13352.

A Team-Based Approach Toward Risk Factors of Atrial Fibrillation

Rajeev Kumar Pathak, MBBS, PhD[a],*,
Sreevilasam Pushpangadhan Abhilash, MD, DM[a],
Jeroen M. Hendriks, RN, MSc, PhD[b,c]

KEYWORDS

- Atrial fibrillation • Modifiable risk factors • Correctable risk factors • Comprehensive AF treatment
- Novel models of care delivery

KEY POINTS

- There are nonmodifiable, modifiable, and reversible risk factors for atrial fibrillation (AF).
- By preventing and treating modifiable risk factors, we can improve the overall outcomes in patients with AF.
- This may be best delivered within an integrated care approach, a collaborative practice model in which multiple specialists collaborate, aiming to improve outcomes in AF.

INTRODUCTION

Atrial fibrillation (AF) is the most prevalent sustained arrhythmia, with evidence from epidemiologic data confirming the emergence of AF as a global epidemic.[1] Various cardiometabolic risk factors such as obesity, hypertension, diabetes mellitus, physical inactivity, and sleep apnea have been independently shown to increase incidence of AF, with the risk of AF increasing exponentially with each additional risk factor.[2] Moreover, a recent study has shown that AF when associated with cardiac risk factors has a more progressive course.[3] Many of these risk factors are modifiable with lifestyle intervention strategies.

Catheter ablation of AF is an effective therapy for drug-refractory symptomatic AF.[4,5] However, reports of the long-term outcomes of AF ablation demonstrate attrition in success with time.[6] Studies have associated cardiac risk factors with the more frequent recurrence of AF.[7] AF management has thus become a complex process requiring a comprehensive focus on the rhythm and symptom management, prevention of thromboembolic complications, treatment of underlying heart disease, and aggressive targeting of modifiable cardiovascular risk factors.[8,9] In this review, the authors discuss the role and benefits of risk factor modification in sinus rhythm maintenance and a team-based integrated approach in risk factor modification as the fourth pillar of AF care.

RISK FACTORS FOR ATRIAL FIBRILLATION

The risk factors for AF can be broadly divided into nonmodifiable, modifiable, and reversible factors. Although little can be done about nonmodifiable risk factors, a thorough search for modifiable risk factors and initiating treatment as early as possible can reduce morbidity and improve overall outcomes. For this reason, AF management should

[a] Australian National University and Canberra Hospital, Canberra, Australian Capital Territory, Australia; [b] Centre for Heart Rhythm Disorders (CHRD), South Australian Health and Medical Research Institute (SAHMRI), University of Adelaide and Royal Adelaide Hospital, Adelaide, Australia; [c] Caring Futures Institute, College of Nursing and Health Sciences, Flinders University, Adelaide, Australia
* Corresponding author. Cardiac Electrophysiology Unit, Department of Cardiology, Canberra Hospital, Yamba Drive, Garran, Australian Capital Territory 2605, Australia.
E-mail address: rajeev.pathak@canberraheartrhythm.com.au

Card Electrophysiol Clin 13 (2021) 257–262
https://doi.org/10.1016/j.ccep.2020.11.008

no longer only focus on clinical end points such as prevention of heart failure or stroke but should have a more holistic approach including timely detection and optimal treatment of risk factors and underlying conditions.[5] Importantly, patients with AF have different risk factor profiles, and interventions aiming at risk factor management should be tailored to individual needs.

MODIFIABLE RISK FACTORS

Cardiac metabolic risk factors keep each other's company. Obesity clusters with other cardiovascular risk factors including impaired glucose tolerance, dyslipidemia, hypertension, and sleep apnea, all associated with an increased AF risk in the general population. In fact, with each additional risk factor the risk of AF and its progression increases proportionately, reaching exponential levels.[10] In addition, physical inactivity, smoking, and excessive alcohol intake are some of the other well-known modifiable risk factors. Targeting these risk factors as early as possible would not only prevent or reverse AF progression but also might potentially improve the underlying conditions themselves, resulting in lesser number of strokes and other cardiovascular adverse events.[3]

OBESITY

Obesity is associated with a greater incidence of developing AF, and this relationship is dynamic in nature.[11,12] Weight loss reduces risk of new AF and also recurrence of AF. Weight loss and aggressive risk factor management through a physician-led clinic resulted in a significant 60% reduction in AF burden over 15 months. This was associated with significant reduction in symptom severity and reduced number and duration of AF episodes on ambulatory monitoring.[13] The sustainability of this process was confirmed in the Long-Term Effect of Goal-Directed Weight Management in an Atrial Fibrillation Cohort (LEGACY) study. The benefit of weight loss was dose dependent, with 10% weight loss being associated with 6-fold greater probability of AF-free survival as compared with the patients who stayed obese.[14] The benefits of aggressive risk factor management extend to patients undergoing ablation. In the Aggressive Risk Factor Reduction Study for Atrial Fibrillation and Implications for the Outcome of Ablation (ARREST-AF) cohort study, postablation patients with body mass index greater than 27 kg/m^2 and at least one additional risk factor were allocated to either a structured weight loss program and aggressive risk factor management or a routine care. Risk factor management

determined outcomes of AF ablation with 87% patients having arrhythmia-free survival after multiple procedures in the interventional arm as compared with 17% in the control arm.[15]

PHYSICAL INACTIVITY

The complementary benefits of cardiorespiratory fitness, in addition to weight loss, have been demonstrated in the CARDIO-FIT study in which cardiorespiratory fitness was improved by gradually increasing the frequency, intensity, time, and type of exercise. Individuals who gained greater than or equal to 2 METS in cardiorespiratory fitness, in addition to weight loss, had a 2-fold greater freedom from AF than weight loss alone.[16] However, the relationship between the amount of exercise and incident AF does not seem to be linear but U-shaped,[17] and this was demonstrated in the Cardiovascular Health Study, where individuals doing moderate-intensity exercise developed less AF than those doing high-intensity exercise or no exercise.[18]

OBSTRUCTIVE SLEEP APNEA

Obstructive sleep apnea (OSA) is one of the novel risk factors for AF. Patients with OSA have a significantly higher risk of developing AF, especially those with severe disease. Recent studies show continuous positive airway pressure (CPAP) can significantly improve OSA symptoms and reduce occurrence of AF.[19] It seems that these beneficial effects of CPAP are achieved through modulation of neurohumoral activation, leading to decreased markers of inflammation and oxidative stress. In addition, treatment with CPAP also affects other risk factors that promote AF. In patients with moderate to severe OSA and the metabolic syndrome, just 3 months of CPAP could lower systolic and diastolic blood pressures and partially reverse metabolic abnormalities.[20] This result serves to highlight the interdependence of modifiable risk factors and the need for a comprehensive approach to their management.

HYPERTENSION AND GLYCEMIC CONTROL

Hypertension is a well-established risk factor for the development of AF. However, there is paucity of clinical studies specifically examining the treatment of hypertension as an intervention for existing AF. The RACE 3 trial, where patients with early persistent AF and mild-to-moderate heart failure were randomized to causal treatment of AF and HF alone versus targeted treatment with mineralocorticoid receptor antagonists, statins, angiotensin-converting enzyme inhibitors, or angiotensin receptor blockers with a blood pressure target of less than 120/80 mm Hg led to significantly improved sinus rhythm at 1 year.[21] Similarly, the evidence for glycemic control and management of dyslipidemia in managing arrhythmia is less robust. The pathophysiologic mechanisms implicated in promoting AF in individuals with diabetes are complex and include autonomic, electrical, and structural remodeling of the atria associated with glycemic fluctuations. Taking all these findings together, the vicious combination of AF and diabetes warrants timely evaluation and appropriate treatment.

EXCESSIVE ALCOHOL INTAKE AND SMOKING

Several studies have also looked at the association between chronic alcohol consumption and incident AF. Framingham Heart Study showed that heavy alcohol consumption (more than 3 drinks/day) was associated with a significantly increased risk of development of AF.[22] It was observed that there was a linear dose–response relationship between alcohol intake and risk of AF, with a significant 8% increase in the relative risk of incident AF for each standard drink per day compared with no drinks a day.[23] Abstinence from alcohol has been demonstrated to reduce arrhythmia recurrences in regular drinkers with AF.[24] In addition, The ARIC study showed that current smoking accounted for about 10% of incident AF.[25] Smoking cessation is strongly recommended, and it should be a priority of every primary care physician to motivate patients to join smoking cessation and health awareness programs.

Treatment of modifiable risk factors is a cost-effective approach.[26] Risk factor management is now a fundamental element of comprehensive management of AF that is recommended by international AF management guidelines.[5] The risk factor management in the LEGACY and the ARREST-AF cohort study was achieved through a separate physician-led specialized clinic, and this is an excellent model to replicate in primary care settings. Given the encouraging data on integrated AF care interventions, a dedicated multidisciplinary AF clinic systematically coordinating the patient care according to current guidelines is the key, and this will improve adherence to guidelines in a cost-effective fashion.[26]

TEAM-BASED APPROACH AND COMPREHENSIVE MANAGEMENT OF ATRIAL FIBRILLATION

Given the multifaceted character of AF and the necessary comprehensive treatment, AF management is considered complex and may require changes in the care delivery process as well. Novel models of care have been introduced to manage patients with chronic and complex conditions such as AF. Integrated care has been identified as a suitable approach to manage patients with AF and is currently the recommended AF treatment approach.[5] Integrated AF care consists of 4 indispensable fundamentals: (1) *comprehensive care:* as described earlier, this refers to an overall treatment and patients' access to all suitable treatment options. (2) *Multidisciplinary team approach:* based on the required comprehensive treatment and the complexity of AF management, the question raises whether this can be appropriately addressed by one single health care professional. Specialized AF clinics has been developed to establish a close collaboration between nurses and cardiologists with a clear division of tasks; the nurse may focus on providing patient education and coordination of care, whereas the cardiologist would be responsible for the medical treatment.[27] Based on the individual patient case, treatment teams can be expanded with multiple specialists as well as generalists that can be involved in the management of AF, working in a collaborative practice model to jointly manage the patient with AF. As such, the role of the internist is significant in diagnosing and treating underlying cardiovascular conditions such as hypertension and diabetes mellitus. Also, the role of the primary care physician (PCP) within such approaches is crucial and 2-fold; firstly, the PCP serves as the gate keeper and is often the initial contact for the patient with AF seeking care. The PCP is responsible for initiating AF treatment (eg, rate control) and referring the patient to cardiology services where appropriate, for complete diagnostic investigation and comprehensive treatment accordingly. Secondly, PCP services are crucial in the follow-up of patients with stable AF, which may include assessment of symptoms, adherence to treatment regimen, and the evaluation of risk factors and support in lifestyle modification in these patients. Coordination of these services and defining where best to provide the care based on the concept "right care at right place" is crucial and requires significant communication processes to prevent fragmentation. (3) *Patient involvement:* naturally, patients should be involved in their care process and empowered in their role. This can be achieved by applying a patient-centered approach, which is respectful of and responsive to individual patient values, needs, and preferences, inviting patients to be involved in the treatment decision-making, while providing evidence-based treatment.[28] However, before patients are able to take on such crucial roles and closely work with the treatment team, they should be educated about the condition, symptoms, treatment options, and about what they can add to improve their outcomes. The power of education is enriching and has recently been demonstrated by the Home-based and Learning Program for AF.[29] This trial demonstrated significant reductions in unplanned hospital admissions by providing education to patients with AF in the safety of their home. Nurses and pharmacists trained in the method of structured educational visiting performed these educational visits by delivering 4 key messages that were considered most applicable in AF: the importance of taking AF medicines as prescribed to reduce symptoms and the risk of stroke; stroke medicines can reduce the risk of stroke significantly; applying a healthy lifestyle to reduce the risk of AF, and the availability of a personal action plan (completed by the patient's cardiologist or PCP) for patients to follow during an episode of AF.[30] (4) *Use of technology:* there is multiple technology applications available to support integrated care in AF. Specific patient applications are available to provide structured education and to support patients in self-managing their condition. Also, decision support technology, based on the latest evidence provided by international practice guidelines, may be used to guide treatment decisions within the treatment team.[31]

Several trials have investigated the effectiveness of specialized AF clinics wherein comprehensive AF treatment is administered by a multidisciplinary team. An initial trial reported improved guideline adherent treatment within a specialized and integrated AF approach.[8] Moreover, the trial showed significant reductions in cardiovascular hospitalization and mortality (hazard ratio [HR]: 0.65; 95% confidence interval [CI] 0.45 to 0.93; $P = .017$), as well as all-cause mortality (HR: 0.44, 95% CI 0.23 to 0.85; $P = .014$) in favor of the integrated AF clinic compared with usual care provided by one physician alone.[32] Also, this approach demonstrated to be cost-effective compared with usual care.[33] A systematic review and meta-analysis confirmed these findings and demonstrated reduced cardiovascular hospitalization (odds ratio [OR] 0.58, 95% CI 0.44–0.77, $P = .0002$) and all-cause mortality (OR 0.51, 95% CI 0.32–0.80, $P = .003$) when applying an integrated AF care approach, compared with usual care, however did not demonstrate significant reductions in AF-related hospitalizations (OR 0.82, 95% CI 0.56–1.19, $P = .29$) or the occurrence of cerebrovascular events (OR 1.00, 95% CI 0.48–2.09, $P = 1.00$). Finally, a recently performed multicentre randomized controlled trial, however, demonstrated no significant difference between patients who received care within a specialized AF approach compared with usual care, for the composite endpoint of cardiovascular hospitalization and mortality (HR: 0.85, 95% CI 0.69–1.04, $P = .12$).[34] In a prespecified subgroup analysis, however, results were not consistent with an HR of 0.52 (95% CI 0.37–0.71) in experienced centers (meaning experience with a specialized AF clinic) and of 1.24 (95% CI 0.94–1.63) in less experienced centers (P for interaction <0.001).

Although current evidence points in the direction of specialized integrated models, given their superiority in improving hospitalization and mortality, many questions remain about the implementation of optimal models and settings, to provide comprehensive AF treatment in a patient-centered, multidisciplinary setting. Further research is required to answer these important questions.

SUMMARY

AF is the most prevalent sustained cardiac arrhythmia and has significant morbidity and mortality associated with. There are nonmodifiable, modifiable, and correctable factors of AF, and primary care physician can play a crucial role in identifying and treating these risk factors. Common cardiovascular risk factors such as hypertension, diabetes mellitus, coronary artery disease, obesity, obstructive sleep apnea, physical inactivity, and alcoholism as well as underlying conditions such as heart failure and renal dysfunction significantly contribute to the development of AF. These risk factors can lead to the development of an abnormal atrial substrate, which translates into disease progression, recurrences, and poorer outcomes. However, therapeutic interventions targeting AF risk factors have been shown to improve arrhythmia outcomes, and specialized clinics in primary care centers is a cost-effective and valid approach. Targeting modifiable risk factors should be an essential "fourth pillar" of AF care alongside appropriate anticoagulation and rate and rhythm control. The delivery of such comprehensive AF care may be best performed within an integrated specialized setting, following a patient-centered and multidisciplinary team approach. Optimal and timely management targeting these conditions is feasible, reduces AF, and improves quality of life.

CLINICS CARE POINTS

- Therapeutic interventions targeting AF risk factors have been shown to improve arrhythmia outcomes. Targeting modifiable risk factors should be an essential "fourth pillar" of AF care alongside appropriate anti-coagulation and rate and rhythm control.

- Integrated specialized services have been demonstrated effective and suitable to provide comprehensive AF management, while applying patient-centered care provided by a multidisciplinary team.

DISCLOSURE

Dr R.K. Pathak reports having received research funding from Medtronic, Abbott Medical, Boston Scientific, and Biotronik.

REFERENCE

1. Wong CX, Brooks AG, Leong DP, et al. The increasing burden of atrial fibrillation compared with heart failure and myocardial infarction: a 15-year study of all hospitalizations in Australia. Arch Intern Med 2012;172(9):739–41.
2. Chamberlain AM, Agarwal SK, Ambrose M, et al. Metabolic syndrome and incidence of atrial fibrillation among blacks and whites in the Atherosclerosis Risk in Communities (ARIC) Study. Am Heart J 2010; 159(5):850–6.
3. Middeldorp ME, Pathak RK, Lau DH, et al. PREVEntion and regReSsive Effect of weight-loss and risk factor modification on Atrial Fibrillation: the REVERSE-AF study-Authors' reply. Europace 2019; 21(6):990–1.
4. Calkins H, Kuck KH, Cappato R, et al. 2012 HRS/EHRA/ECAS expert consensus statement on catheter and surgical ablation of atrial fibrillation: recommendations for patient selection, procedural techniques, patient management and follow-up, definitions, endpoints, and research trial design: a report of the Heart Rhythm Society (HRS) Task Force on Catheter and Surgical Ablation of Atrial Fibrillation. Heart rhythm 2012;9(4):632–696 e21.
5. Group NCAFGW, Brieger D, Amerena J, Attia J, et al. National Heart Foundation of Australia and the Cardiac Society of Australia and New Zealand: Australian Clinical Guidelines for the Diagnosis and Management of Atrial Fibrillation 2018. Heart Lung Circ 2018;27(10):1209–66.
6. Weerasooriya R, Khairy P, Litalien J, et al. Catheter ablation for atrial fibrillation: are results maintained at 5 years of follow-up? J Am Coll Cardiol 2011; 57(2):160–6.
7. Mohanty S, Mohanty P, Di Biase L, et al. Impact of metabolic syndrome on procedural outcomes in patients with atrial fibrillation undergoing catheter ablation. J Am Coll Cardiol 2012;59(14):1295–301.
8. Hendriks JL, Nieuwlaat R, Vrijhoef HJ, et al. Improving guideline adherence in the treatment of atrial fibrillation by implementing an integrated chronic care program. Neth Heart J 2010;18(10):471–7.
9. Mahajan R, Pathak RK, Thiyagarajah A, et al. Risk factor management and atrial fibrillation clinics: saving the best for last? Heart Lung Circ 2017; 26(9):990–7.
10. Chao TF, Ambrose K, Tsao HM, et al. Relationship between the CHADS(2) score and risk of very late recurrences after catheter ablation of paroxysmal atrial fibrillation. Heart Rhythm 2012;9(8):1185–91.
11. Wang TJ, Parise H, Levy D, et al. Obesity and the risk of new-onset atrial fibrillation. JAMA 2004; 292(20):2471–7.
12. Pathak RK, Mahajan R, Lau DH, et al. The implications of obesity for cardiac arrhythmia mechanisms and management. Can J Cardiol 2015;31(2): 203–10.
13. Abed HS, Wittert GA, Leong DP, et al. Effect of weight reduction and cardiometabolic risk factor management on symptom burden and severity in patients with atrial fibrillation: a randomized clinical trial. JAMA 2013;310(19):2050–60.
14. Pathak RK, Middeldorp ME, Meredith M, et al. Long-term effect of goal-directed weight management in an atrial fibrillation cohort: a long-term follow-up study (LEGACY). J Am Coll Cardiol 2015;65(20): 2159–69.
15. Pathak RK, Middeldorp ME, Lau DH, et al. Aggressive risk factor reduction study for atrial fibrillation and implications for the outcome of ablation: the ARREST-AF cohort study. J Am Coll Cardiol 2014; 64(21):2222–31.
16. Pathak RK, Elliott A, Middeldorp ME, et al. Impact of CARDIOrespiratory FITness on arrhythmia recurrence in obese individuals with atrial fibrillation: the CARDIO-FIT Study. J Am Coll Cardiol 2015;66(9): 985–96.
17. Elliott AD, Mahajan R, Pathak RK, et al. Exercise training and atrial fibrillation: further evidence for the importance of lifestyle change. Circulation 2016;133(5):457–9.
18. Mozaffarian D, Furberg CD, Psaty BM, et al. Physical activity and incidence of atrial fibrillation in older adults: the cardiovascular health study. Circulation 2008;118(8):800–7.
19. Naruse Y, Tada H, Satoh M, et al. Concomitant obstructive sleep apnea increases the recurrence

of atrial fibrillation following radiofrequency catheter ablation of atrial fibrillation: clinical impact of continuous positive airway pressure therapy. Heart Rhythm 2013;10(3):331–7.

20. Sharma SK, Agrawal S, Damodaran D, et al. CPAP for the metabolic syndrome in patients with obstructive sleep apnea. N Engl J Med 2011;365(24): 2277–86.

21. Rienstra M, Hobbelt AH, Alings M, et al. Targeted therapy of underlying conditions improves sinus rhythm maintenance in patients with persistent atrial fibrillation: results of the RACE 3 trial. Eur Heart J 2018;39(32):2987–96.

22. Lloyd-Jones DM, Wang TJ, Leip EP, et al. Lifetime risk for development of atrial fibrillation: the Framingham Heart Study. Circulation 2004;110(9):1042–6.

23. Larsson SC, Drca N, Wolk A. Alcohol consumption and risk of atrial fibrillation: a prospective study and dose-response meta-analysis. J Am Coll Cardiol 2014;64(3):281–9.

24. Voskoboinik A, Kalman JM, De Silva A, et al. Alcohol abstinence in drinkers with atrial fibrillation. N Engl J Med 2020;382(1):20–8.

25. Huxley RR, Lopez FL, Folsom AR, et al. Absolute and attributable risks of atrial fibrillation in relation to optimal and borderline risk factors: the Atherosclerosis Risk in Communities (ARIC) study. Circulation 2011;123(14):1501–8.

26. Pathak RK, Evans M, Middeldorp ME, et al. Cost-effectiveness and clinical effectiveness of the risk factor management clinic in atrial fibrillation: the CENT Study. JACC Clin Electrophysiol 2017;3(5): 436–47.

27. Hendriks JM, de Wit R, Vrijhoef HJ, et al. An integrated chronic care program for patients with atrial fibrillation: study protocol and methodology for an ongoing prospective randomised controlled trial. Int J Nurs Stud 2010;47(10):1310–6.

28. Barry MJ, Edgman-Levitan S. Shared decision making–pinnacle of patient-centered care. N Engl J Med 2012;366(9):780–1.

29. Hendriks JM, Brooks AG, Rowett D, et al. Home-based education and learning program for atrial fibrillation: rationale and design of the HELP-AF Study. Can J Cardiol 2019;35(7):846–54.

30. Gallagher C, Rowett D, Nyfort-Hansen K, et al. Patient-Centered educational resources for atrial fibrillation. JACC Clin Electrophysiol 2019;5(10): 1101–14.

31. Kotecha D, Chua WWL, Fabritz L, et al. European Society of Cardiology smartphone and tablet applications for patients with atrial fibrillation and their health care providers. Europace 2018;20(2):225–33.

32. Hendriks JM, de Wit R, Crijns HJ, et al. Nurse-led care vs. usual care for patients with atrial fibrillation: results of a randomized trial of integrated chronic care vs. routine clinical care in ambulatory patients with atrial fibrillation. Eur Heart J 2012;33(21): 2692–9.

33. Hendriks J, Tomini F, van Asselt T, et al. Cost-effectiveness of a specialized atrial fibrillation clinic vs. usual care in patients with atrial fibrillation. Europace 2013;15(8):1128–35.

34. Wijtvliet E, Tieleman RG, van Gelder IC, et al. Nurse-led vs. usual-care for atrial fibrillation. Eur Heart J 2020;41(5):634–41.

Lifestyle as a Risk Factor for Atrial Fibrillation

Celine Gallagher, RN, MSc, PhD[a], Melissa E. Middeldorp, PhD[a],
Jeroen M. Hendriks, RN, MSc, PhD[a,b], Dennis H. Lau, MBBS, PhD[a],
Prashanthan Sanders, MBBS, PhD[a,*]

KEYWORDS

- Lifestyle • Atrial fibrillation • Risk factors • Risk factor modification • Health behavior change

KEY POINTS

- Modifiable cardiovascular risk factors contribute substantially to the growing incidence of atrial fibrillation.
- The modification of cardiovascular risk factors can lead to a decreased incidence of atrial fibrillation and a decreased disease burden in the prevalent atrial fibrillation population.
- An understanding of health behavior change techniques can assist clinicians in facilitating effective modification of cardiovascular risk factors through lifestyle change.

INTRODUCTION

Atrial fibrillation (AF) is associated with significant morbidity and mortality, in addition to increasing health care burden.[1–3] Opportunities to decrease the growing incidence of this condition have become an urgent public health priority. Although there are several nonmodifiable risk factors for AF development, including advancing age and genetics, a growing body of evidence has identified numerous lifestyle factors associated with incident AF. Importantly, owing to the modifiable nature of these risk factors, significant opportunity exists to improve their management in a bid to curtail the growing incidence of this condition and subsequent rising tide of AF-related health care resource utilization.

In this article, we focus on the evidence linking modifiable cardiovascular risk factors with incident AF. We focus on common modifiable cardiovascular risk factors including obesity, hypertension, diabetes, physical inactivity, alcohol intake, and smoking. These risk factors are highly prevalent in developed countries and contribute substantially to the growing AF burden. Moreover, optimal control of these modifiable cardiovascular risk factors is associated with a substantial decrease in the risk of developing AF.[4] Although the lifetime risk of AF development in those aged greater than 55 years in the presence of 1 or more modifiable risk factors, including smoking, excessive alcohol intake, hypertension, diabetes, and a history of heart failure or myocardial infarction, is 1 in 3, a substantial risk reduction of 1 in 5 is evident in those with optimal control of these risk factors.[4] The presence of 3 modifiable risk factors—overweight or obesity, smoking, and alcohol intake—accounted for an almost 3-fold difference in the risk of developing AF in another cohort study, highlighting the role of modifiable risk factors in the etiology of the development of this arrhythmia.[5] Furthermore, there is strong evidence to suggest that, even in those at high genetic risk, optimal control of cardiovascular risk factors significantly decreases the risk of AF development.[6] It is therefore an urgent public health

[a] Department of Cardiology, Centre for Heart Rhythm Disorders, University of Adelaide, Royal Adelaide Hospital, Port Road, Adelaide, South Australia 5000, Australia; [b] College of Nursing and Health Sciences, Flinders University, Bedford Park, South Australia 5042 Australia
* Corresponding author. c/o Department of Cardiology, Centre for Heart Rhythm Disorders, Royal Adelaide Hospital, Port Road, Adelaide, South Australia 5000, Australia.
E-mail address: prash.sanders@adelaide.edu.au
Twitter: @PrashSanders (P.S.)

Card Electrophysiol Clin 13 (2021) 263–272
https://doi.org/10.1016/j.ccep.2020.11.013

priority to develop effective strategies to curtail adverse growing trends in common modifiable cardiovascular risk factors, driven by suboptimal lifestyle choices, including obesity and diabetes, which have demonstrated steep upward trajectories in recent decades.[7]

The modification of lifestyle factors through risk factor reduction programs has shown promise in decreasing AF burden in those with prevalent AF. Several studies have highlighted the effectiveness of simultaneously targeting multiple cardiovascular risk factors in decreasing AF burden and health care resource use, in addition to the cost effectiveness of this strategy.[8–10] However, to date, few studies have demonstrated the effectiveness of comprehensive cardiovascular risk factor modification in decreasing the risk of incident AF. This article reviews the evidence for the role of primary and secondary prevention cardiovascular risk factor management programs on the development and progression of AF. Additionally, we focus on the theory underpinning health behavior change and review practical strategies for implementing a risk factor modification program in the AF population.

HYPERTENSION

Owing to its widespread prevalence, hypertension remains the strongest population attributable risk factor for incident AF, as discussed in Dennis H. Lau and colleagues' article, "Hypertension, Prehypertension, Hypertensive Heart Disease and AF," in this issue. Over 50 years of follow-up in the Framingham cohort has demonstrated an increasing prevalence of treatment for hypertension, with this risk factor associated with the highest population attributable risk for AF development at 19.5%.[11] This is similar to the Atherosclerosis Risk In Communities (ARIC) study, which places the population-attributable risk of hypertension at 21.6%.[12] Estimates of the prevalence of this risk factor in AF studies to date range from 49% to 90%, highlighting the importance of targeting this risk factor to decreased the growing incidence of this condition.[13] Moreover, the opportunity to intervene to reduce this burden may be earlier than thought, with prehypertensive levels of 130 to 139 mm Hg systolic associated with an increased risk of AF development.[14] Blood pressure trajectories over time are also likely to significantly influence the risk of AF. In the Framingham study, the presence of baseline hypertension was associated with an approximate doubling of AF risk over 15 years of follow-up, regardless of increasing or decreasing blood pressure trajectories over time.[15] Similar results were observed

in the Tromsø study, where persistently elevated systolic blood pressure levels over time in females, regardless of increasing or decreasing trajectories, was associated with an approximate doubling of risk of AF development compared with those with stable blood pressure levels.[16] This effect was not as evident in the male population, where baseline hypertension with a decreasing systolic blood pressure trajectory over time was not associated with a risk of AF development, suggesting that sex differences may be present for this risk factor.[16]

Despite this finding, optimal targets to decrease the onset of AF and improve outcomes in those with the condition, remain unknown. Adverse events have been demonstrated with poorly controlled hypertension in AF populations. In the Outcomes Registry for the Better Treatment of AF (ORBIT AF), each 5 mm Hg increase in systolic blood pressure over follow-up was associated with a 5% increase in stroke or transient ischemic attack (hazard ratio [HR], 1.05; 95% confidence interval [CI], 1.01–1.08; $P = .01$), a 5% increase in the risk of myocardial infarction (HR, 1.05; 95% CI, 1.00–1.11; $P = .04$) and a 3% increase in major bleeding events (HR, 1.03; 95% CI, 1.00–1.06; $P = .04$).[17] In the Rivaroxaban versus Warfarin for non-valvular Atrial Fibrillation (ROCKET-AF) study, a similar increase in risk was observed with each 10 mm Hg increase in baseline blood pressure associated with an increased risk of stroke or systemic embolism (HR, 1.07; 95% CI, 1.02–1.13).[18]

OBESITY

Growing trends in overweight and obesity have reached pandemic proportions. It is estimated that by 2030 approximately 38% of the world's population will be obese.[19] These trends are likely to be fueling the growing epidemic of AF. As discussed in Rajiv Mahajan and Christopher X. Wong's article, "Obesity and Metabolic Syndrome in Atrial Fibrillation: Cardiac and Non-Cardiac Adipose Tissue in Atrial Fibrillation," in this issue, obesity has demonstrated a strong and consistent association with AF development in numerous epidemiologic studies. In the Framingham cohort, involving 5282 participants with a mean follow-up of 13.7 years, each 1 unit increase in body mass index (BMI) was associated with a 4% increase in risk of AF development.[20] Moreover, over 50 years of follow-up, an increasing prevalence of obesity, defined as a BMI of 30 kg/m² or greater, from 27.3% in the 1958 to 1967 cohort to 35.4% in the 1998 to 2007 cohort was noted ($P<.001$ for trend).[11] In the 1998 to 2007 cohort, 72.3% of the cohort that developed AF were either overweight or obese, highlighting the highly prevalent nature of this risk factor. Furthermore, compared with individuals with a normal BMI, obesity was associated with a 52% and 46% increase in risk of incident AF for males and females, respectively, after adjustment for confounders.[20] A meta-analysis exploring obesity and the risk of incident AF in 9 cohort studies of 157,518 individuals demonstrated a 29% increase in AF risk (odds ratio, 1.29; 95% CI, 1.23–1.36) with each 5 unit increase in BMI.[21]

Importantly, BMI change over time may also act to modulate both the risk in development of AF and progression to more permanent forms of the arrhythmia. In the Women's Health Study, those who developed obesity over 5 years of follow-up exhibited a 41% increase in the risk of developing AF (HR, 1.41; 95% CI, 1.05–1.90; P = .02), compared with those who maintained a BMI of less than 30 kg/m^2.[22] Furthermore, in a cohort of individuals with paroxysmal AF, BMI independently predicted progression to permanent AF in 3248 individuals over 5 years of follow-up, with a 54% increase in risk in those who were obese (defined as a BMI of $\geq$30 kg/m^2; HR, 1.54; 95% CI, 1.2–2.0; P = .0004) and an 87% increase in those who were severely obese (defined as a BMI of $\geq$35 kg/m^2; HR. 1.87; 95% CI, 1.4–2.5; P<.0001).[23] The HUNT study highlighted the importance of BMI change over time on AF risk, with a 5 kg/m^2 increase in BMI over 40 years of follow-up, conferring a 3-fold increase in risk of AF development.[24] Owing to its increasing incidence and widespread prevalence, targeting obesity as both a primary and secondary prevention measure, is likely to result in significant improvements in AF outcomes. Targeting obesity is also important owing to its strong association with other risk factors known to increase the risk of AF development, including diabetes, hypertension, and sleep apnea.[25,26]

DIABETES

As discussed in Satoshi Higa and colleagues' article, "Diabetes and Endocrine Disorders (Hyper-/Hypothyroidism) as Risk Factors for Atrial Fibrillation," in this issue, diabetes has demonstrated a correlation with AF in most, but not all, large-scale epidemiologic studies. An increase in the risk of AF of approximately one-third has been demonstrated in various studies,[27–29] although a longer duration and poorer glycemic control are also likely to be important factors in risk of AF development.[30] In a Swedish study of 71,483 individuals, although

type 2 diabetes was associated with incident AF in an age- and sex-adjusted model, this effect became nonsignificant once adjusted for BMI.[31] In this study, an increased risk of AF was only observed in those with a duration of type 2 diabetes of more than 20 years, conferring a 44% increase in risk (HR, 1.44; 95% CI, 1.02–2.04).[31] Intensive control of diabetes, targeting a hemoglobin A1c of less than 6% compared with a target of 7.0% to 7.9%, has not been shown to reduce the incidence of AF.[32] However, in established AF, incremental increases in the hemoglobin A1c level have been associated with a greater risk of ischemic stroke.[33]

PHYSICAL INACTIVITY

Moderate levels of physical activity are associated with a reduction in risk of incident AF, with each additional metabolic equivalent gained during exercise testing associated with a 7% decrease in risk.[34] In an older population of 5446 individuals greater than 65 years of age, moderate intensity physical activity was associated with a 28% decrease in the risk of AF development (HR, 0.72; 95% CI, 0.58–0.89), an effect that was not evident at either low or high intensity levels.[35] Increasing levels of leisure time physical activity have also been associated with a decreased risk of incident AF in several studies.[36,37] However, questions remain over higher levels of physical activity with numerous studies demonstrating a heightened risk of AF in endurance athletes.[38,39] Sex differences may also be apparent with a recently published study of 402,406 UK biobank participants demonstrating a decreased risk of incident AF across all levels of physical activity for females, with a heightened risk observed at vigorous activity levels for males (HR, for 5000 metabolic equivalent minutes per week: 1.12; 95% CI, 1.01–1.25).[40] Importantly, this level is significantly above what the majority of the general population is able to achieve and should not deter clinicians from recommending physical activity as a part of a comprehensive primary prevention strategy for incident AF.

In the established AF population, exercise has also demonstrated benefit, although it is clear that more research is required in this area. In those with permanent AF, regular physical activity has been associated with improved health-related quality of life and a lower resting heart rate.[41,42] Short-term aerobic training has also demonstrated improved patient outcomes in individuals referred for catheter ablation for paroxysmal or persistent AF, with a decreased AF burden, improved quality of life, left atrial function, and peak oxygen consumption in the intervention group compared with controls.[43]

ALCOHOL

The role of alcohol and smoking is discussed in detail in Andres Klein and colleagues' article, "Social Risk Factors and Atrial Fibrillation," in this issue. In brief, high levels of alcohol intake have demonstrated a consistent association with incident AF across most studies. This finding has been demonstrated in several meta-analyses, although the threshold for increased risk remains uncertain.[44–46] After excluding case control studies, which may lead to an overestimation of risk, sex differences are apparent, with moderate levels of alcohol intake associated with a heightened AF risk in males but not females.[44]

In the established AF population, high levels of alcohol intake (>27 standard drinks per week) have been associated with an increased mortality risk in males but not females.[47] However, an increased risk of thromboembolism has been observed in females consuming more than 20 standard drinks per day.[47] After catheter ablation, an increased risk of AF recurrence has been observed in individuals consuming alcohol on a daily basis.[48] Atrial remodeling is thought to play a significant contributory role, with greater amounts of low-voltage zones in those consuming larger quantities of daily alcohol, and hence a greater risk of failure.[48] Recently, a greater likelihood of freedom from atrial arrhythmia was observed after catheter ablation in those advised to abstain from alcohol altogether in a randomized controlled trial.[49]

SMOKING

Data are conflicting concerning the risk of incident AF attributable to smoking. Although numerous epidemiologic studies have not demonstrated any association with AF,[27,50,51] others have described an association with current smoking with risk estimate increases ranging from 32% to 200%.[52–54] This finding may be due to variations across studies in numbers of daily cigarettes smoked or habit duration; or it may be due to baseline differences across populations. One meta-analysis found a 23% increase in the risk of AF attributable to current smoking.[55] More recently, another meta-analysis of 29 cohort and case-control studies demonstrated a heightened AF risk for current (relative risk [RR], 1.32; 95% CI, 1.12–1.56) and former smokers (RR, 1.09; 95% CI, 1.00–1.18), with each additional 10 cigarettes smoked per day conferring a 14% risk increase (RR, 1.14; 95% CI, 1.10–1.20).[56] A greater likelihood of failure after ablation for persistent AF has also been identified in smokers with nonpulmonary vein triggers, compared with nonsmokers.[57]

In established AF, current cigarette smoking has been associated with numerous adverse events including increased all-cause mortality (RR, 1.82; 95% CI, 1.33–2.49; $P = .0002$), cardiovascular death (RR, 1.54; 95% CI, 1.31–1.81; $P<.00001$), and major bleeding events (RR, 1.93; 95% CI, 1.08–3.47; $P = .03$).[58] However, no impact on the risk of stroke or thromboembolism was observed in a meta-analysis.[58] Cigarette smoking is also a known contributor to atherogenesis, endothelial dysfunction, and promotion of a heightened prothrombotic state, all of which are unfavorable in the setting of AF.[59]

HEALTH BEHAVIOR CHANGE

Health behavior change is a complex process. Lifestyle habits are developed and sustained, often over long periods of time, making it challenging for many patients to think about changing them and for clinicians to empower them to do so. Additionally, many patients may not have the knowledge to identify behaviors that require modification to achieve optimal outcomes. Effective health behavior change consultations move away from paternalistic models of care delivery to incorporating the patient as an active team member. Although there are several underpinning health behavior change theories, a commonly applied model—the transtheoretical model of change—identifies 5 key stages of the change process (precontemplation, contemplation, planning, action, and maintenance).[60] Assessment by the clinician of each individual's stage is an important factor in facilitating progress to action and maintenance phases.[60] Once a behavior has been identified, the determination of an individual's importance and confidence in achieving the desired change is essential to ensuring that information given is appropriately targeted to equip the patient to both value the change (importance), and to understand how to effectively achieve the desired result (confidence).[60] Identifying barriers to achieving change is another essential component to achieving optimal outcomes and often emerges during discussions concerning confidence in achieving the proposed health behavior change.

Several other theories of health behavior change have also been developed including the health belief model,[61] self-determination theory,[62] the theory of planned behavior,[63] and temporal self-regulation theory.[64] Despite the plethora of theories available, there is little evidence to support the superiority of any single strategy in achieving effective change. Many are hampered by low-quality evidence supporting their use, creating uncertainty about optimal models to support behavior change. Despite this finding, several theories share common elements including an assessment of readiness to change, determination of the value placed on change by the individual, or reward from achieving the desired result, and addressing underlying beliefs and identifying barriers to achieve meaningful health behavior change. These elements are critical components to the successful implementation of effective cardiovascular risk factor management programs.

RISK FACTOR MODIFICATION FOR INCIDENT ATRIAL FIBRILLATION

Few programs have examined the role of cardiovascular risk factor management for the prevention of AF development. To date, only 1 study has examined the impact of an intensive lifestyle intervention on the risk of developing AF in individuals with type 2 diabetes. The intervention randomized 5065 individuals to an intensive lifestyle intervention, focused on caloric restriction and improving physical activity levels, or to diabetic education and support groups.[65] After a mean follow-up of 9 years, the intensive lifestyle intervention did not result in a decreased AF incidence compared with the group receiving diabetic education and support. This finding may be, in part, due to the relatively modest weight loss achieved in the intervention group of this study and the subsequent lack of impact observed on the incidence of AF. There may be other contributory factors, including lower use of cardioprotective medications in the intervention group compared with the education and support groups.[65] The primary prevention of AF through lifestyle modification and aggressive management of cardiovascular risk factors remains an understudied field with further research in this area urgently required.

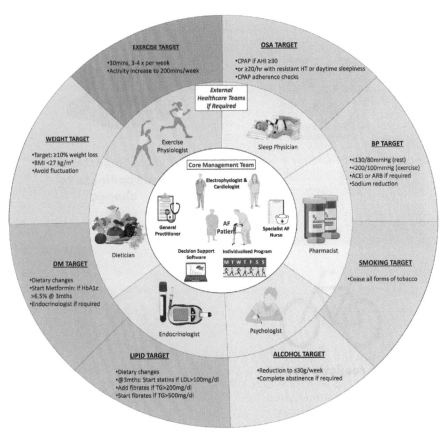

Fig. 1. Targets for cardiovascular risk factor management in the population with prevalent AF. ACEI, angiotensin-converting enzyme inhibitors; AHI, apnea–hypopnea index; ARB, angiotensin receptor blockers; CPAP, continuous positive airway pressure; DM, diabetes mellitus; HT, hypertension; LDL, low-density lipoprotein cholesterol; OSA, obstructive sleep apnea; TG, triglycerides. (*Created with* BioRender.com.)

RISK FACTOR MODIFICATION IN PREVALENT ATRIAL FIBRILLATION

In contrast with the primary prevention field, the role of cardiovascular risk factor management in AF populations has asserted itself as an essential component of comprehensive AF care delivery, demonstrating efficacy in decreasing the burden and progression of AF. A randomized controlled trial of 150 symptomatic overweight and obese AF patients, in which the intervention arm participated in a weight reduction and comprehensive risk factor management program, resulted in improved subjective and objective AF burden, in addition to beneficial cardiac remodeling.[8] In a series of Australian observational studies, comprehensively addressing multiple risk factors in a dedicated physician-led clinic resulted in a greater likelihood of freedom from AF in overweight and obese individuals at both short- and long-term follow-up (**Fig. 1** for components of this program).[9,66] Additionally, this strategy was also associated with a decreased likelihood of progression to more permanent forms of the arrhythmia and a greater likelihood of reversal, with incremental increases in weight loss.[67] Another randomized controlled trial exploring the use of a cardiac rehabilitation program that incorporated education and exercise as well as regular clinic appointments with a specialist nurse, in addition to prespecified pharmacotherapy (mineralocorticoid antagonists, angiotensin-converting enzyme inhibitors, and/or angiotensin receptor blockers and statins) was also associated with a greater likelihood of maintenance of sinus rhythm after 12 months of follow-up in 245 patients with early persistent AF and mild to moderate heart failure undertaking a rhythm control strategy (odds ratio, 1.77; 95% CI, 1.02–3.05).[68] However, the treatment of a single isolated risk factor (hypertension) did not result in greater freedom from AF in 184 patients undertaking catheter ablation for AF, suggesting the need for a comprehensive approach to cardiovascular risk factor management.[69]

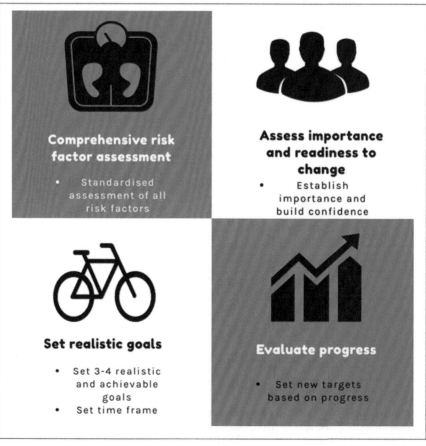

Fig. 2. Application of health behavior change techniques in AF. (*Created with* BioRender.com.)

HOW TO IMPLEMENT A RISK FACTOR MODIFICATION PROGRAM

Little evidence exists to guide clinicians in the delivery of comprehensive cardiovascular risk factor management programs for the prevention of incident AF. Owing to a lack of research in this field, optimal targets for individual risk factors are unclear. At this stage, primary prevention recommendations should be adopted until the development of a rigorous evidence base in this area occurs. Several international guidelines exist to guide clinicians in primary prevention measures, although differing recommendations across guidelines can make it a challenging field for the clinician to navigate. Moreover, primary prevention cardiovascular guidelines are largely geared toward the prevention of ischemic disease, with little guidance for the primary prevention of AF.[70,71] However, an assessment of overall cardiovascular risk to guide pharmaceutical treatment, the concomitant management of multiple risk factors, and the use of clinicians skilled in health behavior change techniques are likely to result in reduced risk of AF development.

In the established AF population, a greater evidence base exists for simultaneous targeting of multiple cardiovascular risk factors to decrease AF burden, frequency, and progression. Evidence to date would suggest that this is process optimally undertaken in a dedicated clinic, separate from medical management of the arrhythmia. A full suite of options to assist in optimizing cardiovascular risk factor profiles are required, with empowerment of the individual to self-monitor and manage their condition a critical component to its success. The role of patient education concerning their condition is essential to improve outcomes and to establish importance for the individual in the health behavior change process.[72] Tools including the use of a food diary, exercise record, home blood pressure monitoring, an AF symptom diary, monitoring of downloads from continuous positive airway pressure machines, and referral to other members of the multidisciplinary team may all be useful and have been successfully applied in cardiovascular risk factor modification programs in AF populations.[9,66] Underpinning successful health behavior change, and in accordance with the well-established chronic care model, is a move away from paternalistic models of care delivery to the patient as an active team member.[73] The involvement of family and caregivers is essential. The importance of setting realistic goals (generally 3–4 at any 1 time) and regular consultations to monitor progress and reassess targets is crucial. Finally, a cohesive and consistent message from all members of the health care team regarding the importance of lifestyle modification is critical to its success. An infographic of the essential components of a holistic cardiovascular risk factor management program in AF is depicted in **Fig. 2**.

SUMMARY

The emergence of AF as one of the greatest health care challenges of this century has led to an urgent need to develop strategies to both prevent onset of the condition and to improve outcomes in the prevalent population. Lifestyle factors play an important role in the incident and prevalent AF populations, although optimal targets for risk factors are yet to be determined. The optimization of cardiovascular risk factor profiles is likely to lead to reduced development of AF with further research, specifically evaluating comprehensive risk factor reduction programs, required in the primary prevention field. In the prevalent AF population, the simultaneous targeting of cardiovascular risk factors in a dedicated clinic has demonstrated improved patient outcomes and reduced the burden and progression of AF. It is clear that lifestyle factors play a critical role in the etiology and progression of AF, with aggressive cardiovascular risk factor management an essential pillar in combating the growing burden of this condition.

CLINICS CARE POINTS

- Modifiable risk factors should be simultaneously targeted to reduce both development and progression of AF.
- Due to its strong association with other risk factors, and AF development and progression, overweight and obesity should be aggressively managed.
- In the established AF population, a dedicated clinic to simultaneously manage all cardiovascular risk factors has demonstrated reduced disease burden and progression.
- The use of health behavior change techniques, including goal setting and regular feedback, is essential to success.
- Team based care, inclusive of the primary care physician, and empowerment of the individual to play an active role in their management, is critical to optimization of risk factor profiles and subsequent improved outcomes.

FINANCIAL DISCLOSURE

Drs C. Gallagher and M.E. Middeldorp are supported by a Postdoctoral Fellowship from the

University of Adelaide. Dr J.M. Hendriks is supported by a Future Leader Fellowship from the Heart Foundation of Australia. Dr D.H. Lau is supported by the Robert J. Craig Lectureship from the University of Adelaide and by a Mid-Career Fellowship from The Hospital Research Fund. Dr P. Sanders is supported by a Practitioner Fellowship from the National Health and Medical Research Council of Australia and by the National Heart Foundation of Australia.

CONFLICT OF INTEREST DISCLOSURES

Dr J.M. Hendriks reports that the University of Adelaide has received on his behalf lecture and/or consulting fees from Medtronic and Pfizer/BMS. Dr D.H. Lau reports that the University of Adelaide receives on his behalf lecture and/or consulting fees from Biotronik, Bayer, Medtronic, Abbott Medical, Boehringer Ingelheim, and MicroPort. Dr P. Sanders reports having served on the advisory board of Medtronic, Abbott Medical, Boston Scientific, PaceMate, and CathRx. Dr P. Sanders reports that the University of Adelaide receives on his behalf lecture and/or consulting fees from Medtronic, Abbott Medical, and Boston Scientific. Dr P. Sanders reports that the University of Adelaide receives on his behalf research funding from Medtronic, Abbott Medical, Boston Scientific, and MicroPort. The remaining authors have nothing to disclose.

REFERENCES

1. Chugh SS, Havmoeller R, Narayanan K, et al. Worldwide epidemiology of atrial fibrillation: a global burden of disease 2010 study. Circulation 2014; 129(8):837–47.
2. Freeman JV, Wang Y, Akar J, et al. National trends in atrial fibrillation hospitalization, readmission, and mortality for Medicare beneficiaries, 1999-2013. Circulation 2017;135(13):1227–39.
3. Gallagher C, Hendriks JM, Giles L, et al. Increasing trends in hospitalisations due to atrial fibrillation in Australia from 1993 to 2013. Heart 2019;105(17): 1358–63.
4. Staerk L, Wang B, Preis SR, et al. Lifetime risk of atrial fibrillation according to optimal, borderline, or elevated levels of risk factors: cohort study based on longitudinal data from the Framingham Heart Study. BMJ 2018;361:k1453.
5. Di Benedetto L, Michels G, Luben R, et al. Individual and combined impact of lifestyle factors on atrial fibrillation in apparently healthy men and women: the EPIC-Norfolk prospective population study. Eur J Prev Cardiol 2018;25(13):1374–83.
6. Weng LC, Preis SR, Hulme OL, et al. Genetic predisposition, clinical risk factor burden, and lifetime risk of atrial fibrillation. Circulation 2018;137(10): 1027–38.
7. Casagrande SS, Menke A, Cowie CC. Cardiovascular risk factors of adults age 20-49 years in the United States, 1971-2012: a series of cross-sectional studies. PLoS One 2016;11(8):e0161770.
8. Abed HS, Wittert GA, Leong DP, et al. Effect of weight reduction and cardiometabolic risk factor management on symptom burden and severity in patients with atrial fibrillation: a randomized clinical trial. JAMA 2013;310(19):2050–60.
9. Pathak RK, Middeldorp ME, Meredith M, et al. Long-term effect of goal-directed weight management in an atrial fibrillation cohort: a long term follow-up study (LEGACY). J Am Coll Cardiol 2015;65(20): 2159–69.
10. Pathak RK, Evans M, Middeldorp ME, et al. Cost-effectiveness and clinical effectiveness of the risk factor management clinic in atrial fibrillation: the CENT study. JACC Clin Electrophysiol 2017;3(5): 436–47.
11. Schnabel RB, Yin X, Gona P, et al. 50 year trends in atrial fibrillation prevalence, incidence, risk factors, and mortality in the Framingham Heart Study: a cohort study. Lancet 2015;386(9989):154–62.
12. Huxley RR, Lopez FL, Folsom AR, et al. Absolute and attributable risks of atrial fibrillation in relation to optimal and borderline risk factors: the Atherosclerosis Risk in Communities (ARIC) study. Circulation 2011;123(14):1501–8.
13. Manolis AJ, Rosei EA, Coca A, et al. Hypertension and atrial fibrillation: diagnostic approach, prevention and treatment. Position paper of the Working group 'hypertension arrhythmias and Thrombosis' of the European Society of hypertension. J Hypertens 2012;30(2):239–52.
14. Conen D, Tedrow UB, Koplan BA, et al. Influence of systolic and diastolic blood pressure on the risk of incident atrial fibrillation in women. Circulation 2009;119(16):2146–52.
15. Rahman F, Yin X, Larson MG, et al. Trajectories of risk factors and risk of new-onset atrial fibrillation in the Framingham Heart Study. Hypertension 2016; 68(3):597–605.
16. Sharashova E, Wilsgaard T, Ball J, et al. Long-term blood pressure trajectories and incident atrial fibrillation in women and men: the Tromsø Study. Eur Heart J 2020;41(16):1554–62.
17. Vemulapalli S, Inohara T, Kim S, et al. Blood pressure control and cardiovascular outcomes in patients with atrial fibrillation (from the ORBIT-AF registry). Am J Cardiol 2019;123(10):1628–36.
18. Vemulapalli S, Hellkamp AS, Jones WS, et al. Blood pressure control and stroke or bleeding risk in anticoagulated patients with atrial fibrillation: results

from the ROCKET AF Trial. Am Heart J 2016;178: 74–84.

19. Hruby A, Hu FB. The epidemiology of obesity: a big picture. PharmacoEconomics 2015;33(7):673–89.

20. Wang TJ, Parise H, Levy D, et al. Obesity and the risk of new-onset atrial fibrillation. JAMA 2004; 292(20):2471–7.

21. Wong CX, Sullivan T, Sun MT, et al. Obesity and the risk of incident, post-operative, and post-ablation atrial fibrillation. JACC Clin Electrophysiol 2015; 1(3):139–52.

22. Tedrow UB, Conen D, Ridker PM, et al. The long- and short-term impact of elevated body mass index on the risk of new atrial fibrillation in the Women's Health Study. J Am Coll Cardiol 2010;55(21): 2319–27.

23. Tsang TS, Barnes ME, Miyasaka Y, et al. Obesity as a risk factor for the progression of paroxysmal to permanent atrial fibrillation: a longitudinal cohort study of 21 years. Eur Heart J 2008;29(18):2227–33.

24. Feng T, Vegard M, Strand LB, et al. Weight and weight change and risk of atrial fibrillation: the HUNT study. Eur Heart J 2019;40(34):2859–66.

25. Bertomeu-Gonzalez V, Moreno-Arribas J, Esteve-Pastor MA, et al. Association of body mass index with clinical outcomes in patients with atrial fibrillation: a report from the FANTASIIA registry. J Am Heart Assoc 2020;9(1):e013789.

26. Benjamin EJ, Levy D, Vaziri SM, et al. Independent risk factors for atrial fibrillation in a population-based cohort. The Framingham Heart Study. JAMA 1994;271(11):840–4.

27. Kannel WB, Wolf PA, Benjamin EJ, et al. Prevalence, incidence, prognosis, and predisposing conditions for atrial fibrillation: population-based estimates. Am J Cardiol 1998;82(8a):2n–9n.

28. Perez MV, Wang PJ, Larson JC, et al. Risk factors for atrial fibrillation and their population burden in post-menopausal women: the Women's Health Initiative Observational Study. Heart 2013;99(16):1173–8.

29. Huxley RR, Filion KB, Konety S, et al. Meta-analysis of cohort and case-control studies of type 2 diabetes mellitus and risk of atrial fibrillation. Am J Cardiol 2011;108(1):56–62.

30. Dublin S, Glazer NL, Smith NL, et al. Diabetes mellitus, glycemic control, and risk of atrial fibrillation. J Gen Intern Med 2010;25(8):853–8.

31. Larsson SC, Wallin A, Hakansson N, et al. Type 1 and type 2 diabetes mellitus and incidence of seven cardiovascular diseases. Int J Cardiol 2018;262:66–70.

32. Fatemi O, Yuriditsky E, Tsioufis C, et al. Impact of intensive glycemic control on the incidence of atrial fibrillation and associated cardiovascular outcomes in patients with type 2 diabetes mellitus (from the Action to Control Cardiovascular Risk in Diabetes Study). Am J Cardiol 2014;114(8):1217–22.

33. Saliba W, Barnett-Griness O, Elias M, et al. Glycated hemoglobin and risk of first episode stroke in diabetic patients with atrial fibrillation: a cohort study. Heart Rhythm 2015;12(5):886–92.

34. Qureshi WT, Alirhayim Z, Blaha MJ, et al. Cardiorespiratory fitness and risk of incident atrial fibrillation: results from the henry ford exercise testing (FIT) project. Circulation 2015;131(21):1827–34.

35. Mozaffarian D, Furberg CD, Psaty BM, et al. Physical activity and incidence of atrial fibrillation in older adults: the Cardiovascular Health Study. Circulation 2008;118(8):800–7.

36. Everett BM, Conen D, Buring JE, et al. Physical activity and the risk of incident atrial fibrillation in women. Circ Cardiovasc Qual Outcomes 2011; 4(3):321–7.

37. Drca N, Wolk A, Jensen-Urstad M, et al. Physical activity is associated with a reduced risk of atrial fibrillation in middle-aged and elderly women. Heart 2015;101(20):1627–30.

38. Abdulla J, Nielsen JR. Is the risk of atrial fibrillation higher in athletes than in the general population? A systematic review and meta-analysis. Europace 2009;11(9):1156–9.

39. Andersen K, Farahmand B, Ahlbom A, et al. Risk of arrhythmias in 52 755 long-distance cross-country skiers: a cohort study. Eur Heart J 2013;34(47): 3624–31.

40. Elliott AD, Linz D, Mishima R, et al. Association between physical activity and risk of incident arrhythmias in 402 406 individuals: evidence from the UK Biobank cohort. Eur Heart J 2020;41(15):1479–86.

41. Hegbom F, Stavem K, Sire S, et al. Effects of short-term exercise training on symptoms and quality of life in patients with chronic atrial fibrillation. Int J Cardiol 2007;116(1):86–92.

42. Osbak PS, Mourier M, Kjaer A, et al. A randomized study of the effects of exercise training on patients with atrial fibrillation. Am Heart J 2011;162(6):1080–7.

43. Malmo V, Nes BM, Amundsen BH, et al. Aerobic interval training reduces the burden of atrial fibrillation in the short term: a randomized trial. Circulation 2016;133(5):466–73.

44. Gallagher C, Hendriks JML, Elliott AD, et al. Alcohol and incident atrial fibrillation - a systematic review and meta-analysis. Int J Cardiol 2017;246:46–52.

45. Larsson SC, Drca N, Wolk A. Alcohol consumption and risk of atrial fibrillation: a prospective study and dose-response meta-analysis. J Am Coll Cardiol 2014;64(3):281–9.

46. Kodama S, Saito K, Tanaka S, et al. Alcohol consumption and risk of atrial fibrillation: a meta-analysis. J Am Coll Cardiol 2011;57(4):427–36.

47. Overvad TF, Rasmussen LH, Skjoth F, et al. Alcohol intake and prognosis of atrial fibrillation. Heart 2013;99(15):1093–9.

48. Qiao Y, Shi R, Hou B, et al. Impact of alcohol consumption on substrate remodeling and ablation outcome of paroxysmal atrial fibrillation. J Am Heart Assoc 2015;4(11):e002349.

49. Voskoboinik A, Kalman JM, De Silva A, et al. Alcohol abstinence in drinkers with atrial fibrillation. N Engl J Med 2020;382(1):20–8.

50. Frost L, Hune LJ, Vestergaard P. Overweight and obesity as risk factors for atrial fibrillation or flutter: the Danish Diet, Cancer, and Health Study. Am J Med 2005;118(5):489–95.

51. Psaty BM, Manolio TA, Kuller LH, et al. Incidence of and risk factors for atrial fibrillation in older adults. Circulation 1997;96(7):2455–61.

52. Krahn AD, Manfreda J, Tate RB, et al. The natural history of atrial fibrillation: incidence, risk factors, and prognosis in the Manitoba Follow-Up Study. Am J Med 1995;98(5):476–84.

53. Heeringa J, Kors JA, Hofman A, et al. Cigarette smoking and risk of atrial fibrillation: the Rotterdam Study. Am Heart J 2008;156(6):1163–9.

54. Chamberlain AM, Agarwal SK, Folsom AR, et al. Smoking and incidence of atrial fibrillation: results from the Atherosclerosis Risk in Communities (ARIC) study. Heart Rhythm 2011;8(8):1160–6.

55. Zhu W, Yuan P, Shen Y, et al. Association of smoking with the risk of incident atrial fibrillation: a meta-analysis of prospective studies. Int J Cardiol 2016; 218:259–66.

56. Aune D, Schlesinger S, Norat T, et al. Tobacco smoking and the risk of atrial fibrillation: a systematic review and meta-analysis of prospective studies. Eur J Prev Cardiol 2018;25(13):1437–51.

57. Cheng WH, Lo LW, Lin YJ, et al. Cigarette smoking causes a worse long-term outcome in persistent atrial fibrillation following catheter ablation. J Cardiovasc Electrophysiol 2018;29(5):699–706.

58. Zhu W, Guo L, Hong K. Relationship between smoking and adverse outcomes in patients with atrial fibrillation: a meta-analysis and systematic review. Int J Cardiol 2016;222:289–94.

59. Morris PB, Ference BA, Jahangir E, et al. Cardiovascular effects of exposure to cigarette smoke and electronic cigarettes: clinical perspectives from the prevention of cardiovascular disease section Leadership Council and Early Career Councils of the American College of Cardiology. J Am Coll Cardiol 2015;66(12):1378–91.

60. Prochaska JO, Velicer WF. The transtheoretical model of health behavior change. Am J Health Promot 1997;12(1):38–48.

61. Rosenstock IM, Strecher VJ, Becker MH. Social learning theory and the health belief model. Health Educ Q 1988;15(2):175–83.

62. Ryan RM, Deci EL. Self-determination theory and the facilitation of intrinsic motivation, social development, and well-being. Am Psychol 2000; 55(1):68–78.

63. Ajzen I. The theory of planned behaviour: reactions and reflections. Psychol Health 2011;26(9):1113–27.

64. Hall PA, Fong GT. Temporal self-regulation theory: a model for individual health behavior. Health Psychol Rev 2007;1(1):6–52.

65. Alonso A, Bahnson JL, Gaussoin SA, et al. Effect of an intensive lifestyle intervention on atrial fibrillation risk in individuals with type 2 diabetes: the Look AHEAD randomized trial. Am Heart J 2015;170(4): 770–7.e5.

66. Pathak RK, Middeldorp ME, Lau DH, et al. Aggressive risk factor reduction study for atrial fibrillation and implications for the outcome of ablation: the ARREST-AF cohort study. J Am Coll Cardiol 2014; 64(21):2222–31.

67. Middeldorp ME, Pathak RK, Meredith M, et al. PREVEntion and regReSsive Effect of weight-loss and risk factor modification on Atrial Fibrillation: the REVERSE-AF study. Europace 2018;20(12): 1929–35.

68. Rienstra M, Hobbelt AH, Alings M, et al. Targeted therapy of underlying conditions improves sinus rhythm maintenance in patients with persistent atrial fibrillation: results of the RACE 3 trial. Eur Heart J 2018;39(32):2987–96.

69. Parkash R, Wells GA, Sapp JL, et al. Effect of aggressive blood pressure control on the recurrence of atrial fibrillation after catheter ablation: a randomized, open-label clinical trial (SMAC-AF [substrate modification with aggressive blood pressure control]). Circulation 2017;135(19):1788–98.

70. Arnett DK, Blumenthal RS, Albert MA, et al. 2019 ACC/AHA guideline on the primary prevention of cardiovascular disease: a report of the American College of Cardiology/American heart association Task Force on clinical practice guidelines. Circulation 2019;140(11):e596–646.

71. Piepoli MF, Hoes AW, Agewall S, et al. 2016 European guidelines on cardiovascular disease prevention in clinical practice: the Sixth Joint Task Force of the European Society of Cardiology and other Societies on cardiovascular disease prevention in clinical Practice (constituted by representatives of 10 societies and by invited experts)Developed with the special contribution of the European association for cardiovascular prevention & rehabilitation (EACPR). Eur Heart J 2016;37(29):2315–81.

72. Gallagher C, Rowett D, Nyfort-Hansen K, et al. Patient-centered educational resources for atrial fibrillation. JACC Clin Electrophysiol 2019;5(10): 1101–14.

73. Wagner EH, Austin BT, Von Korff M. Organizing care for patients with chronic illness. Milbank Q 1996; 74(4):511–44.